ORTHOPAEDIC INFECTION

Diagnosis and Treatment

RAMON B. GUSTILO, M.D.
Chairman, Department of Orthopaedic Surgery,
Hennepin County Medical Center;
Professor of Orthopaedics,
University of Minnesota, Minneapolis

ROBERT P. GRUNINGER, M.D.
Director, Microbiology Laboratory,
Hennepin County Medical Center;
Assistant Professor, Department of Laboratory
Medicine and Pathology, Department of Medicine,
University of Minnesota, Minneapolis

DEAN T. TSUKAYAMA, M.D.
Director, Musculoskeletal Sepsis Unit,
Hennepin County Medical Center;
Assistant Professor of Medicine,
University of Minnesota, Minneapolis

W.B. SAUNDERS COMPANY   **1989**
Harcourt Brace Jovanovich, Inc.
Philadelphia   London   Toronto   Montreal   Sydney   Tokyo

W. B. SAUNDERS COMPANY
Harcourt Brace Jovanovich, Inc.

The Curtis Center
Independence Square West
Philadelphia, PA 19106

Library of Congress Cataloging-in-Publication Data

Orthopaedic Infection: Diagnosis and Treatment / [edited by] Ramon B. Gustilo.
   p. cm.
  ISBN 0-7216-2341-7
   1. Musculoskeletal system — Infections — Treatment.   I. Gustilo, Ramon B.
  [DNLM: 1. Antibiotics — therapeutic use. 2. Bacterial Infections. 3. Bone Diseases —
therapy. 4. Joint Diseases — therapy. 5. Muscular Diseases — therapy. WE 140 C9758]
RC925.5.C87 1989
616.7 — dc19
DNLM/DLC
for Library of Congress   89-5978
  ISBN 0-7216-2341-7   CIP

Editor: Edward Wickland
Designer: Terri Siegel
Production Manager: Peter Faber
Manuscript Editor: Carol Robins
Illustration Coordinator: Walt Verbitski
Indexer: Kathy Garcia
Cover Designer: Ellen Bodner

Orthopaedic Infection: Diagnosis and Treatment   ISBN 0-7216-2341-7

Last digit is the print number: 9 8 7 6 5 4 3 2 1

This book is dedicated to our clinical and research faculty, residents, and nurses, in appreciation of their contributions in caring for the patients of the Musculoskeletal Sepsis Unit of Hennepin County Medical Center and Metropolitan–Mount Sinai Medical Center.

Contributors

QUENTIN N. ANDERSON, M.D.
Assistant Professor of Radiology, University of Minnesota Medical School, Minneapolis. Head, Department of Radiology, Hennepin County Medical Center; Active Staff, Hennepin County Medical Center and Metropolitan–Mount Sinai Medical Center, Minneapolis.
Radiographic Evaluation of Inflammatory Bone Disease

ELIN BARTH, M.D., Ph.D.
Moore-Lunsford Chair of Orthopedic Research, University of South Carolina School of Medicine, Columbia, South Carolina.
Microbial Adhesion and the Pathogenesis of Biomaterial-Centered Infections; Microbes, Metals, and Other Nonbiological Substrata in Man: Substratum and Substrate Factors in Infection

JOSEPH E. CLINTON, M.D.
Assistant Chief, Department of Emergency Medicine, Hennepin County Medical Center, Minneapolis, Minnesota.
Puncture Wounds by Inanimate Objects and Mammalian Bite

LEO J. deSOUZA, M.B., F.R.C.S. Ed., F.R.C.S.(C)
Assistant Professor of Orthopaedic Surgery, University of Minnesota Medical School, Minneapolis. Attending Staff, Hennepin County Medical Center and Metropolitan Medical Center, Minneapolis. Consulting Staff, Methodist Hospital, Minneapolis.
Infection of the Spine

ANTHONY G. GRISTINA, M.D.
Professor, Section of Orthopedic Surgery, Bowman Gray School of Medicine, Winston-Salem, North Carolina. Staff, North Carolina Baptist Hospital, Winston-Salem.
Microbial Adhesion and the Pathogenesis of Biomaterial-Centered Infections; Microbes, Metals, and Other Nonbiological Substrata in Man: Substratum and Substrate Factors in Infection

ROBERT P. GRUNINGER, M.D.
Assistant Professor, Departments of Laboratory Medicine and Pathology, University of Minnesota Medical School, Minneapolis. Chief, Microbiology Laboratory, Hennepin County Medical Center; Associate Pathologist, Director of Clinical Microbiology, Infectious Disease Consultant, Chair, Infection Control Committee, University of Minnesota Medical Center, Minneapolis.
Diagnostic Microbiology in Bone and Joint Infections; Antibiotic-Impregnated PMMA Beads in Bone and Prosthetic Joint Infections; Fungal Infections in Bones and Joints

DAVID R. P. GUAY, Pharm.D.
Assistant Professor, College of Pharmacy, University of Minnesota, Minneapolis. Clinical Scientist, The Drug Evaluation Unit, Department of Medicine, Hennepin County Medical Center, Minneapolis.
Antibiotic Therapy of Chronic Osteomyelitis

RAMON B. GUSTILO, M.D.
Professor of Orthopaedic Surgery, University of Minnesota, Minneapolis. Chairman, Department of Orthopaedics, Hennepin County Medical Center, Minneapolis. Staff, Hennepin County Medical Center and Metropolitan–Mount Sinai Medical Center, Minneapolis.
Evolving Concepts in the Treatment of Musculoskeletal Sepsis; Management of Open Fractures; Management of Acutely Infected Fractures; Management of Infected Nonunion; Management of Chronic Osteomyelitis; Management of Infected Total Hip Replacement; Management of Infected Total Knee Replacement

CLAUDE R. HITCHCOCK, M.D., Ph.D.
Emeritus Professor of Surgery, University of Minnesota Medical School, Minneapolis. President, Minneapolis Medical Research Foundation, Inc. Emeritus Chief of Surgery, Hennepin County Medical Center, Minneapolis.
Gas Gangrene; Non-clostridial Necrotizing Skin and Soft Tissue Infections

LIBERATO A. C. LEAGOGO, M.D.

Instructor, Orthopedic Surgery, University of the Philippines, Manila. Staff, Makati Medical Center Philippine Orthopaedic Institute, Inc., Manila.
Management of Infected Total Hip Replacement

JOHN E. LONSTEIN, M.D.

Clinical Associate Professor, Department of Orthopaedics, University of Minnesota, Minneapolis. Attending Staff, Minnesota Spine Center and Riverside Medical Center, Minneapolis; Cerebral Palsy Spine and Spine Services and Gillette Children's Hospital, St. Paul.
Management of Postoperative Spine Infections

ROBERT L. MERKOW, M.D.

Assistant Professor of Orthopaedics, Department of Orthopaedic Surgery, University of Minnesota, Minneapolis. Attending Orthopaedic Surgeon, Hennepin County Medical Center, Minneapolis, Minnesota. Chief, Department of Orthopedic Surgery, Metropolitan–Mount Sinai Medical Center, Minneapolis.
Hand Infections

ANTONIO M. MONTALBAN, M.D.

Assistant Chairman and Assistant Professor, Department of Orthopaedics, University of the Philippines, Manila. Staff, Philippine General Hospital, Manila.
Mycobacterial Infections of Bones and Joints

RAYMOND T. MORRISSY, M.D.

Clinical Professor of Orthopaedics, Emory University, Atlanta. Medical Director and Chief of Orthopaedics, Scottish Rite Children's Hospital, Atlanta.
Septic Arthritis in Children; Acute Hematogenous Osteomyelitis

J. PHILLIP NELSON, M.D.

Active Staff, St. Luke's Hospital, Denver, Colorado.
Prevention of Postoperative Infection by Airborne Bacteria

GEORGE PELTIER, M.D.

Clinical Assistant Professor, University of Minnesota School of Medicine, Minneapolis. Active Staff, Hennepin County Medical Center and Metropolitan–Mount Sinai Medical Center; Courtesy Staff, Riverside Medical Center; Fairview-Southdale Hospital; Abbott Northwestern Hospital; Minneapolis Children's Medical Center, Minneapolis.
Sacral Pressure Sores

PHILLIP K. PETERSON, M.D.

Professor of Medicine, University of Minnesota Medical School, Minneapolis. Chief, Infectious Diseases, Department of Medicine, Hennepin County Medical Center, Minneapolis.
Bone and Joint Infections in Immunocompromised Patients; Antibiotic Therapy of Chronic Osteomyelitis

RAFAEL S. RECTO, M.D.

Professor, Department of Orthopaedics, University of the Philippines, Manila. Director, National Orthopedics Hospital, Philippines. Staff, Philippine General Hospital, Manila.
Mycobacterial Infections of Bones and Joints

PETER A. SCHLESINGER, M.D., F.A.C.P.

Assistant Professor of Medicine, University of Minnesota, Minneapolis. Attending Physician, Division of Rheumatology, Department of Medicine, Hennepin County Medical Center, Minneapolis.
Nonsuppurative Infectious Arthritis

STEVEN L. SHORE, M.D.

Associate Clinical Professor of Pediatrics, Emory University School of Medicine, Atlanta. Chief, Infectious Disease Division, Scottish Rite Children's Hospital, Atlanta.
Septic Arthritis in Children; Acute Hematogenous Osteomyelitis

MARGARET L. SIMPSON, M.D.

Assistant Professor of Medicine, University of Minnesota, Minneapolis. Member, Department of Medicine, Division of Infectious Disease, Hennepin County Medical Center, Minneapolis.
Mycobacterial Infections of Bones and Joints; Septic Arthritis in Adults

DEAN T. TSUKAYAMA, M.D.

Assistant Professor of Medicine, University of Minnesota Medical School, Minneapolis. Medical Director, Musculoskeletal Sepsis Unit, Hennepin County Medical Center, and Metropolitan–Mount Sinai Medical Center, Minneapolis.
Antibiotic-Impregnated PMMA Beads in Bone and Prosthetic Joint Infections; Bone and Joint Infections in Immunocompromised Patients; Antibiotic Therapy of Chronic Osteomyelitis

THOMAS F. VARECKA, M.D.

Assistant Professor of Medicine, Department of Orthopaedic Surgery, University of Minnesota, Minneapolis. Chief, Hand Section, Hennepin County Medical Center, Minneapolis.

Soft Tissue Coverage in Open Fractures

LAWRENCE X. WEBB, M.D.

Assistant Professor, Section of Orthopedic Surgery, Bowman Gray School of Medicine, Winston-Salem, North Carolina. Staff, North Carolina Baptist Hospital, Winston-Salem.

Microbial Adhesion and the Pathogenesis of Biomaterial-Centered Infections; Microbes, Metals, and Other Nonbiological Substrata in Man: Substratum and Substrate Factors in Infection

BARBARA WICKLUND, B.S., M.T. (A.S.C.P.)

Staff, Musculoskeletal Sepsis Unit, Metropolitan – Mount Sinai Medical Center, Minneapolis, Minnesota.

Antibiotic-Impregnated PMMA Beads in Bone and Prosthetic Joint Infections

DAVID N. WILLIAMS, M.B., Ch.B., F.R.C.P.

Clinical Associate Professor, University of Minnesota Medical School, Minneapolis. Staff, Methodist Hospital, and Park Nicollet Medical Center, Minneapolis.

Antibiotic Penetration into Bones and Joints; Antibiotic Prophylaxis in Bone and Joint Surgery

Foreword

It is almost 20 years since I discovered, while a medical student on orthopedic surgery, that it took at least six weeks of intensive antibiotic therapy to cure chronic osteomyelitis. This was surprising. At about the same time, I saw my first patient with necrotizing cellulitis die. The case fatality rate of this infectious disease was over 50 percent. This was astonishing. Shortly thereafter, I learned that infections of prosthetic joints necessitated removal of the prosthesis. This was perplexing. The intervening 20 years have witnessed an exhilarating development of more potent antibiotics and advanced surgical and medical technologies. Yet, the serious morbidity and mortality associated with many musculoskeletal infections have not changed much. It is no wonder that medical students appear even more incredulous.

This is not to say that there has not been substantial progress in this area of surgery and medicine. Indeed, the many contributors to this book have demonstrated how much has been learned about these infections in recent years. The microbial factors responsible for the tenacity of orthopedic infections are being elegantly unraveled. The microbiology and radiology departments continue to develop new techniques to aid in diagnosis. And, we do have improved methods of prevention and treatment of these infections.

This book bears testimony to the great fund of knowledge regarding musculoskeletal infections. It is also a tribute to the inspirational leadership of one of its editors, Ramon Gustilo. His insatiable, scholarly interest in the problems of orthopedic infections, by itself, places him in a somewhat unique class of orthopedic surgeons. The diversity of backgrounds of his many colleagues who have contributed to this book demonstrates the infectious nature of his enthusiasm for the field and also underscores his belief that continued progress demands an interdisciplinary approach. Because of this diversity, this volume will serve as an important reference book for the orthopedic surgeon, infectious diseases specialist, general surgeon, rheumatologist, and clinical microbiologist.

PHILLIP K. PETERSON

Contents

Ramon B. Gustilo, M.D.

1

Evolving Concepts in the Treatment of Musculoskeletal Sepsis

From Hippocrates to Galen, to Louis Pasteur, to Lister, and many others that follow, the search for "miraculous substance" and surgical treatment to eradicate wound sepsis incessantly continues. In spite of twentieth century advances in medicine and surgery, wound sepsis following emergency and elective surgery, i.e., open fractures, joint replacements, osteomyelitis, septic arthritis, and gas gangrene, is a dreadful complication that challenges the ingenuity and patience of every physician and surgeon. Moreover, the patient suffers prolonged morbidity, economic loss, and oftentimes permanent disability.

During the last decade, there have been several medical and technological advances that affect the traditional approach in the management of musculoskeletal sepsis; however, surgery, as is true in the past, remains the primary treatment. This implies radical debridement of infected tissues, complete evacuation of pus, and achievement of a viable environment not conducive to bacterial growth. As Louis Pasteur once said, "it is not the bacteria, but the terrain where it grows"; it is important to remember this in the control or eradication of wound sepsis. What has changed during the last decade in the surgical treatment of wound sepsis is the understanding and knowledge of when, why, and how much has to be debrided and the ability to reconstruct soft tissue and skeletal defects following radical surgery. Repeated debridement is mandatory to achieve a vascular and viable environment. The learning process of effective surgical debridement

comes through fully understanding the disease process and is acquired only by repeated experience in treating musculoskeletal sepsis.

Antibiotics for almost every bacteria known to man, along with the knowledge of which ones, when to use them, how much to give, and how long to give them, have added a quantum leap in the treatment of musculoskeletal sepsis. Working closely with infectious disease consultants, we have become able to give antibiotics appropriately and effectively with minimal side effects. Working together as a team allows us to treat difficult cases that before had resulted in prolonged morbidity, amputation, and even loss of life. The advances in making early diagnosis, in the microbiology of identifying bacteria, and in sophisticated sensitivity studies make antibiotic therapy and prophylaxis more effective and safer than ever before. The advance of local antibiotic beads that provide a very high local concentration of antibiotics where they are needed has been very effective in treating difficult cases, obviating the toxicity of prolonged parenteral antibiotic therapy. This is particularly true in the administration of aminoglycosides for gram-negative or mixed infection over a 2-week period. The unsettled question remains: How long must antibiotics be given in different types and stages of musculoskeletal sepsis?

Fracture stability reduces wound sepsis, and fracture instability promotes wound sepsis. The understanding of the relationship of fracture stability and sepsis has advanced and contributed greatly to our success of treating infected fractures and nonunion. The old concept—that the presence of metal in infected fractures absolutely necessitates its removal—is no longer true, provided that

From the Department of Orthopaedic Surgery, Hennepin County Medical Center, Minneapolis, Minnesota.

1

fracture stability is maintained. The formation of glycocalyx in implants renders antibiotic therapy in infected joint prostheses ineffective against the infecting organism. The discovery of glycocalyx has provided new and very important information as to why the prosthesis has to be removed because of failure to control sepsis in spite of prolonged antibiotic therapy and repeated surgery. This is in contrast to an infected fracture in which healing can proceed in spite of the presence of metal and continuing infection, provided that it is under control and that stability is maintained.

Our current knowledge of wound healing and of the pathogenesis of wound sepsis through sterile operating environment, i.e., air filter, air-flow exchange, or personal attire and movement as well as antibiotic prophylaxis, has been shown to definitely reduce wound sepsis. Our knowledge of wound healing in clean, contaminated, and infected wounds provides the surgeon with the timing and type of wound closure to use. Sophisticated wound coverage, i.e., microvascular and local flaps, is a great advance in surgical technology in converting a complex wound problem to a simple one with much less morbidity. Early bone grafting in infected open fracture and infected nonunion, at the right time, in spite of low-grade infection, was heresy in the past, yet contemporary surgical practice, based on a decade of clinical experience and good results, suggests that in a controlled infected but viable environment, cancellous bone grafting stimulates vascular formation and promotes fracture and wound healing in spite of sepsis.

The understanding of deficiencies and the risk of sepsis in the immunosuppressed patients undergoing emergency or elective surgery affecting wound healing requires strict adherence to meticulous surgical technique and appropriate antibiotic prophylaxis. The knowledge of nutritional requirements as they affect healing, particularly in chronic sepsis, in a debilitated or polytrauma patient adds another dimension in therapeusis and prophylaxis in wound sepsis that was not recognized a decade ago. Probably the best example and most difficult problem facing the orthopedic surgeon today is an infected joint replacement in an elderly patient. The problems are poor soft tissue, bone loss, mixed infection, general debility, and poor cardiovascular status. The surgical approach is complex and difficult. The morbidity is prolonged, with tremendous financial drain and lifelong disability. Without question, a multidisciplinary approach is required, i.e., one utilizing an orthopedic surgeon and infectious disease internist specialist.

We have come a long way in the treatment of musculoskeletal sepsis; however, old and new problems keep developing and remain a continuing challenge. This book is written by experts in the various fields of musculoskeletal sepsis in an attempt to provide information regarding current concepts in the pathogenesis and treatment of musculoskeletal sepsis.

Anthony G. Gristina, M.D.
Elin Barth, M.D.
Lawrence X. Webb, M.D.

CHAPTER

2

Microbial Adhesion and the Pathogenesis of Biomaterial-Centered Infections

PROLOGUE

"Although I am now 50 years old, I have uncommonly well-preserved teeth because it is my custom every morning to rub my teeth very hard with salt."

After that, he wrote, he cleaned between his teeth with a quill and then polished them with a cloth. When he scraped a bit of white debris from between his teeth, mixed it with rain water, and stuck it in a little tube on the needle of his microscope, he saw for the first time salivary pellicle, dental plaque, and adhesive microcolonies of polymicrobial, mixed oral flora, including *Streptococcus mutans, Streptococcus salivaris, Streptococcus sanguis,* enterococci, *Lactobacillus* species, *Bacteroides* species, and other larger microorganisms. Thus the story begins.

The year was 1682; the man, Antony Leeuwenhoek, was the janitor/lens grinder of Delft, Holland.[1] It was 250 years later that marine microbiologists noted microbial attachment to surfaces and 290 years until microbiologists began to understand the molecular mechanisms of microbial attachment, adhesion, aggregation, and microcolony formation.[2, 3] It was also 290 years later that Gibbons elucidated the mechanisms of microbial adhesion by *S. mutans,* plaque formation, and dental caries and tremendous interest was directed to these same phenomena in infectious diseases.[2]

From the Section on Orthopedic Surgery, Bowman Gray School of Medicine, Winston-Salem, North Carolina.

INTRODUCTION

This chapter discusses the relevant mechanisms in adhesion; biofilm-mediated, biomaterial-centered infections; and osteomyelitis. This report also presents the results of a continuing study of bacterial adhesion to biomaterials and to compromised tissues; describes the probable relationship of bacterial colonization within a coherent biofilm on foreign-body surfaces and compromised tissues to the protection of those bacteria from antibacterial agents and host defense mechanisms; indicates that adhesive bacteria with a biofilm may be, in some cases, incompletely detected by routine sampling methods; and, last, discusses the clinical and therapeutic significance of microbial adhesion. Chapter 3 details the mechanisms and physicochemistry of the interactions between microbes, metals, other nonbiologic substrata and man.

MICROBIAL ADHESION AND AGGREGATION IN NATURE AND MAN

Adhesion and aggregation involve interactions between microorganisms and surfaces (substrata) in an ambient fluid milieu. The surface may be inorganic or organic, "inert" or reactive, devitalized or animate; the organisms of the same or different species; the cell types prokaryocytes or eukaryocytes, interacting or cross-acting; and the environment, any that supports life forms (Fig. 2–1).

An almost universal feature is a connecting physicochemical microenvironment that acts

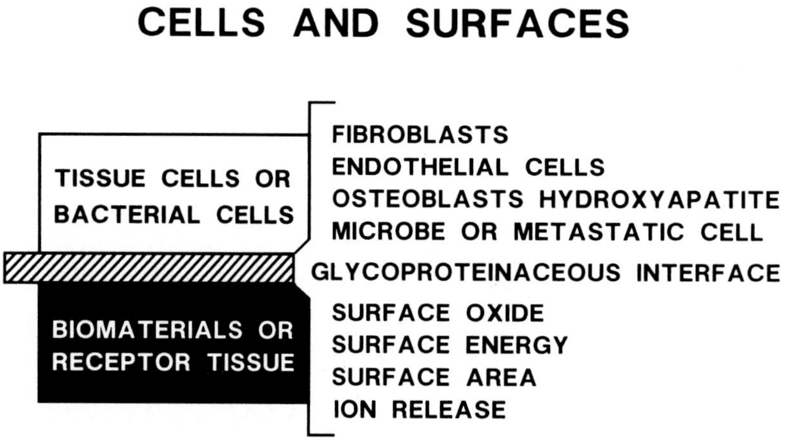

CELLS AND SURFACES

FIGURE 2–1. Bacteria, tissue cells, and metastatic cells have similar, though individually specific, destinies, in that they are adhesive for receptors on a conditioned substratum. The surface characteristics of the biomaterial or receptor tissue and glycoproteinaceous interface (derived from the ambient fluid milieu) also direct adhesion of available bacteria and normal or metastatic tissue cells.

as a communicating or conducting milieu and that is composed of features and elements of the systems involved and a continuum or matrix of bacterial origin composed of complex, hydrated, anionic, acidic polysaccharides and glycoproteins, "the slime or biofilm."

Adhesion to, and colonization of, substrata is a fundamental characteristic of most bacteria and is the actual state of the majority of microbes in natural environments and in health or disease in man. In natural habitats, proliferating microcolonies of mixed organisms on surfaces form slippery films called "slime layers." These thickened layers of slime or biofilm, mixed with environmental debris, may form a biomat or biomass and are a ubiquitous feature of life-supporting environments.[3-6]

Some species of bacteria have highly evolved strategies for colonization of eukaryocytic substrata, which results in gastrointestinal, urinary, respiratory, and musculoskeletal infections. In general, however, undamaged eukaryocytic cells show an amazing resistance to pathogenic bacteria, except for host-specific and site-specific pathogens in certain diseases. At sites of externalization of host tissue, special membrane cells, fluids, and mechanical strategies serve to protect higher animals. At these sites and along the surfaces of the organ systems involved (e.g., the skin, respiratory system, and gastrointestinal tract), a de facto collaboration or symbiosis exists with friendly bacteria that usually prevents colonization by pathogens.

ADHESION AND AGGREGATION IN DISEASE

The pathogenesis of osteomyelitis can best be understood in terms of microbial adhesion based on findings made in studies of bacterial ecosystems in nature and of bacterial behavior in certain tissue-centered diseases as well as in infections centered about biomaterials and foreign bodies. Insights derived from the mechanisms of prokaryocyte (bacterial) adhesion to surfaces are also relevant to tissue (eukaryotic) integration with biomaterial surfaces, to organ-specific metastases of neoplastic cells and to the ontogeny or the ultimate destiny of eukaryotic cells.[5-12]

BACTERIAL ADHESION IN BIOMATERIAL-CENTERED INFECTIONS

In 1963, studies by one of the authors suggested that internal fixation devices and dead bone provided a structural framework along which microorganisms (*Staphylococcus aureus* and *Staphylococcus epidermidis*) could colonize and propagate and that all foreign bodies or biomaterials tested demonstrated similar qualities (Fig. 2–2).[13, 14] Subsequently, in 1972, Bayston and Penny described the excessive production of a mucoid substance as a possible factor in the colonization of Holter shunts by *S. epidermidis*.[15] In 1976, surface effects and sequestration of ions from biometals and biomaterials were suggested as factors in the behavior of bacteria that colonized foreign bodies and biomaterials. It was noted that some reactive metals inhibited bacterial growth, but that growth was abundant adjacent to "inert" materials, such as stainless steel, Vitallium, nylon, and methylmethacrylate.[16] Studies in 1979 first demonstrated bacterial adhesion and biofilm-mediated polymicrobial infections in tissue and internal fixation devices from infected surgical wounds.[17-20] Reports in 1981 and

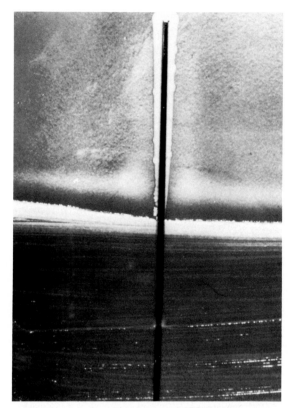

FIGURE 2–2. Bacterial propagation along Vitallium. The inoculated portion of the agar plate is at the bottom of the illustration. The organism is *Staphylococcus aureus*. (Reprinted with permission from Gristina et al: An *in vitro* study of bacterial response to inert and reactive metals and to methyl methacrylate. J Biomed Mater Res 10:273–281, 1976.)

1982 indicated slime or biofilm-mediated colonization on plastic catheters by *S. epidermidis*.[21, 22]

Several studies have clearly implicated adhesive slime-producing bacteria as causal agents in biomaterial, foreign body, and osteomyelitis infections.[8, 9, 16, 18–29] Millions of biomaterial components have been permanently or temporarily implanted. These include joint replacements; heart valves; vascular prostheses; cardiac pacemakers; mesh-fabric devices; dental implants; transcutaneous, transmucosal, and intravascular catheters; and sutures. A profoundly disturbing complication of the use of many of these devices is resistant, recurrent, frequently catastrophic, and always costly infection. For example, an infected total joint, internal fixation device, or vascular prosthesis almost always results in reoperation, amputation, osteomyelitis, or death.

Fundamental to the pathogenesis of biomaterial-centered sepsis is adhesion to and colonization of the surfaces of biomaterials, producing a foreign body locus or center of infection that cannot be cleared by antibiotics or intact host defenses until the biomaterial substratum is removed.

When nonliving substrata (biomaterial devices and some tissue transplants) are introduced into mammalian hosts, they may become favored sites for adhesive colonization, especially in the immunocompromised patient. For example, total joints or internal fixation devices, intravenous catheters, heart valves, vascular grafts, allografts, and almost all permanently or temporarily inserted transcutaneous or deep biomaterials may develop biofilm-mediated infections that are resistant to antibiotics and host defenses and tend to persist until the biomaterial or foreign body is removed.

PATHOGENIC SEQUENCE IN SUBSTRATUM-INDUCED INFECTION

Relevant to morbidity, prevention, and treatment, there emerges a hypothetical concept that progression to clinical infection in biomaterial-related disease in normal or immunosuppressed patients involves the maturation of an inoculum of known pathogens (*S. aureus, Escherichia coli*) or the transformation of nonpathogens (*S. epidermidis*) to a septic focus of slime-producing virulent organisms (Fig. 2–3). This maturation or transformation appears to occur in the presence of, and to be potentiated by, the surface of biomaterials. Biofilm-mediated adhesion and colonization by bacteria occurs at the skin surface in the presence of suture materials, tissue-traversing transcutaneous devices or transmucosal devices, at contaminated deep implant sites, and after sufficient exposure time (days to weeks). The bacteria in this form have acquired a new pathogenic potential. If prolonged presence of the device is required or allowed, local infection and/or distant seeding may occur. In infections of deep implants, early or late contamination, adhesion, and colonization may occur either at surgery or later, by seeding from skin abscesses, infected skin sutures, dental caries, or infected organ systems. In early or late disease, whether or not accepted pathogens or normally noninvasive bacteria such as *S. epidermidis* are present, the interaction of potentially adhesive slime-producing strains and biomaterial surfaces may result in successful

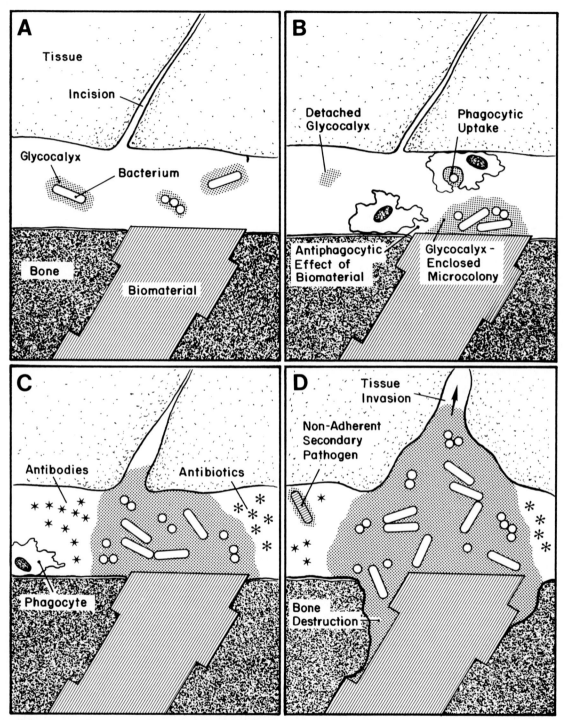

FIGURE 2–3. Diagrammatic evolution of an infection associated with a prosthetic biomaterial. Initially, bacteria are introduced into the wound *(A)*; they express their natural tendency to adhere *(B)* to an inert surface, on which they are protected by the antiphagocytic effect of the biomaterial and on which they form as microcolonies within a biofilm that protects them from phagocytic uptake and from nonimmune antibacterial serum factors. When the bacterial microcolony has burgeoned to a greater size *(C)*, the ion-exchange function of its glycocalyx affords a measure of protection from antibiotics and appears to protect the bacteria from both bactericidal and opsonizing antibodies. In the later stages of this infection *(D)*, the pathogens may cause destruction of bone and other tissue changes, and the colonies may shed secondary pathogens that, being for some reason less adhesive, are not necessarily representative in number, type, or pathogenicity of the adhesive colonies and may therefore confuse the diagnostic picture by dominating aspirates and other routine microbiologic samples. (Reprinted with permission from Gristina AG, Costerton JW: Bacterial adherence and the glycocalyx and their role in musculoskeletal infection. Orthop Clin North Am 15:517–535, 1984.)

colonization and clinical infection with morbid consequences.

INFECTION IN OSTEOMYELITIS

Osteomyelitis shares characteristics with other infections caused by adhesive bacteria: traumatized, dead, or compromised tissue is frequently involved; the disease is resistant to antibiotic therapy and to natural host defense mechanisms; polymicrobial infections are often present; and the disease tends to persist until dead tissue or sequestrum is removed.[31-35] With these features in mind, we have investigated bacterial adhesion on bone and surrounding tissues in resistant cases of osteomyelitis.

In general, osteomyelitis presents as an acute disease characterized by bone destruction and septicemia or as a chronic indolent infection of osseous structures featuring recurrent purulent drainage from resistant foci, which are often centered on residual dead bone or sequestrum. There are reports of unique bacterial forms and of site-specific and patient-specific clinical presentations. The etiology of acute, chronic, and regional osteomyelitis is certainly multifactorial, and all variables interlock to provide specific clinical sequences. At the initiation of each sequence, an inoculum of bacteria and a susceptible focus are required. Microbial delivery may be provided by direct contamination (as in trauma or an operation) or by immediate or delayed hematogenous or contiguous spreading. The concept of site specificity of the bacteria would appear to apply in trauma in the presence of compromised tissue or biomaterials, for particular microbes, or in certain patient groups.[32-41]

ADHESION IN OSTEOMYELITIS

Electron microscopic studies of acute and chronic osteomyelitic bone specimens indicate that infecting organisms also use bone as a substratum for adhesive biofilm-mediated colonization (Fig. 2–4).[32] In addition to bone primarily involved in osteomyelitis, bone adjacent to biomaterial implants may be secondarily involved by contiguous spread from the infected joint space or colonized biomaterial.[24, 31]

Traumatized, ischemic, or devitalized bone secondary to fractures, bone grafts, or allografts, as well as adjacent damaged tissues, may also act as infection-inducing foreign bodies.

An especially critical clinical setting frequently occurs in trauma and after biomaterial or total joint surgery when nonbiological devices (biomaterials, total joints, and internal fixation metals) are juxtaposed to traumatized and damaged tissues — a format that in essence can double susceptibility to infection and that the clinical literature, prior to the use of prophylactic antibiotics, supported.[41, 42]

TRAUMA IN OSTEOMYELITIS

Morrissy has demonstrated that trauma causes site localization in osteomyelitis.[36] Localization of septic emboli at hematoma sites has been considered probable. Platelets and fibrin specifically may represent sites of adhesion or act as receptors for bacterial adhesins. Damage to endothelial cells may expose fibronectin or other receptors for bacteria. The role of fibronectin as a mediator of microbial adhesion at sites of tissue trauma should be further studied. Hook has located receptor sites on *S. aureus* for collagen, suggesting a mechanism for the affinity of this important pathogen for bone in osteomyelitis.[43] Damaged blood vessel endothelial linings at trauma sites may allow microbial adhesion to exposed laminin in basement membranes, another possible mechanism for site localization and abscess formation in osteomyelitis.[7, 9, 19, 29, 32, 43–45]

ADHESION TO TISSUES

Studies by Costerton and colleagues,[6] Ofek and Beachey,[8] Christensen and others,[9] and Gibbons and van Houte[46] indicate that in man in certain diseases, bacteria colonize, propagate, infect, and resist host defenses by a complex of mechanisms that involve adhesion to target surfaces or cells, as in burns and cystic fibrosis (*Pseudomonas aeruginosa*), soft tissue trauma (*S. aureus*), gonococcal infections (*Neisseria gonorrhoeae*), endocarditis (*S. sanguis* and *S. mutans*), gastroenteritis (*E. coli*), and dental caries (*S. mutans*).

FACTORS IN MICROBIAL ADHESION, AGGREGATION, AND BIOFILM FORMATION

- Molecular mechanisms in adhesion
- The bacteria
- Polysaccharides and biofilm
- Conditioning films

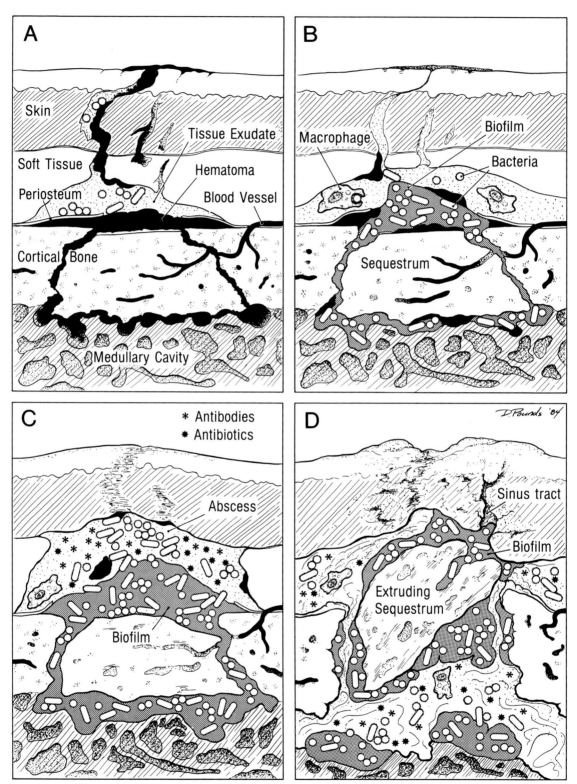

FIGURE 2–4. The sequence of pathogenesis in osteomyelitis.

A, Initial trauma produces soft tissue destruction and bone fragmentation, as well as wound contamination by bacteria. In closed wounds, contamination may occur by hematogenous seeding.

Legend continued on opposite page

Molecular Mechanisms in Adhesion

Initial attachment (*reversible nonspecific adhesion*) is dependent on the general physical characteristics of the bacterium, the fluid interface, and the substratum. Within the effective range of these phenomena, initial attachment of bacteria may be partially predictable, based on particle size, charge, and the relative hydrophobicity between the bacterium fluid phase and surface. *Specific irreversible adhesion,* which occurs after initial attachment, suggests time-dependent, biosynthetic chemical processes that in part depend on specific protein adhesin-receptor interactions as well as on carbohydrate polymer synthesis. Exopolysaccharides are vital for subsequent cell-to-cell aggregation and the sequestration of nutrients from the substratum and adjacent milieu.[3, 10, 32, 47-50]

The basic mechanisms of bacterial adhesion are dependent not only on the bacterial polymer but also on substratum and host factors. Studies in the marine, dental, and medical literature of certain diseases and of infections centered on biomaterials and of osteomyelitis have suggested the following progression.[43] Bacteria may arrive randomly at the surface of a biomaterial, foreign body, or osseous substrata by direct contamination, contiguous spread (as from adjacent epithelial cells or via transcutaneous prostheses) or by hematogenous seeding (e.g., heart valves, joint replacements, osteomyelitis).

The bacterial surface charge is negative, as are most substrata surfaces; however, isoelectric points of materials at the surface liquid interface can vary with pH and tissue damage caused by surgery, trauma, or infection.[51-53] Corrosion also alters pH and charge.[53] The common charges of the microbe and substratum tend to repel each other; however, van der Waals forces at the secondary minimum (approximately 10 nm) effectively position a particle or bacterium near the surface. At closer ranges, repulsion is maximal until the primary minimum is entered (2 to 3 nm) where attraction occurs.[10] New studies indicate that hydrophobic forces are exerted at distances as great as 15 nm, and at 8 to 10 nm are ten to 100 times as great as van der Waals forces.[48] Some degree of hydrophobicity exists for many bacteria and most surfaces.[10, 54] Attractive hydrophobic interactions tend to overcome repulsion and position bacteria at the primary minimum (Fig. 2–5). When a bacterium is within 1 nm or in surface contact, as demonstrated in transmission electron microscopy (TEM) preparation of *S. epidermidis* (Fig. 2–6), it is conceivable that chemical bonding occurs.

Subsequent to, or concomitant with, initial attachment, specific fimbrial adhesins and substratum receptors may interact if they are present in the particular biological system, as in bacteria-to-tissue cell pathogenesis.[10]

Proteinaceous adhesins (fimbriae) then form strong bonds with glycoproteinaceous surface residues or the cell receptors that are available in almost all biological systems. Exopolysaccharides also bind to the surface glycoproteins or function in cell-to-cell aggregation, further consolidating adhesion, microcolony, and biofilm formation. If other environmental conditions, such as temperature, nutrients (substrates), antagonists, and cation balance are favorable, bacterial propagation occurs (Fig. 2–7). Biomaterials, foreign bodies, and devitalized tissue and bone in a biological environment are passive and susceptible substrates due to the fact that, unlike normal tissues, they are not protected by normal intact eukaryotic exopolysaccharide polymers.[32, 44] Indeed, they are passive only in the sense that they are inanimate and do not resist infection; rather, they are physicochemically active and may encourage infection.[44]

Additional factors further influence the establishment of bacterial biofilms on favorable substrata. These include fluid graphics, pH, surface configuration of the substratum, tensions at fluid and surface interfaces, glycoproteinaceous residua on surfaces (which provide

---

FIGURE 2-4. *Continued.*

B, As the infection progresses, bacterial colonization occurs within a protective exopolysaccharide biofilm. The biofilm is particularly abundant on the devitalized bone fragment, which acts as a passive substratum for colonization.

C, Host defenses are mobilized against the infection, but are unable to penetrate, or be effective in the presence of, the biofilm.

D, Progressive inflammation and abscess formation eventually result in the development of a sinus tract and, in some cases, ultimate extrusion of the sequestrum that is the focus of the resistant infection.

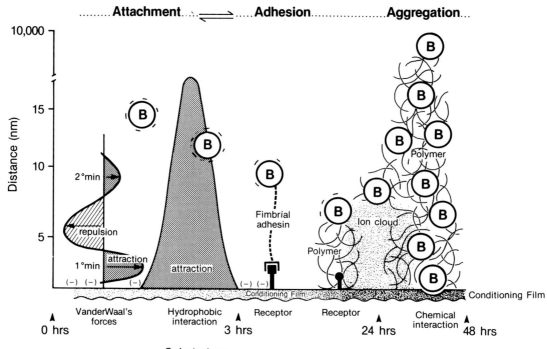

FIGURE 2-5. Molecular sequence in bacterial (B) attachment, adhesion, and aggregation to substratum. (Reprinted with permission from Gristina AG et al: Biomaterial specificity, molecular mechanisms and clinical relevance of *S. epidermidis* and *S. aureus* infections in surgery. In Proceedings of Symposium on Pathogenicity and Clinical Significance of Coagulase-Negative Staphylococci. Heppenheim, Germany. Copyright 1987, by Gustav Fischer–Verlag, Stuttgart.)

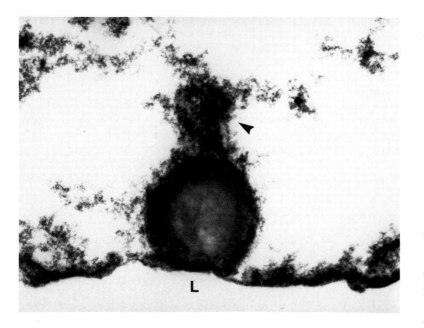

FIGURE 2-6. Transmission electron microscopy of *S. epidermidis* (SE-360) (ruthenium-red stain) on the surface of a soft contact lens (L). Note direct surface contact with a minimum of polysaccharide at contact interface and the aggregation of polysaccharides (arrow). (Reprinted with permission from Gristina AG et al: Biomaterial specificity, molecular mechanisms and clinical relevance of *S. epidermidis* and *S. aureus* infections in surgery. In Proceedings of the Symposium on Pathogenicity and Clinical Significance of Coagulase-Negative Staphylococci. Heppenheim, Germany. Copyright 1987, by Gustav Fischer–Verlag, Stuttgart.)

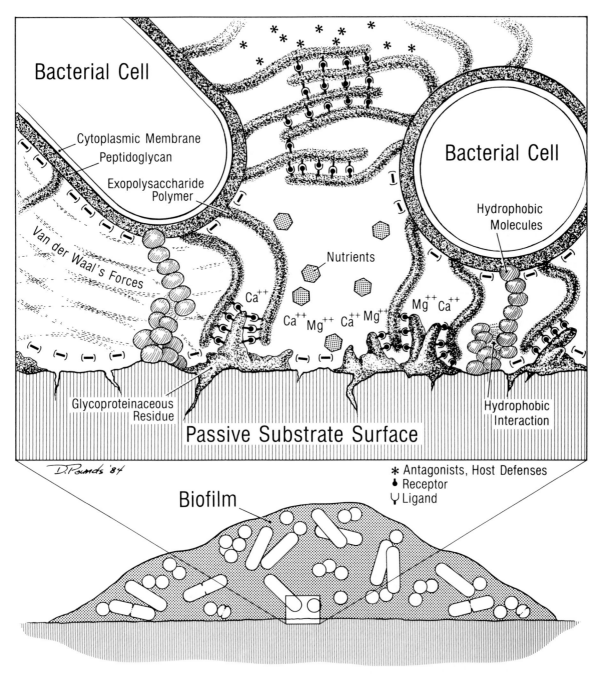

FIGURE 2–7. Mechanism of bacterial adhesion. At specific distances, the initial repelling forces between like charges on the surfaces of bacteria and substrate are overcome by attracting van der Waal's forces and hydrophobic interactions between molecules occurs. Under appropriate conditions, there is extensive development of exopolysaccharide polymers, allowing ligand-receptor interaction and pertinaceous binding of the bacteria to the substrate. This interaction depends on ions and nutrients present in the microzone. (Reprinted with permission from Gristina AG et al: Adherent bacterial colonization in the pathogenesis of osteomyelitis. Science 228:990–993, 1985.)

exopolysaccharide bonding sites), availability of nutrients and cations, the growth phase of each prokaryocytic cell, and competition by other organisms.[55-58] The effect of surface area of substrata, such as biomaterials or devitalized bone, remains to be investigated. It seems logical to assume that, all other factors being equal, random contact between bacterial cells and substrata increases as surface area increases.[32]

Bacteria

Adhesion is a general property of almost all bacteria and is dependent upon an intricate and sometimes exquisitely specific series of events based on determinants and characteristics of the bacteria, the substratum to be colonized, and the intervening ambient fluid milieu or environment.

Generally, the bacteria involved are accepted pathogens, such as *S. aureus, P. aeruginosa* or *E. coli.* However, in immunocompromised patients or in association with particular substrata or under optimized conditions, selection of normally autochthonous bacteria or nonpathogens may occur.

Bacteria in tissue adhesion are as follows: *N. gonorrhoeae,* pelvic and urinary inflammatory disease; *E. coli,* human diarrhea; *P. aeruginosa,* respiratory disease and cystic fibrosis; *S. mutans,* dental disease and endocarditis; and *S. aureus* and *S. sanguis,* surgical and soft tissue infections.[9]

The two most studied bacteria with regard to biomaterial-centered infections and osteomyelitis are *S. epidermidis* and *S. aureus,* respectively.

BACTERIA IN BIOMATERIAL SEPSIS

Our studies and those of others have most frequently isolated *S. epidermidis* and *S. aureus.* Additional organisms isolated include *E. coli,* peptococci, *P. aeruginosa, P. mirabilis,* and beta-streptococci.[9, 44] The variety of organisms recovered is increasing as awareness increases and methodology improves.

S. epidermidis, usually thought of as a nonpathogenic commensal human skin saprophyte, has emerged as a serious pathogen in biomaterial-related infections. Masur and Johnson[25] and others have listed *S. epidermidis* as a leading cause of infections in prostheses, shunts, and implants.[23, 41] Orthopedic reviews have also pointed out the pathogenic potential of *S. epidermidis.* Also disturbing is the fact that *S. epidermidis* is not only a significant biomaterial-associated pathogen but is emerging as a leading organism in nosocomial infections, especially those in immunosuppressed patients.[59-64]

BACTERIA IN OSTEOMYELITIS

S. aureus is the most common pathogen isolated in chronic osteomyelitis. Studies of adult osteomyelitis by Cierny and Mader have shown an incidence of polymicrobial infection approaching 75 percent.[35] The most common pathogens were *S. aureus; Pseudomonas* species; *Enterococcus* species; *S. epidermidis;* and *Streptococcus, Bacillus,* and *Proteus* species. Acute osteomyelitis also commonly involves *S. aureus.* Also included are patient-specific (age, immune status, drug abuse) and site-specific species such as *Salmonella* in hemoglobinopathy, *Pseudomonas* species in heroin addicts, *Candida* and *Aspergillus* species in host defense problems and intravenous access devices, group B streptococci in neonates, *Haemophilus influenzae* in children, and anaerobes in diabetes.[59]

POLYMICROBIAL COLONIZATION

Isolation of multiple organisms from biomaterial, compromised soft tissue, and osteomyelitic infections is occurring with increasing frequency. Our studies indicate that polymicrobial infections occur in more than half of the cases in this group. This is especially so when the infection is chronic, is produced by an open wound or burn, or is centered about a biomaterial device that communicates with the skin or external environment in some way. Multiple organism infections are seen even more commonly in chronic osteomyelitis centered on dead bone or communicating with the surface via a sinus tract.[19, 26, 27, 55] However, polymicrobial infections are a frequent feature of biomaterial sepsis and osteomyelitis, even in the absence of a sinus tract. Syntrophic mixed colonies within a biofilm envelope may share aerobic and anaerobic metabolic pathways and substratum nutrients to their mutual advantage.

Extracellular Polymers — The "Slime" and Biofilm

THE SLIME

The exopolysaccharide "slime" produced by bacteria is probably one of the pivotal factors responsible for the behavior of biomaterial-centered infections. The complex exopolysaccharide acts as an ion exchange resin for enhanced nutrition; moderates susceptibility to phagocytosis and response to antibodies; and functions in later stages of surface adhesion, aggregation, and polymicrobial interaction. In general, exopolysaccharides are composed of neutral monosaccharides such as D-glucose, D-galactose, L-fucose, and L-rhamnose and contain amino sugars and sialic acid. Our studies of S. epidermidis indicate the presence of mannose.[65] Polysaccharides are linear and branched polymers varying in length and compositions. In any case, these and other constituents vary between and within species. The extracellular polysaccharide substance of "slime-producing" strains of S. epidermidis is a loose amorphous material composed of a range of low- and high-molecular-weight polymers associated in large part through ionic interactions.[5, 31, 44, 66–69]

Currently, only the monomeric carbohydrate moieties and several amino acids in the exopolysaccharide slime of S. epidermidis have been described. In a report by Ichiman and Yoshida, glucose, galactose, glycerol, hexosamine, phosphorus, glycine, alanine, and phenylalanine have been described as major components of slime.[70] These S. epidermidis strains were randomly selected from clinical specimens unrelated to biomaterial infections. These types of studies are useful in a preliminary way to define the general nature of the material. However, because these average compositional studies are usually done prior to any size or charge fractionation of individual polymers comprising the mixture, the fine structures of the polymers remain to be elucidated. These studies are necessary and essential as a first step in defining the role of the complex exopolysaccharide material and its relationship to bacterial cell adhesion, its resistance to phagocytosis, and the bactericidal activity of mammalian defense cells. Extraction and characterization studies of the chemical composition of the extracapsular slime are now under way in our laboratory.

THE BIOFILM

Shortly after attachment and adhesion (3 to 4 hours or sooner), as growth and propagation accelerate and if colony conditions are optimal, extracellular polysaccharide polymers are produced that provide additional adhesion to surfaces and function in coaggregation to daughter cells or to cells of other species in consortia formation and polymicrobial infection. Production of polysaccharide and polymer function varies with species, growth phase, and nutrient conditions. Polysaccharide polymer integrity is dependent on available cations such as Ca^{++} and Mg^{++}. The aggregated accumulation of polysaccharides, bacteria, and bacterial microcolonies, of the same or different species, and environmental and host products forms the biofilm.

The biofilm matrix formed by the exopolysaccharide polymers serves not only as an adhesive mechanism but also appears to be virulence-related. In addition, the biofilm has been shown to confer resistance to host defense mechanisms and may also impede the effective penetration of antibiotics. Accumulated biofilm may eventually fragment and detach as inocula, secondary to hemodynamic forces (about heart valves or catheters) or trauma (at joint replacements, internal fixation devices or dental and soft tissue abscesses). Inocula of pathogens in biofilm represent a source of and explanation for hematogenous septic emboli, distant seeding, and secondary infection. The pertinaceous nature of the biofilm appears to be a major factor in the persistence of many chronic orthopedic infections.[26, 31, 32, 44, 47, 50, 68, 71]

Glycoproteinaceous Conditioning Films

Glycoproteinaceous conditioning films, derived from fluid or matrix phases containing fibronectin, osteonectin, fibrinogen, collagen, and other proteins, almost immediately coat a biomaterial or tissue substratum and provide receptor sites for bacterial or tissue adhesion.[71] The specific role of each of the macromolecular constituents of this layer will differ for each organism or tissue cell type. Glycoproteinaceous films on a biomaterial surface have been shown to inhibit the osseointegration of titanium implants and glass ceramic implants. Fibronectin has discrete binding sites for S. epidermidis and S. aureus and this implies a role in mediating infection.[72–75]

Studies of interfacial phenomenon by Baier have indicated the dramatic influence of initial surface free energy and state of cleanliness of implanted materials on the adsorption of conditioning films and the subsequent adhesion of host tissue cells and bacterial cells.[57, 58] The tenacity of cellular binding is directed by the protein dominated conditioning film. Glyco-proteinaceous conditioning films contain co-valently bound, short-chain, "bush-like" sugar groups that serve as receptors for bacterial ligands.[57, 58]

Silicon- and stearate-covered surfaces offer low-energy factors (surface energy range, 22 dynes/cm^2) for poor adhesion. Radiofrequency glow discharge treated stainless steel, chrome, cobalt, and titanium offer high surface energy and bioadhesion. Controlled experiments defining the relationship of bacterial exopolysaccharides to substratum surface energy and to fluid medium qualities and constituents are needed.[57, 58]

CLINICAL STUDIES

Clinical Review (S. epidermidis, S. aureus)

Our review of the clinical literature (Table 2–1) indicates that S. epidermidis appears to be the principal isolate from infections in a biomaterials setting that contains polymers and that S. aureus remains the predominant pathogen associated with metals, compromised tissues, surgical wounds, and osteomyelitis.[27, 28, 41, 42, 44, 61, 76–78]

Metallic, internal fixation device–associated infections, in the absence of methylmethacrylate or other polymers, appear to be dominated by S. aureus and gram-negative bacteria.[42]

Total joint infections (biomaterials: Vitallium, high density polyethylene and methylmethacrylate) predominantly involve S. epidermidis and secondarily involve S. aureus. Intravascular catheters, transperitoneal catheters, neurosurgical shunts, and aortofemoral grafts share a common major pathogen, S. epidermidis.[77]

Intravascular devices, such as heart valves and aortofemoral grafts, are subject to a high rate of infection. The major pathogen of these polymer prostheses is S. epidermidis.[23]

Transcutaneous or transmucosal devices, such as intravenous and peritoneal dialysis catheters, frequently become infected if left indwelling for any length of time. Most transcutaneous devices are of polymer composition, with the exception of traction or fixation pins of stainless steel. The principal pathogen for polymeric transcutaneous devices is S. epidermidis. In contrast, the principal reported pathogen for metallic transcutaneous devices is S. aureus, which occurs in 80 percent of infected cases using external (percutaneous) fixation pins of stainless steel. This is relevant and unexpected because the pins directly traverse a saturated S. epidermidis environment.[41, 42, 77]

Soft contact lenses are fabricated from hydrophilic methylpolymers. After P. aeruginosa, S. epidermidis is the second most common cause of hydrophilic soft contact lens–induced bacterial keratitis.[78]

Osteomyelitis infrequently involves S. epidermidis, except when associated with other organisms (S. aureus and gram-negative bacteria consortia formation).

Direct Studies and Identification of Pathogenic Bacteria in Situ on Biomaterials

CLINICAL RETRIEVAL (METHODS)

Methods have been abridged. For details, see the study by Gristina and associates.[44]

From 1979 through 1986, 171 specimens were retrieved and aerobically and anaerobi-

TABLE 2–1. Biomaterial-Centered Infection* (S. Epidermidis and S. Aureus)

Surface Material	Category	No. of Cases	S. epidermidis	S. aureus
Polymer	Hickman catheters Endotracheal tubes Sutures	102	64.4%	33%
Polymer + metal	Total joints	5	50.1%	33.2%
Metal	Osteosyntheses Transcutaneous pins	21	14.4%	57.2%
Tissue	Septic joints	23	18%	39%
Bone	Osteomyelitis	20	20%	50%

* Percentages represent numbers of cases which involved S. epidermidis or S. aureus, including polymicrobial retrievals. The remaining percentages are composed of other organisms and negative cultures.
Courtesy of Wake Forest University Medical Center, 1979–1986.

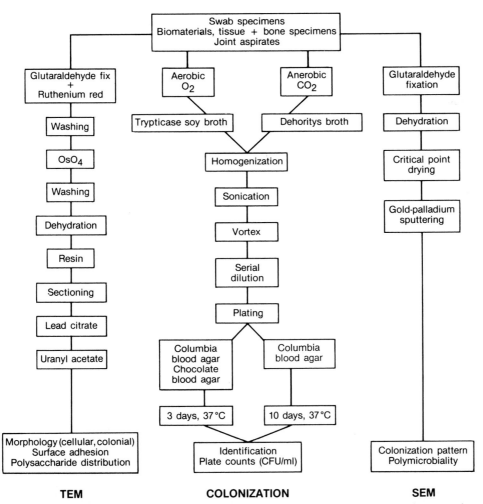

FIGURE 2–8. Evaluation procedures for clinical retrievals comprising swab specimens, biomaterials, tissue and bone specimens, and joint aspirates are shown. Specimens were processed for transmission electron microscopy (TEM), microbial identification and quantification (COLONIZATION), and scanning electron microscopy (SEM).

cally cultured. Selected specimens were examined by transmission and scanning electron microscopy (SEM) (Fig. 2–8).

CULTURING TECHNIQUES

For Aerobic Cultures. Biomaterials, bone, and tissue specimens were placed in 10 ml of phosphate-buffered saline (PBS), pH 7.2. Bone and tissue specimens were homogenized in a tissue grinder. All specimens were sonicated for 5.5 minutes at 37° C. After "vortexing" for 30 seconds, the bacterial suspensions were serially diluted with PBS to a concentration of 10^{-6} and cultured on Schaedler's blood agar and chocolate blood agar plates at 37° C for 3 days.[24, 31, 44]

For Anaerobic Cultures. Specimens were prepared similarly but in a CO_2–N_2 atmosphere. Dehority's broth was used instead of PBS. Dilutions were cultured on anaerobic blood agar plates for 10 days at 37° C within an anaerobic jar.[24, 31, 44]

SCANNING ELECTRON MICROSCOPY

Specimens were fixed in glutaraldehyde, dehydrated in ethanol, and critically point-dried according to standard procedures. They were sputtered with a 100 Å thick gold-palladium layer and examined in a Philips 501 SEM.[24, 31, 44]

TRANSMISSION ELECTRON MICROSCOPY

Specimens were fixed in glutaraldehyde, dehydrated in ethanol, stained with ruthenium-red followed by OsO_4, dehydrated in propylene oxide, embedded in Epon Resin and sectioned. The sections were then stained with uranyl acetate and lead citrate, stabilized with a carbon layer 50 Å thick and examined in a Philips EM-400 TEM.[24, 31, 44]

Results: Direct Studies, Identification, Morphology (Scanning and Transmission Electron Microscopy)

The review of our data at the Bowman Gray School of Medicine in the retrieval of 171 infected biomaterial specimens indicates that *S. epidermidis* predominates as an adhesive colonizer of polymers. *S. aureus* is a principal pathogen for metallic and compromised tissue substrata associated with surgical wounds, trauma, and osteomyelitis (Table 2 – 1).

The direct examination of biomaterials, tissues, and osteomyelitic bone from infections showed that the causative bacteria grew in polysaccharide biofilms and were adhesive to the surfaces of biomaterials and tissues in 75 percent of the cases. This high rate of recovery of adhesive biofilm-mediated growth suggested that the process commonly occurs in the presence of a foreign body or biomaterial-related infection. Scanning electron microscopy showed that the infecting bacteria grew in coherent microcolonies in an extensive adhesive biofilm (Fig. 2 – 9). Transmission electron microscopy showed this biofilm to have a gelatinous matrix that contained bacterial and host cells (Fig. 2 – 10). Because of the adhesive mode of growth of the infecting organisms, accurate microbiological sampling was difficult. The analysis of joint fluids, wound exudates, or swabs of infected sites often yielded growth of only one species from what was frequently a polymicrobial population (two thirds of cases), based on biomaterial scrapings, tissue homogenates, and electron microscopic studies.[24]

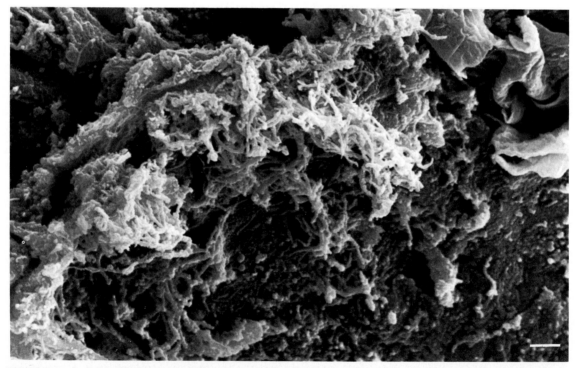

FIGURE 2 – 9. Scanning electron microscopy of the intradermal portion of a steel staple shows part of the very thick bacterial biofilm that developed on the surface of this device. Rod-shaped bacterial cells surrounded by amorphous intracellular material are clearly discernible within a very thick biofilm. The white bar indicates 5 μm. (Reprinted with permission from Gristina AG et al: Bacterial colonization of percutaneous sutures. Surgery 98:12 – 18, 1985.)

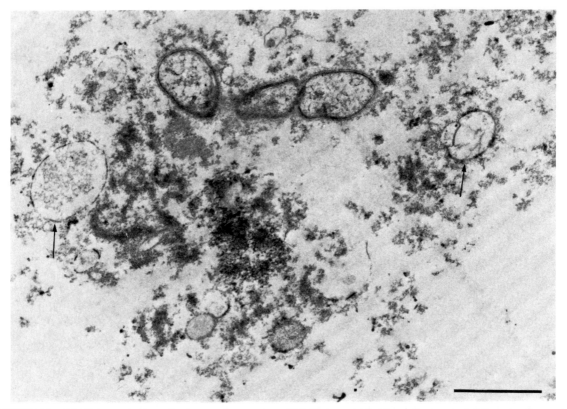

FIGURE 2–10. Transmission electron microscopy of biofilm material from the synovial tissue adjacent to an infected tibia. A microcolony consisting of gram-negative, rod-shaped bacteria, and many partially lysed bacterial cells whose outer cell walls are missing (arrows) can be seen. Bar = 1 μm.

The coherent properties of the adhesive biofilms that are found on surfaces in these infections may prevent detection of truly representative organisms. Therefore, antibiotics that are chosen may not be effective against all of the bacterial species present in biofilm infections.

Laboratory Studies

IN VITRO STUDY (METHODS)

Methods have been abridged. For details, see the study by Gristina and co-workers.[44]

Comparative Colonization of Biomaterials. Comparative colonization of the *S. epidermidis* (SE-360 strain [Yoshida] and an *S. aureus* stain (SA-WF1, retrieved from a biomaterial infection), was performed on standard-sized discs of Vitallium, 35 Multiphase Nickel Cobalt Chromium alloy, 316 stainless steel, and polymethylmethacrylate (PMMA). The biomaterials were exposed to standardized bacterial suspensions of Log phase slime-producing

mutants for 1, 4, 8, 16, 20, 24, 28, and 48 hours at 37° C. Then sonication, serial dilution, and culturing on blood agar plates for 24 hours at 37° C were performed and colony-forming unit (CFU) disc of adhesive cells determined.

Colonization of Hydrophilic Contact Lenses. The lenses used consisted of 62 percent polymacon and 38 percent water, by weight. Log phase bacterial suspensions of *S. epidermidis* (SE-360), a clinical isolate of *P. aeruginosa* (PA-WF1), a clinical isolate of *S. epidermidis* from an infected eye (SE-WF1), and a clinical isolate of *S. aureus* (SA-WF1) in trypticase soy broth with gluconic acid were used. The lenses were incubated in flasks in 20 ml of bacterial suspension (2.5×10^7 organisms per ml).[44]

Energy Dispersive X-ray Analysis (EDXA). Specimens for EDXA (biomaterial —polymeric soft contact lens; bacteria—*S. epidermidis* and *P. aeruginosa*) were prepared as for SEM and as above, but sputtered with a layer of carbon 200 Å thick instead of with gold-palladium. The EDXA permits elemental analysis of an extremely small area (100 nm in diameter) when used in conjunction with SEM. Using the characteristic x-ray emission generated from a sample during SEM examination, EDXA analyzes x-ray energy levels (each element having its own level) and intensity.[28]

Comparative Colonization of Biomaterials (S. epidermidis, S. aureus). Initial attachment time for *S. epidermidis* was significantly ($p <$ 0.05) longer than for *S. aureus* for all materials (4 hours for *S. epidermidis* versus 1 hour for *S. aureus*). Slime production was evident after 4 hours of incubation for both strains. Peak colo-

nization time for all bacteria versus biomaterials combinations was 24 hours. *S. epidermidis* showed significantly greater preference for polymers than metals, whereas the opposite was the case for *S. aureus*. The absolute maximum CFU/disc was found for *S. epidermidis* on PMMA (1.6×10^8 at 24 hours).

SEM and TEM of Bacteria-to-Polymer Interface (S. epidermidis [SE-360] and P. aeruginosa [PA-WF1]). The number of colonizing bacteria per lens of each strain did not differ significantly. SEM showed a discontinuous colonization pattern for both microbes, with the density of organisms within each colony increasing from the edge to the center. This pattern is consistent with that of clonal colony establishment from the initial inoculum (Fig. 2–11). TEM showed that *Pseudomonas* and *S. epidermidis* were both suspended above, and in direct contact with, the surface of the lens. However, direct contact was more typical of *Staphylococcus* and rare for *Pseudomonas* (see Fig. 2–6).[65]

Energy Dispersive X-ray Analysis (EDXA) of Bacteria-to-Polymer (Soft Contact Lens) Interface, S. epidermidis (SE-360) and S. aureus (SA-WF1). Carbon, aluminum, chlorine, silicon, phosphorus, calcium, and iron were found in the polysaccharide part of the 8-micron thick bacterial film on the lens (Fig. 2–12). Traces of chlorine and silicon may represent the embedding resin and plastic grid, respectively. The spectra for SE-360 and SA-WF1 did not differ.

DISCUSSION

The "Race for the Surface"

At the moment of implantation, a biomaterial is a ready site for competitive bacterial or tissue colonization. Its free energy sites are awaiting satisfaction by the first available colonizers, either bacteria or host cells (Fig. 2–13). In the case of metals, if the first colonizing cells are tissue and a secure bond is established, subsequent colonizers have to deal with a living, integrated cell surface, one that, if not subsequently traumatized or altered, is basically resistant to bacterial colonization by virtue of its viability, intact cell membranes, surface polysaccharides, and available host defense mechanisms.[29, 43, 79] Many biological polymers have an initial surface-free energy that is essentially antiadhesive for tissue cells.[74] However, polymers of high hydrophobicity are proadhesive for many bacterial pathogens

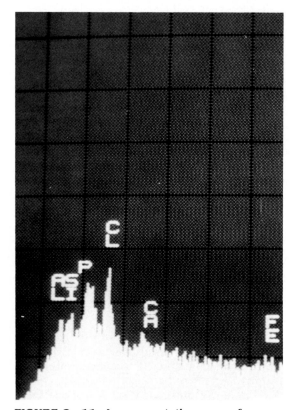

FIGURE 2–11. A representative scan of energy dispersive x-ray microanalysis of bacterial biofilm (SE-360) on a soft contact lens. Carbon (C), aluminum (Al), silicon (Si), chlorine (Cl), calcium (Ca), and iron (Fe) were found and analyzed in sequential areas in 2-micron steps from the surface. Each area scanned measured $2 \times 2 \mu^2$. (Reprinted with permission from Gristina AG et al: Biomaterial specificity, molecular mechanisms and clinical relevance of *S. epidermidis* and *S. aureus* infections in surgery. In Proceedings of the Symposium on Pathogenicity and Clinical Significance of Coagulase-Negative Staphylococci. Heppenheim, Germany. Copyright 1987, by Gustav Fischer–Verlag, Stuttgart.

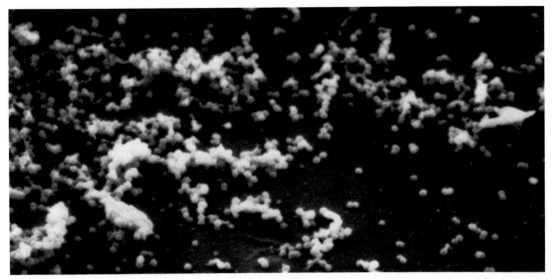

FIGURE 2 – 12. Scanning electron micrograph illustrating colonization pattern. Central from the edge (left), bacterial clusters are more frequent and organisms within the clusters are interconnected by the flocculent-appearing slime.

that readily adhere to their surfaces in *in vitro* test environments.[54] *In vivo,* available bacteria may defeat the host tissue cells in the race for the polymer's surface and thus cause infection, instead of tissue integration, of the polymer. Once bacterial adhesion has occurred, it is unlikely that tissue cells will be able to displace these primary colonizers to occupy and integrate the surface.

The Biofilm and the Microenvironment

The role of polysaccharide polymers requires further specific study, for they are abundant in almost all bacteria surface interrelationships, in natural ecosystems, and in healthy and diseased animals. Our studies show copious and confluent bridging between bacteria and substratum surfaces. It is likely, by virtue of physical mass and anionic charge, that the bacterial envelope and polymer aggregate, which form the biofilm, produce a microenvironment (microzone) that is shielded, to a degree, from host defenses and antagonists. The microenvironment may develop climatic qualities of its own, such as pH, ion, nutrient, and toxin concentrations, and may also provide colony cohesiveness and receptivity for consortial organisms through specific polymer interaction (Figs. 2 – 7 and 2 – 14).[31, 32, 44, 55, 80]

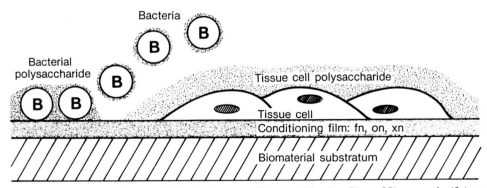

FIGURE 2 – 13. Implanted biomaterial substratum with conditioning film of fibronectin (fn), osteonectin (on), or other proteins (xn). The surface may be colonized by bacteria (B) or tissue cells. If successful tissue colonization occurs first, available energy sites, receptors, or both are satisfied and bacterial adhesion is less likely.

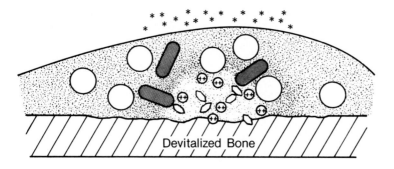

Bacteria (aerobic, anerobic)
Biofilm
Microzone
Ions (Ca++, Mg++)
Metabolites
* Antagonists and Host Defenses

FIGURE 2–14. In osteomyelitis, polymicrobial colonization with aerobic and anaerobic bacteria occurs. The bacterial polymer aggregate may form a microzone with climatic qualities of its own regarding metabolite and ion concentrations and may to a degree act as a barrier to antagonists.

For those bacteria directly in contact with or near the surface, utilization of potential substrates, metabolites, molecules, or ions from the substratum and at their envelope becomes crucial. Middle layers of organisms will be dependent on diffused molecules from the substrata or adjacent environment or on metabolites produced by pioneer colonizers. Outer layers will absorb ambient factors.

Our preliminary EDXA studies indicate the presence of iron, calcium, silicon, chlorine, phosphorus, and aluminum at the surface and within the biofilm. These initial studies are not quantitative, nor can they, for the area involved, discriminate precisely between cells or polysaccharides.

Our TEM studies indicate that the polysaccharide was localized in the regions between bacteria and that a number of the *S. epidermidis* appeared to be directly on the surface of the polymer without significantly interspersed polysaccharide. This suggests that for *S. epidermidis,* the polysaccharide functions significantly in cell-to-cell aggregation and also that *S. epidermidis* surface chemical interaction may be occurring. On the other hand, our studies of *P. aeruginosa* have shown abundant polysaccharide interspersed between the bacteria and the polymer surface.[65]

Polysaccharide biofilm may also impede antibiotic penetration. Our studies indicate a 2 Log+ increase in the antibiotic level required to maintain minimal inhibitory concentration (MIC) and minimal bactericidal concentration (MBC) values for a biofilm-enclosed *S. epider-*

midis strain on the surface of stainless steel when challenged with tobramycin as compared with MIC and MBC values from original suspension cultures (non-biofilm enclosed of the same organisms) (Gristina et al, unpublished data) (Fig. 2–15). These findings also suggest selection for more adhesive or ultimately antibiotic resistant organisms.

Substratum Direction of Adhesion

BONE

Bone is a composite structure composed of calcium hydroxyapatite crystals and a collagen matrix grossly similar to synthetic composites or to partially crystalline polymers. Dead, devitalized bone is inanimate, thus providing a passive substratum for bacterial colonization and ultimate incorporation of its proteinaceous and mineral constituents as metabolites.[32, 44, 53]

Traumatized bone, devoid of normal periosteum and blood supply, represents a site of crystalline and collagen exposure. We have suggested that surfaces and/or crystalline structures may accelerate microbial metabolism as well as provide bacterial metabolites and receptors, thereby allowing a lesser infecting inoculum of bacteria to act as a pioneer colonizer. At the traumatized or exposed site of bone, crystal faces representing open or unsatisfied Ca^{++} and PO_4^{---} bonds are available as free energy sites for binding with bacterial surfaces (Fig. 2–16). Bacteria *(S. aureus)* also have receptors for collagen, which is ubiquitous in bone and tissues and may also be available and receptive at sites of trauma, especially when normal cell membranes and surfaces are disturbed or when host defenses are diminished by ischemia or other causes.[43, 44, 53, 81]

SOFT TISSUE

Soft tissue (traumatized) is represented by amorphous organic fragments of cellular tissue and matrices, is rich in microbial nutrient material, and provides a surface for colonization. Inanimate, passive, and fertile traumatized tissues are unable to resist colonization.

ALLOGRAFTS

Allografts represent a particularly large mass of dead bone and cartilage that have clinically demonstrated a 14 percent rate of infection.[82] This suggests that masses of dead bone are logical sites for colonization and infection.

ENDOTHELIAL CELLS

Endothelial cells are surrounded by a well-developed glycocalyx. Studies have indicated that when this outer polysaccharide margin is traumatized by viruses, toxins, or inflammation, fibronectin receptor sites are exposed.[82] We have suggested that these sites are then susceptible to bacterial adhesion, colonization, and the development of vascular infection. This may explain in part S. epidermidis and other bacterial colonization and infection of aortofemoral graft vascular junctions. We also suggest that endothelial damage may be a factor in site localization by trauma or by septic emboli in osteomyelitis. Healthy endothelial cell tissue cultured and seeded over vascular graft polymer surfaces might protect against bacterial adhesion or thrombogenic events.[29, 32, 45]

PLATELETS

Gram-positive bacteria, S. aureus, Streptococcus pyogenes, S. mutans, and S. sanguis, which are the most common causes of bacterial endocarditis, bind to fibronectin, fibrin, or platelets. Trauma to natural heart valves or conditioning of plastic valves by fibronectin, fibrin, and platelet vegetations may be the initial and pivotal step in the colonization of heart valves. Platelets used as a bridge may allow bacterial binding to damaged tissues. This is also a possible mechanism in trauma-induced osteomyelitis.[9]

Metals, Polymers, and Ceramics As Substrata

An in-depth discussion of these substrata is held in the following chapter.

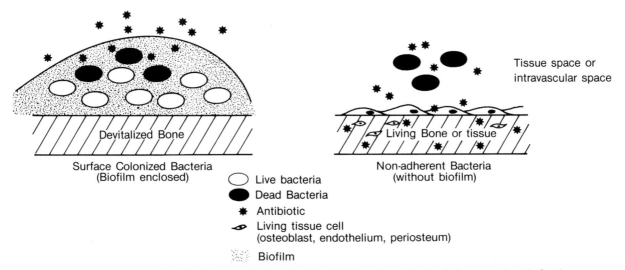

FIGURE 2 – 15. Antibiotic effectiveness is blocked by biofilm about bacteria in organized infection on the surface of a sequestrum or biomaterial substratum. Free-floating bacteria, not protected by biofilm, are more susceptible to standard antibiotic levels, which reach organisms via normal circulation or tissues.

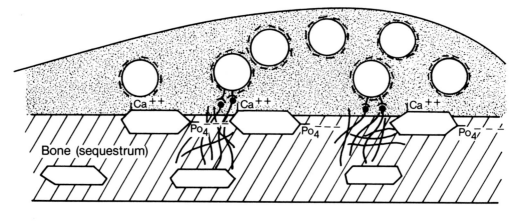

Ca⁺⁺   Exposed unsatisfied bonds of hydroxyapatite (HAP)
         ⋏   Collagen receptor
         ❘   Active site of collagen fibers
         ◯   Bacteria
              Biofilm
         ⬭   HAP crystal

FIGURE 2–16. Dead bone consisting of hydroxyapatite crystals within a collagen meshwork is colonized by slime-producing bacteria interacting with charged, unsatisfied binding sites on the crystal surface. Collagen receptors on the bacterial surface interact with active sites on the collagen fibers.

SUMMARY

The Bacteria

S. aureus is the major pathogen in biometal, bone and joint, and soft tissue infections, but is associated to a lesser degree with polymer-sited infections. *S. aureus* may also participate in concert with *S. epidermidis* and gram-negative organisms.

By clinical studies, *S. epidermidis* shows a predilection to cause infection in association with biomaterial surfaces, especially when the biomaterial is a polymer or when a polymer is a component of a complex device. Our *in vitro* studies also verify preferential adhesion to the surfaces of polymers. Similar findings have been presented by other investigators.[30] *S. epidermidis* is also a factor in polymicrobial infections associated with other substrata, such as metals, compromised bone, and tissues; however, in those cases, it appears to act as a co-pathogen and frequently augments, or is augmented by, other organisms. Immuno-compromised patients are also subjected to *S. epidermidis* infections, especially when biomaterials are present. The frequency of laboratory identification of *S. epidermidis* should increase as its pathogenic potential is understood.

Genesis and Pathogenesis

Bacteria in natural habitats, certain tissue diseases, biomaterial-centered infections, and osteomyelitis have a common survival mode based on adhesive colonization of substrata. In osteomyelitis, compromised tissues and bone provide that substratum. The interaction of physical and biological factors then allows bacterial attachment and adhesion. Proteinaceous appendages, polysaccharide polymers, surfaces, and milieu substances interact and intermix to form an aggregate of bacteria and polysaccharides in a biofilm. Additional symbiotic species may joint in syntrophic consortia and in certain locations may present as a polymicrobial infection. Nutrition and resistance to host defenses and antibiotics are enhanced by the biofilm. Within this biofilm, microzones of optimized conditions may develop and the infection stabilizes or even spreads and characteristically cannot be adequately treated until the substratum is removed. Thus, bacterial adhesion and its denominators direct the pathogenesis of osteomyelitis and biomaterial infections.

The high rate of identification of biofilm-mediated bacterial adhesion in studies of osteomyelitis and infected biomaterials suggests that the adhesive mode of growth is ubiquitous and is the natural state of bacterial existence in this type of infection. The observed tendency of osteomyelitis and biomaterial-related infections to persist until removal of the foreign-body nidus suggests, at least in part, a causal relationship between the natural, biofilm mode of bacterial existence and the cause and persistence of these infections.

The coherent properties of adhesive biofilms that are found on surfaces in these infections may prevent truly representative organisms from detaching in sufficient numbers to be detected completely and consistently by simple aspiration and routine culture techniques. Therefore, antibiotics that are chosen on the basis of results of such methods may not be effective against all of the bacterial species involved in these biofilm infections.

Biomaterial, damaged-tissue and biofilm-mediated resistant infections are not only a threat to the patient with a total joint arthroplasty or internal fixation device; they also present a danger to every patient who harbors any type of biomaterial, allograft, organ transplant, or artificial organ.

Defensive and Therapeutic Strategies

A novel defensive strategy may be to make biomaterial surfaces proadhesive to encourage rapid colonization by healthy tissue cells (endothelium, bone, soft tissue), which tend to resist colonization and infection and allow normal defense mechanisms to operate. Antiadhesive surfaces, though seemingly a clever approach, are neutralized by conditioning films and have in effect already been defeated by an infinite number of experiments in nature. Antibiotics that interfere with bacterial polymer synthesis and adhesive mechanisms, and which penetrate biofilm or are delivered by the substratum, should be effective. Blocking or saturating analogs are an appropriately sophisticated approach that should be studied and may provide an effective countermeasure.

EPILOGUE

Antony Leeuwenhoek did not lose his teeth until he was 80 and remained a productive scientist until his death at 91. He attributed his excellent dental health to his habit of brushing his teeth with salt and the very hot coffee that he had for breakfast (a combination of hypertonic saline, heat, and tannic acid — three antibacterial agents). Antony Leeuwenhoek, the first of the microbe hunters, was also first in "the race for the surface."

Acknowledgment

The authors gratefully acknowledge the assistance of Dr. Quentin N. Myrvik, Dr. Jon C. Lewis, and Dr. M. Madison Slusher in the preparation of this chapter; Cindy Clark for manuscript preparation; and Toni Meador for editorial assistance.

References

1. de Kruif P: Microbe Hunters. New York, Blue Ribbon Books, 1926, p 17.
2. Gibbons RJ, van Houte J: Bacterial adherence and the formation of dental plaques. In Beachey EH, ed: Bacterial Adherence. New York, Chapman and Hall, 1980, pp 61–104.
3. Fletcher M: Effect of solid surfaces on the activity of attached bacteria. In Savage DC, Fletcher M, eds: Bacterial Adhesion. New York, Plenum Press, 1985, pp 339–362.
4. Jones HC, Roth IL, Sanders WM III: Electron microscopic study of a slime layer. J Bacteriol 99:316–325, 1969.
5. Costerton JW, Irvin RT, Cheng K-J: The bacterial glycocalyx in nature and disease. Ann Rev Microbiol 35:299–324, 1981.
6. Costerton JW, Marrie TJ, Cheng K-J: Phenomena of bacterial adhesion. In Savage DC, Fletcher M, eds: Bacterial Adhesion. New York, Plenum Press, 1985, pp 3–43.
7. Lopes JD, dos Reis M, Brentani RR: Presence of laminin receptors in Staphylococcus aureus. Science 229:275–277, 1985.
8. Ofek I, Beachey EH: General concepts and principles of adherence in animals and man. In Beachey EH, ed: Bacterial Adherence. New York, Chapman and Hall, 1980, pp 1–31.
9. Christensen GD, Simpson WA, Beachey EH: Adhesion of bacteria to animal tissues: Complex mechanisms. In Savage DC, Fletcher M, eds: Bacterial Adhesion. New York, Plenum Press, 1985, pp 279–305.
10. Jones GW, Isaacson RE: Proteinaceous bacterial adhesins and their receptors. Crit Rev Microbiol 10:229–260, 1984.
11. Nicolson GL, Winkelhake JL: Organ specificity of blood-borne tumour metastasis determined by cell adhesion. Nature 255:230–232, 1975.
12. Kieran MW, Longnecker BM: Organ specific metastasis with specific reference to avian systems. Cancer Metastasis Rev 2:165–182, 1983.
13. Gristina AG, Rovere GD: An in vitro study of the effects of metals used in internal fixation on bacterial growth and dissemination. J Bone Joint Surg 45A:1104, 1963.
14. Gristina AG, Rovere GD: An in vitro study of the effects of metals used in internal fixation on bacterial growth and dissemination. In Orthopaedic Research Society (Book of Abstracts). Miami Beach, 1963, pp 3–4.
15. Bayston R, Penny SR: Excessive production of mucoid substances in staphylococcus SIIA: a possible factor in colonisation of Holter shunts. Dev Med Child Neurol (Suppl) 27:25–28, 1972.
16. Gristina AG, Rovere GD, Shoji H, Nicastro JF: An in

vitro study of bacterial response to inert and reactive metals and to methylmethacrylate. J Biomed Mater Res 10:273–281, 1976.

17. Gristina AG, Costerton JW, Leake E, Kolkin J, Wright MJ: Bacteria and their relationship to biomaterials. Orthop Trans 5:332, 1981.

18. Gristina AG, Kolkin J: Current concepts review: total joint replacement and sepsis. J Bone Joint Surg 63A:128–134, 1983.

19. Gristina AG, Kolkin J, Leake E, Costerton JW, Wright MJ: Bacteria and their relationship to biomaterials. In Book of Abstracts. First World Biomaterials Conference. Vienna, European Society for Biomaterials, April 1980, Vol 2, p 39.

20. Gristina AG, Costerton JW: Bacterial adherence to biomaterials: The clinical significance of its role in sepsis. In Anderson JM, ed: Biomaterials '84 Transactions. Second World Congress on Biomaterials. Washington, DC, Society for Biomaterials, April 1984, Vol 7, p 175.

21. Christensen GD, Simpson WA, Bisno AL, Beachey EH: Adherence of slime-producing strains of *Staphylococcus epidermidis* to smooth surfaces. Infect Immun 37:318–326, 1982.

22. Peters G, Locci R, Pulverer G: Microbial colonization of prosthetic devices. II. Scanning electron microscopy of naturally infected intravenous catheters. Zentralbl Bakter Mikrobiol Hyg B 173:293–299, 1981.

23. Bandyk DF, Berni GA, Thiele BL, Towne JB: Aortofemoral graft infections due to *Staphylococcus epidermidis.* Arch Surg 119:102–107, 1984.

24. Gristina AG, Costerton JW: Bacterial adherence to biomaterials and tissue: the significance of its role in clinical sepsis. J Bone Joint Surg 67A:264–273, 1985.

25. Masur H, Johnson WD: Prosthetic valve endocarditis. J Thorac Cardiovasc Surg 80:31–37, 1980.

26. Gristina AG, Costerton JW: Bacteria-laden biofilms: a hazard to orthopedic prostheses. Infect Surg 3:655–661, 1984.

27. Sugarman B, Young EJ, eds: Infections Associated with Prosthetic Devices. Boca Raton, Fla, CRC Press, 1984.

28. Schmitt DD, Bandyk DF, Pequet AJ, Malanzoni MA, Towne JB: Mucin production by *Staphylococcus epidermidis:* a virulence factor promoting adherence to vascular grafts. Arch Surg 121:89–95, 1986.

29. Webb LX, Gristina AG, Myers RT, Cordell AR, Hobgood CD, Costerton JW: Inhibition of bacterial adherence by antibacterial surface pretreatment of vascular prostheses. J Vasc Surg 4:16–21, 1986.

30. Merritt K, Turner GE: Adherence of bacteria to biomaterials. Abstract, 11th Annual Meeting of the Society for Biomaterials. San Diego, 1985.

31. Gristina AG, Costerton JW: Bacterial adherence and the glycocalyx and their role in musculoskeletal infection. Orthop Clin North Am 15:517–535, 1984.

32. Gristina AG, Oga M, Webb LX, Hobgood CD: Adherent bacterial colonization in the pathogenesis of osteomyelitis. Science 228:990–993, 1985.

33. Waldvogel FA, Vasey H: Osteomyelitis: the past decade. N Engl J Med 303:360–370, 1980.

34. Hall BB, Fitzgerald RH, Rosenblatt JE: Anaerobic osteomyelitis. J Bone Joint Surg 65A:30–35, 1983.

35. Cierny G, Couch L, Mader J: Adjunction local antibiotics in the management of contaminated orthopaedic wounds. In Final Program: American Academy of Orthopedic Surgeons 54th Annual Meeting, Park Ridge, Ill, 1986, p 86.

36. Morrissy RT, Haynes DW: Acute hematogenous osteomyelitis: a model with trauma as an etiologic agent. Paper presented at the 51st Annual Meeting of the American Academy of Orthopedic Surgeons. Atlanta, February 9–14, 1984.

37. Eismont FJ, Bohlman HH, Prasanna LS, Goldberg VM, Freehofer AA: Pyogenic and fungal vertebral osteomyelitis with paralysis. J Bone Joint Surg 65A:19–29, 1983.

38. Simpson MB Jr, Merz WG, Kurlinski JP, Solomon MH: Opportunistic mycotic osteomyelitis: bone infections due to *Aspergillus* and *Candida* species. Medicine 56:475–482, 1977.

39. Lewis R, Garbach S, Altner P: Spinal *Pseudomonas* chondro-osteomyelitis in heroin users. N Engl J Med 286:1303, 1972.

40. Ortiz-Neu C, Marr JS, Cherubin CE, Neu HC: Bone and joint infections due to *Salmonella.* J Infect Dis 1138:820–828, 1978.

41. Dougherty SH, Simmons RL: Infections in bionic man: the pathobiology of infections in prosthetic devices, part 2. Curr Probl Surg 19:269–318, 1982.

42. Towers AG: Wound infection in an orthopaedic hospital. Lancet 2:379–381, 1965.

43. Speziale P, Raucci G, Visai L, Switalski LM, Tempe R, Hook M: Binding of collagen to *Staphylococcus aureus* strain Cowan 1. J Bacteriol 167:77–81, 1986.

44. Gristina AG, Hobgood CD, Barth E: Biomaterial specificity, molecular mechanisms and clinical relevance of *S. epidermidis* and *S. aureus* infections in surgery. In Pulverer G, Quie PG, Peters G, eds: Pathogenicity and Clinical Significance of Coagulase-Negative Staphylococci. Stuttgart, Gustav Fischer–Verlag, 1987, pp 143–157.

45. Ryan US, Ryan JW, Crutchley DJ: The pulmonary endothelial surface. Fed Proc 44:0013–0019, 1985.

46. Gibbons RJ, van Houte J: Dental caries. In Creger WP, Coggins CH, Hancock EW, eds: Selected topics in the clinical sciences. Ann Rev Med 26:121–136, 1975.

47. Beachey EH: Bacterial adherence: adhesin-receptor interactions mediating the attachment of bacteria to mucosal surfaces. J Infect Dis 143:325–345, 1981.

48. Pashley RM, McGuiggan PM, Ninham BW: Attraction forces between uncharged hydrophobic surfaces: direct measurements in aqueous solution. Science 229:1088–1089, 1985.

49. Pringle JH, Fletcher M, Ellwood EC: Selection of attachment mutants during the continuous culture of *Pseudomonas fluorescens* and their relationship between attachment ability and surface composition. J Gen Microbiol 129:2557–2569, 1983.

50. Fletcher M: Adherence of marine micro-organisms to smooth surfaces. In Beachey EH, ed: Bacterial Adherence. New York, Chapman and Hall, 1980, pp 345–374.

51. Rutter PR, Dazzo FB, Freter E, Gingell D, Jones GW, Kjelleberg S, Marshall KC, Mrozek H, Rades-Rohkohl E, Robb ID, Silverman M, Tylewska S: Mechanisms of adhesion. In Marshall KC, ed: Microbial Adhesion and Aggregation. Berlin, Springer-Verlag, 1984, pp 5–19.

52. Lyklema J: Interfacial electrochemistry of surfaces with biomedical relevance. In Andrade JD, ed: Surface and Interfacial Aspects of Biomedical Polymers, Vol 1. Surface Chemistry and Physics. New York, Plenum Press, 1985, pp 293–334.

53. Mears DC: Materials and Orthopedic Surgery. Baltimore, Williams & Wilkins, 1979.

54. Hogt AH, Dankert J, Hulstaert CE, Feijen J: Cell sur-

face characteristics of coagulase-negative staphylococci and their adherence to fluorinated poly(ethylenepropylene). Infect Immun 51:294–301, 1986.

55. Paerls HW: Influence of attachment on microbial metabolism and growth in aquatic ecosystems. In Savage DC, Fletcher M, eds: Bacterial Adhesion. New York, Plenum Press, 1985, pp 363–400.

56. Gibbons RJ: Adherence of bacteria to host tissue. In Schlesinger D, ed: Microbiology. Washington, DC, American Society for Microbiology, 1977, pp 395–406.

57. Baier RE: Conditioning surfaces to suit the biomedical environment: recent progress. J Biomech Eng 104:257–271, 1982.

58. Baier RE, Meyer AE, Natiella JR, Natiella RR, Carter JM: Surface properties determine bioadhesive outcomes: methods and results. J Biomed Mater Res 18:337–355, 1984.

59. Waldvogel FA: Treatment of osteomyelitis and septic arthritis. Bull NY Acad Med 58:733–749, 1982.

60. Lowy FD, Hammer SM: Staphylococcus epidermidis infections. Ann Intern Med 99:834–839, 1983.

61. Winston DJ, Dudnick DV, Chapin M, Winston GH, Gale RP, Martin WJ: Coagulase-negative staphylococci bacteremia in patients receiving immunosuppressive therapy. Arch Intern Med 143:32–36, 1983.

62. Pegram S, Muss H, McCall C, Cooper R, White D, Richards P, Jackson D, Stuart J, Spurr C, Hopkins J, Capizzi R: A comparative study of moxalactam (M) vs. ticarcillin and tobramycin (TT) in febrile neutropenic cancer patients. Proc ASCO 3:100, 1984.

63. Fitzgerald RH: The infected total hip arthroplasty. In Welch RB, ed: The Hip. Proceedings of the 12th Open Scientific Meeting of the Hip Society. St. Louis. CV Mosby Co 1984, pp 347–358.

64. Henderson K: Infections associated with prostheses, shunts and implants. In Yoshikawa TT, Chow AW, Guze LB, eds: Infectious Diseases: Diagnosis and Management. New York, Wiley Medical, 1980, pp 274–285.

65. Slusher MM, Myrvik QN, Lewis JC, Gristina AG: Extended-wear lenses, biofilm, and bacterial adhesion. Arch Ophthalmol 105:110–115, 1987.

66. Yoshida K, Ichiman Y: Immunological response to a strain of Staphylococcus epidermidis in the rabbit: production of a protective antibody. J Med Microbiol 11:371–377, 1978.

67. Govan JRW, Fyfe JAM: Mucoid Pseudomonas aeruginosa and cystic fibrosis: resistance of the mucoid form to carbenicillin, flucloxacillin and tobramycin and the isolation of mucoid variants in vitro. J Antimicrob Chemother 4:233–240, 1978.

68. Baltimore RS, Mitchell M: Immunologic investigation of mucoid strains of Pseudomonas aeruginosa. J Infect Dis 41:238–247, 1980.

69. Roth IL: Physical structure of surface carbohydrates. In Sutherland IW, ed: Surface Carbohydrates of the Prokaryotic Cell. London, Academic Press, 1977, pp 5–26.

70. Ichiman I, Yoshida K: The relationship of capsular type of Staphylococcus epidermidis to virulence and induction of resistance in the mouse. J Appl Bacteriol 51:229–241, 1981.

71. Govan JRW: Mucoid strains of Pseudomonas aeruginosa: the influence of culture medium on the stability of mucus production. J Med Microbiol 8:513–522, 1975.

72. Vercellotti GM, McCarthy JB, Lindholm P, Peterson PK, Jacob HS, Furcht LT: Extracellular matrix proteins (fibronectin, laminin and type IV collagen) bind and aggregate bacteria. Am J Pathol 120:13–21, 1985.

73. Barth E, Ronningen H, Salheim LF: Comparison of ceramic and titanium implants in cats. Acta Orthop Scand 56:491–495, 1985.

74. Switalski LM, Ryden C, Rubin K, Ljungh A, Hook M, Wadstrom T: Binding of fibronectin to Staphylococcus strains. Infect Immun 42:628–633, 1983.

75. Baier RE: Surface chemical factors presaging bioadhesive events. Ann NY Acad Sci 34–57, 1983.

76. Green SA, Ripley MJ: Chronic osteomyelitis in pin tracks. J Bone Joint Surg 66A:1092–1098, 1984.

77. Fitzgerald RH, Kelly PJ: Infections in the skeletal system. In Simmons RL, Howard RJ, Henriksen AI, eds: Surgical Infectious Diseases. Norwalk, Conn, Appleton-Century-Crofts, 1982, pp 1005–1028.

78. Patrinely JR, Wilhelmus KR, Rubin JM, Key JE 2nd: Bacterial keratitis associated with extended wear soft contact lenses. CLAO J 11:234–236, 1985.

79. Gristina AG, Costerton JW, Webb LX: Microbial adhesion, biofilms and the pathophysiology of osteomyelitis. In D'Ambrosia R, Mavier RL, eds: Orthopedic Infections. Thorofare, NJ, Charles B. Slack, (in press).

80. Brown MRW, Williams P: The influence of environment on envelope properties affecting survival of bacteria in infections. Ann Rev Microbiol 39:527–556, 1985.

81. Gomer R: Surface diffusion. Sci Am 247: 98–109, 1982.

82. Burwell RG, Friedlaender GE, Mankin HJ: Current Perspectives and Future Directions: the 1983 Invitational Conference on Osteochondral Allografts. Clin Orthop July–August (197):141–157, 1985.

Anthony G. Gristina, M.D.
Elin Barth, M.D.
Lawrence X. Webb, M.D.

CHAPTER

3

Microbes, Metals, and Other Nonbiological Substrata in Man

Substratum and Substrate Factors in Infection

INTRODUCTION

General aspects of bacterial adhesion that are common to all substrata and environments were reviewed in Chapter 2. Those concepts form the basis of our discussion of the unique qualities of metals and other nonbiologic substrata that share comparative physicochemical properties.

Most implants, prostheses, or artificial organs are composed of one or more metals or synthetic materials. There are several excellent reviews that detail the many materials involved.[1-3] This presentation focuses on the general characteristics of metals (stainless steel, chrome cobalt, and titanium alloys), polymers (methylmethacrylate [MM] and high-density polyethylene [HDP]), ceramics, and Bioglass and their relevance to microbial colonization. Special problems of complex devices are also discussed.

INITIAL EVENTS IN ADHESION TO METALLIC SURFACES

Almost instantly upon implantation, a biomaterial is coated by elements, macromolecules, and cellular debris, which are ambient to the host site and integral to the surgical procedure. Surface properties of the biomaterial,

artificial organ, or biologic implant in part direct its adsorption affinity and deposition as well as the subsequent qualitative and quantitative composition of the conditioning film. Host proteins, such as collagen, fibronectin, laminin, osteonectin, fibrinogen, fibrin, and thrombin as well as platelets or other cellular elements, are most frequently involved. Deposition, adsorption, layering, and intermixing occur as a time-dependent, physicochemical interaction. Colonizing tissue cells or bacteria (if present) then bind more or less directly, and with varying degrees of physicochemical integration, to substrata via this complex macromolecular layer. There is a potentially high degree of selectivity specific to this interaction. Factors that direct this selectivity include the molecular structure and surface energy of the substrata, fluid environment constituents, intermediary film, and types of pioneer cells involved.

Clean metallic surfaces, especially those of chrome cobalt alloys and titanium, are resistant to corrosion by virtue of their elemental composition, crystalline homogeneity, and the surface oxides that form spontaneously or are created by an accelerated nitric acid passivation process during final production. It is these surface oxides that form the reactive interface with glycoproteinaceous molecules of the conditioning film. Surgical alloys have relatively high surface energy values that encourage tenacious binding of intermediary glycoproteins and colonizing cells.[4-7] Specific environmental proteins interact as coapting agents for pro-

From the Section on Orthopedic Surgery, Bowman Gray School of Medicine, Winston-Salem, North Carolina.

karyocytes and eukaryocytes. Titanium and chrome cobalt alloys allow closer and stronger cellular binding than do polymers or Bioglass.[4-6, 8-10]

DESIGN, FUNCTION, AND ADHESION

The design of many implant devices necessitates that a sector (usually metallic for orthopedic implants and polymeric for vascular devices) of the prosthesis or artificial organ be colonized by host cells. This provides secure fixation or integration (e.g., a total joint replacement requires fixation in bone and should be adhesive for tissue). Another portion (usually polymer) remains intra-articular and, by mechanical design, of a low coefficient of friction and also antiadhesive for tissue. A third portion (MM) is designed to bridge the gap between metal and bone, providing fixation to both and acting as a cement. This latter sector should be adhesive to both metal and bone. However, studies have shown that MM is not adhesive for tissue or bone cells and may provoke an inflammatory response. Methylmethacrylate also provides an excellent substratum for bacterial colonization and may in-

hibit host defenses. Vascular prostheses have similar general design characteristics. Although they may be composed completely of polymers, preferably the hemodynamic portion remains nonadhesive for blood fractions while the peripheral regions are designed for tissue coaptation.

SUBSTRATUM DISRUPTION, BIOFILM, AND MICROZONES

Substratum disruption (before or after bacterial colonization) caused by trauma, wear, corrosion, toxins, viral effects, or bacterial mechanisms establishes environmental conditions that natural selection has prepared microorganisms to opportunize (Fig. 3–1, see also Fig. 2–14). Polymer, metal, and compromised tissue fractions may be utilized directly within the bacterial envelope. For example, metal ions, such as iron, magnesium, chromium, cobalt, and others, are available in trace or greater amounts, especially after corrosion. This process occurs to some degree even with more stable alloys, such as stainless steel, when they are scoured by wear, work, or implantation.

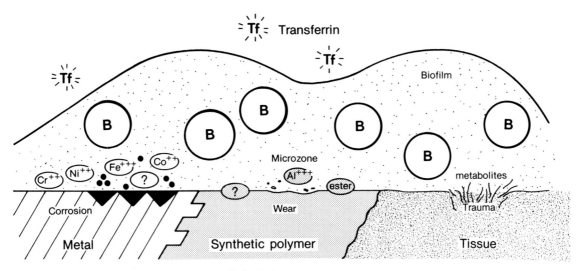

FIGURE 3–1. Surface disruption by wear, corrosion, trauma, or bacterial mechanisms frees metabolites or ions, which are then available to bacteria (B) within a biofilm microenvironment. Within the polysaccharide biofilm, metal ions required by pathogenic bacteria may be shielded from host protein binding complexes (Tf). (See also Figure 2–14.) (Reprinted with permission from Gristina AG, et al: Biomaterial specificity, molecular mechanisms and clinical relevance of *S. epidermidis* and *S. aureus* infections in surgery. Proceedings of the Symposium on Pathogenicity and Clinical Significance of Coagulase-Negative Staphylococci. Heppenheim, Germany. Copyright 1987, by Gustav Fisher–Verlag, Stuttgart.

The microzone is an environmental, metabolic microclimate within the bacterial biofilms wherein optimal conditions may exist and antagonistic environmental factors are blunted by protective bacterial polymers. On biomaterial surfaces within this polysaccharide biofilm, microzone ions are shielded from host protein-binding complexes (lactoferrin, transferrin), which lower iron concentration levels below those usually required by pathogenic bacteria. Iron is linked to virulence and inhibits macrophage function. Mg^{++}, Ca^{++}, and other trace ions stabilize (via acidic groups) the complex polysaccharide polymers in gel formation, thereby enhancing both cell-to-cell and cell-to-surface adhesion and possibly increasing resistance to external antagonists. Some synthetic polymers, such as polyurethane and methylmethacrylate, contain esters that may be metabolized by *Staphylococcus epidermidis*. Traces of aluminum and other substances may also be present from polymer manufacturing processes or contamination.[8, 9, 11–14]

Semantic Comment: ``Inert''

The use of the term "inert" with respect to biomaterials tends to convey a meaning of absolute nonreactivity in a biological system and is basically misleading. Physicochemically, a substance cannot be finitely or absolutely inert vis-à-vis another substance, cell, or organism.[15]

METALS AND ALLOYS

Metals are crystalline structures with regular, repetitive, crystalline lattices. Their mechanical properties are described by their tensile and yield strengths, moduli of elasticity, fracture toughness, hardness, Poisson ratio, compliance curves, and fatigue properties. The addition of small amounts of one or more elements to form an alloy may markedly improve their tensile and yield strength, fracture toughness, fatigue properties, workability, and formability. Alloying can also be an effective means for improving corrosion resistance (Table 3–1).

Failure Modes

In contrast to ceramics and glasses, metals are ductile and, to a certain degree, capable of elastic deformation. There are four modes of failure for metals:

1. Excessive, i.e. plastic, deformation..
2. Fracture, preceded by plastic deformation if the modulus of elasticity is low.
3. Abrasion or erosion, which induce irregularities in the metal surface, thereby forming notches of stress concentration that may initiate a fracture (even though the load may be well below the defined critical load for the material).
4. Chemical attack (i.e., corrosion), which forms pits in the metal surface, followed by stress corrosion fracture.

The patterns of stress-cracking described under (3) and (4) are analogous to the brittle fractures seen in ceramics and glass ceramics. Alloys such as stainless steel, chrome cobalt, and titanium (Ti6Al4V) have a relatively high modulus of elasticity (120 to 180 MN/m^2), compared with that of bone; this high modulus of elasticity, in contrast to that of bone, is responsible for the stress-shielding effect on bone encountered in orthopedic implantation surgery.

Laboratory studies have suggested that failure of metal fixation, which is ultimately based on these previously discussed qualities, may be relevant to increased susceptibility to staphylococcal infections. Work by Merritt and co-workers on *Staphylococcus aureus* and open fractures indicated an increased rate of infection when stable internal fixation was not used; however, paradoxical results occurred when *Proteus mirabilis* was the infecting organism.[16] Further studies may define a causal association specific for each organism and metal based in part on the inability of metals to match the modulus of elasticity of bone, a property that results in stress-shielding changes in normal bone.

SURFACE EFFECTS OF METAL ALLOYS

Metal surfaces represent planar cuts through a crystalline structure and generally exhibit moderate to high surface energies exceeding 40 dynes/cm. The geometric arrangement of metal atoms on the exposed surface plane, and thus the number of unsatisfied bonds, depends on the orientation of the cut surface. Thus, the various surface planes differ in the way they interact with molecules of the adsorbed substance. A clean metallic surface yields high surface free energy and is therefore

TABLE 3–1. Composition and Mechanical Properties of Metal Alloys for Surgical Implants*

	Stainless Steel ASTM F55 or F56 316 or 316 L: Wrought	CO-CR ASTM F75 ASTM F75 (Vitallium, Zimalloy Vinertium, Allivum, Protasul-2): Cast	CO-CR ASTM F90 (Protasul-10:) Wrought
Composition (weight %)			
Carbon	0.08 max. (0.03 max.)	0.35 max.	0.05–0.15
Manganese	2.00 max.	1.0 max.	2.0 max.
Phosphorus	0.03 max	—	—
Sulfur	0.03 max.	—	—
Silicon	0.75 max.	1.00 max.	1.00 max.
Tungsten	—	—	14–16
Cobalt	—	Bal. (57.4–65)	Bal. (46–53)
Chromium	17–20	27–30	19–21
Nickel	10–14	2.5 max.	9–11
Molybdenum	2–4	5–7	—
Iron	Bal. (59–70)	0.75 max.	3.0 max.
Properties			
Hardness	$R_B85–95$	$R_C25–34$	$R_B98–100$
Hardness (CW)†	R_C30	—	R_C65
UTS	80,000 psi	95–105,000	130,000
UTS (CW)	140,000	—	250,000
0.2% YS	35,000	65,000	55,000
0.2% YS (CW)	115,000	—	190,000
Max. strain	55%	8%	50%
Max. strain (CW)	22%	—	10%
Modulus (0.2%)	$17.5–57.5 \times 10^6$ psi	32.5×10^6	$27.5–95 \times 10^6$

	MP35N AMS 5758 Vacuum Remelt: Cast-Wrought	Titanium (Pure) ASTM F67 Cast-Wrought	Titanium 6Al-4V Alloy ASTM F136 Cast-Wrought
Composition (weight %)			
Carbon	0.25 max.	0.10 max.	0.08 max.
Manganese	0.15 max.	—	—
Phosphorus	0.015 max.	—	—
Sulfur	0.01 max.	—	—
Silicon	0.15 max.	—	—
Oxygen	—	0.45 max.	0.13 max.
Cobalt	Bal. (30.25–38)	—	—
Chromium	19–21	—	—
Nickel	33–37	—	—
Molybdenum	9–10.5	—	—
Iron	1.0 max.	0.5 max.	0.25 max.
Aluminum	—	—	5.5–6.5
Vanadium	—	—	3.5–4.5
Titanium	—	Bal. (99+)	Bal. (88.5–92)
Properties			
Hardness	R_C50 (R_C8)	R_B100	Depends on surface finish
UTS	125,000 (325,000) psi	90,000	125,000–130,000
0.2% YS	60,000 (235,000)	80,000	115,000–120,000
Max. strain	70% (10%)	18%	10%
Modulus (0.2%)	$30–117.5 \times 10^6$ psi	40×10^6	60×10^6

* Reprinted with permission from Mears DC: Materials and Orthopedic Surgery. Copyright 1979 by The Williams & Wilkins Company, Baltimore.

† CW indicates the value obtained for maximal cold reduction. Modulus (0.2 percent) is the apparent Young modulus at 0.2 percent strain.

reactive and potentially capable of catalyzing chemical reactions. According to the *random walk theory,* the efficiency of this catalytic activity is defined by the diffusion coefficient. Molecules absorbed to such clean surfaces diffuse about freely as the energy to perform these random movements is directly acquired from the thermal vibrations of the underlying lattice. Therefore, molecular fragments encounter other molecules and interact more frequently than in a free solution. Chemical reactions at such surfaces are accelerated without a significant increase in temperature.[1, 14, 17, 18]

New molecules formed at these surfaces are not strongly bound to the surface and may escape more easily. In nonmetallic crystalline structures, the number of molecules exposed, and thus the numbers available to stimulate chemical interaction, also varies with the angle of the surface cut and the composition of the crystal lattice.

CELL BEHAVIOR ON METAL SURFACES

When a bacterium arrives at a metal surface within van der Waals primary minimum, its envelope and outer membranes are exposed to surface disassociation and molecular activity at distances of approximately 0.25 nm. In effect, chemical interaction occurs with the surface or with macromolecules in the glycoproteinaceous conditioning film. We suggest that increased chemical reactivity and the ready formation of new molecules at surfaces may explain the acceleration of bacterial metabolic processes that result in growth, polysaccharide production, and biofilm and colony formation on specific substrata after they are contaminated by bacteria. Therefore, surface physical and chemical qualities, especially of metals or crystalline substances, may be the triggers for increased metabolic activity and growth phase changes in some bacteria and possibly in eukaryocytes.[14, 15, 18]

THE INORGANIC-BIOTISSUE INTERFACE

When implanted in bone, surgical alloys are always surrounded by a fibrous tissue capsule, although this capsule may be thin. One exception is titanium and its alloys. According to Kasemo, covalent, ionic, or hydrogen bonding may occur at the boundary between the bone tissue and the titanium oxide surface.[4] It is important to realize that it is the chemical qualities of the surface oxide with which the biomolecules interact. The exact composition of the first monolayer has not been identified. However, it is believed that molecular interactions are taking place at distances that approximate chemical bonding (0.25 nm). The sequences involve the same forces (as outlined in Chapter 2) for reversible and irreversible bacterial adhesion. These interactions and affinities are both specific and dynamic.[4, 14] For titanium alloys, a direct bone-implant contact is seen, even at the ultrastructural level. This is called *osseointegration* (Fig. 3–2). For successful osseointegration to occur, the stress transfer perpendicular to the implant surface must exceed any shear forces along this interface.[19] Excessive shear forces will lead to bone resorption and connective tissue formation around the implant even if the implant material is extremely biocompatible.

Bone has been reported to deposit on the surface of titanium implants as if osteoblasts actually colonize the titanium surface and deposit bone in an "implantofugal" manner.[18] We suggest that titanium and titanium alloy surfaces readily and directly colonized by osteoblasts or tissue cells may be protected to a higher degree against colonization by bacterial pathogens.

Clinical Comment: Metallic Total Joint Replacement Without Methylmethacrylate for Fixation

A review of 780 porous, coated total knee replacements (Vitallium and HDP), followed for 6 years, indicated a significantly lower rate of infection than a comparable series with MM (380 cases). There was one late infection in the uncemented series ($2\frac{1}{2}$ years following surgery after a steroid injection, *S. epidermidis*) and three infections in the cemented series (one *S. aureus,* one *S. epidermidis,* and one *Micrococcus* species). A 2-year review of 500 porous coated uncemented total hips revealed no infections. All groups used prophylactic antibiotics (Hungerford DS, 1986, unpublished data). These are preliminary and encouraging data from a group of skilled surgeons. However, it would be premature to regard such data as direct evidence of a lower tendency to infection in the absence of cement until a longer follow-up is conducted and a broader group of patients is

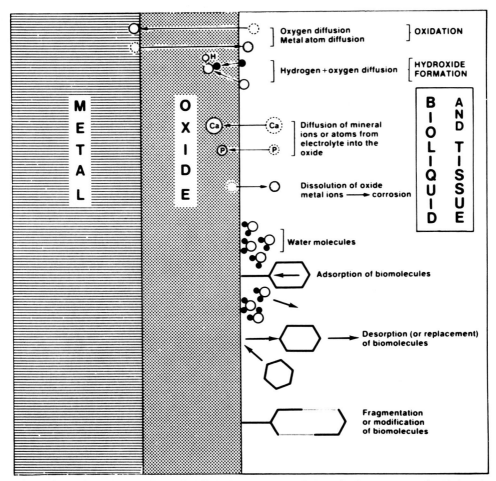

FIGURE 3–2. Schematic illustration of various transport and chemical processes that take place at an implant-biotissue (bioliquid) interface. Note that all direct interaction is between surface oxide and biomolecules and that interaction with metal requires transport of small (atoms, ion) molecular fragments through oxide. (Reprinted with permission from Kasemo B: Biocompatibility of titanium implants: surface science aspects. J Prosthet Dent 49:832–836, 1983.)

examined. Preliminary animal studies suggest a lower rate of infection when metals are implanted without methylmethacrylate. However, the mechanisms for these observations have not been defined.[20]

CERAMICS/GLASS CERAMICS

Ceramics are crystalline structures, as are metals, and are used as dental and orthopedic implants *Bioactive glass ceramics* are composites of crystals dispersed in an amorphous glass phase. There are three categories of ceramics:

1. *Inert, crystalline ceramics* are fine-grained, polymeric 2-Al_2O_3 or Al_2O_3/MgO.

2. *Porous, bioinert ceramics* consist of Al_2O_3, calcium carbonate–bonded aluminas, phosphate-bonded aluminas, or calcium oxide–stabilized zirconia.

3. *Resorbable ceramics* consist of tricalcium phosphate, hydroxyapatite, or calcium aluminates.

Bioactive glass ceramics are brittle and possess poor mechanical properties. They are postulated to react chemically with biological tissue but, at the same time, to be bioinert, i.e., to cause no foreign body reaction and to be nonbiodegradable by the tissues. The main constituent of these materials is silicon oxide interspersed with various crystalline substances.[21]

Bacterial adhesion to ceramics and glass ceramics is likely; however, clinical significance and microbiological characteristics should be studied further before any conclusions can be drawn.

POLYMER SUBSTRATA

Most medical polymers are amorphous. There are three that are in part crystalline: polytetrafluoroethylene (PTFE), polyethylene (HDPE), and polypropylene.[1] Crystalline zones (spherulites) confer rigidity, whereas amorphous zones confer toughness. Increased rates of reaction may occur even on a noncatalytic two-dimensional planar surface because, as the random walk theory indicates, molecular contact is more likely in a planar or membrane system than in a three-dimensional one.[4, 18, 22]

Although high-molecular-weight medical polymers in general are thought to be resistant to bacterial deterioration, polyvinylchloride, for example, contains low-molecular-weight plasticizers (polypropylene sebacate) that are vulnerable to attack by *Pseudomonas aeruginosa* and *Serratia marcescens*.[1] Methylmethacrylate also has a noncrystalline, porous structure that, in effect, provides surface area for diffusion and molecular interaction. Studies have shown that *S. epidermidis* has a higher rate of adhesion to polymers than does *S. aureus*.[14, 23]

Other properties of polymers relevant to bacteria have been discussed in the section on substratum disruption.

Polymer-to-Polymer Interactions

It is possible that bacterial polymers may interact with substratum synthetic polymers after surface disruption by mechanisms similar to their own polysaccharide-to-polysaccharide interaction in bacterial aggregation (Fig. 3–3). Free ions (Ca^{++}, Mg^{++}) interact with acidic groups (carboxyl groups [COO^-], hydroxyl groups [OH^-]) to link polysaccharide chains in helical configurations or linear arrays. Simple neutral nonionic linear and helical interaction may also occur between adjacent long-chain polymers.[12–14]

CORROSION

Substratum corrosion involves a gradual breakdown of the material caused by physical, chemical, or microbiological factors in the environment. "Biodegradation," the corrosion of an implanted biomaterial, is defined as the gradual breakdown of a material, mediated either by specific cellular activity or by the vital activity of the environment.

Ceramics, glass ceramics, and polymers are not completely inert. By definition, these ma-

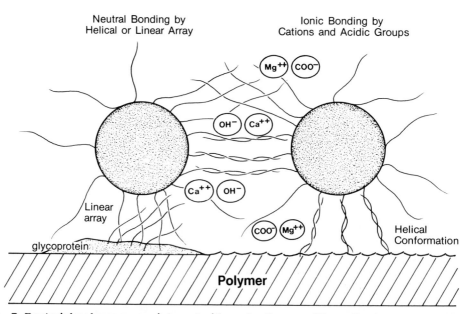

FIGURE 3–3. Bacterial polymers may interact with each other or with synthetic polymers after surface disruption either by neutral or ionic bonding in linear or helical configuration.

terials do not corrode but undergo dissolution. Resorbable ceramics undergo an intentional, balanced biodegradation in order to be replaced by biological tissue. Four special types of metal corrosion should be mentioned:

1. *Crevice corrosion* of metals is a form of occluded "cell" corrosion that results in a severe localized attack of the shielded surface.
2. *Galvanic corrosion* of metals occurs when electric current is generated by contact of dissimilar metals or by contact between certain metals and other substrata or tissues in an electrolyte or physiologic solution.
3. *Fretting corrosion* of metals is brought about by frictional forces between the metal surface and the substratum to which this surface is exposed.[1, 24]
4. *Microbial corrosion* of metals is corrosion by bacteria. It occurs in natural environments and may ultimately be demonstrated *in vivo*. In nature, bacteria possess enzymes that can break down metals. *Pseudomonas* K_2 and plasmid-bearing strains of *Escherichia coli, P. aeruginosa,* and *S. aureus* possess the mercuric reductase enzyme.[25, 26]

Both gram-positive bacteria (*S. epidermidis* and *S. aureus*) as well as gram-negative bacteria (*P. aeruginosa*) are dependent on the availability of metallic ions to maximize virulence. In man, free iron is generally unavailable to pathogens because it is bound by proteins (lactoferrin and transferrin). Metallic corrosion products, such as ionic iron and other metal ions, may increase virulence at biomaterial sites, since they probably become directly available to bacteria within the bacterial envelope (see Fig. 3–1). Within the biofilm microenvironment, they are shielded from binding proteins and are made available to bacterial systems (enterochelin). Iron also inhibits macrophage function. On the other hand, high concentrations of free metallic ions may be toxic to bacteria and tissue cells.[11] This could also occur at corrosion sites.

Several gram-negative rods, including species of *Pseudomonas, Acinetobacter, Flavobacterium,* and *Aeromonas,* can transform volatile lead compounds but not inorganic lead. Furthermore, a wide variety of marine bacteria either oxidize or reduce manganese and may play a role in manganese corrosion. Bacteria do not directly oxidize molybdenum or uranium as they do iron, but some copper sulfide minerals may be directly attacked. The accumulation of metals by microorganisms is not understood, but they do obtain energy from oxidation of inorganic compounds. Many or-

ganisms have cellular components that are highly metal-specific, such as the protein methallothioneim, which is present in the cells of the reticuloendothelial system (RES) in humans. Organisms may degrade sulfide minerals, thereby recovering zinc from sphalerite (ZnS) and lead from galena (PbS).

It appears that microbial metabolic pathways involve the transport and utilization of a series of trace metals, including iron, cobalt, molybdenum, boron, copper, zinc, magnesium, and aluminum. Some of these ions are known as corrosion products from biometals, and some are present in trace amounts on many biomaterials secondary to manufacturing processes.[9]

The types of bacteria that produce corrosion in biometals are generally not found in wounds. However, the influence of trace ions on pathogenesis in wound infection has not been completely studied. In a biomaterial environment, many more organisms appear to be capable of pathogenic processes and it is possible that, for these bacteria singly and in consortia, a corrosive, metabolic pathway exists.[1]

The real question is whether, and which, of the bacterial or nonbacterial corrosion products or trace elements that are present stimulate or inhibit bacterial growth and infection. This remains to be answered by *in vivo* studies.

ARTIFICIAL ORGANS

Artificial organs, e.g., the mechanical heart, present special problems. They are composites of many materials, including metals and polymers. They involve compatibility not only between materials but also between materials and adjacent tissues. Complexity is added by the need for proadhesive sectors (solid system tissue integration) and antiadhesive sectors (fluid environment or hemodynamic system compatibility). Furthermore, there is usually a power conduit that traverses organ space, body cavities, mucous membranes, and skin to the external ambient and microbial environment. The conduit represents a communications pathway not only for the power source but for microbes as well. The surfaces of the artificial organ represent colonization sites for bacteria, with each biomaterial favoring a particular colonizing species. Polymers may favor *P. aeruginosa* and *S. epidermidis*, whereas metals may favor *S. aureus*. The required hemodynamic interactions within the device create fluid eddies and tissue damage, which are favorable to clotting cascades and the initial events of microbial adhesion. The attempted integration of synthetic vessel and natural vasculature creates a site of intimal perturbation and endothelial damage, exposing potential receptor sites for bacterial adhesion. These are significant but not insurmountable problems.

SUMMARY

The organisms have not really changed; the substrata have.

Our studies and clinical review presented in Chapter 2 suggest that at our present level of information and insight, bacteria preferentially colonize specific substrata. *S. aureus* has been associated with biometal and tissue infections. The presence of polymers in a prosthesis or the use of polymers alone appears to allow preferential colonization by *S. epidermidis*. Polymers in certain locations (the eye) appear to select for *P. aeruginosa* and *S. epidermidis*. The organisms involved possess fundamental metabolic mechanisms that optimize their survival on differing substrata. When appropriate substrata are presented, the substratum in effect selects the organism, and if conditions are optimal, an infection results.[14]

The Race for the Surface

When a biomaterial is implanted, there is virtually a "race for the surface" between tissue cells and bacteria. Host defense systems are a vital factor. If the race is won by tissue, the surface is occupied and defended and less available for bacterial colonization. Glycoproteinaceous conditioning films, which immediately coat the surface of biomaterials, tend to frustrate the antiadhesive nature of surfaces and provide receptor sites for bacterial adhesion, as do polysaccharide polymers produced by the first layer of bacterial colonizers.[27, 28] Even in a pure and essentially antiadhesive system, colonization is usually possible by a few bacteria with optimal attachment abilities. These initial colonizers provide a foundation for growth and propagation or for subsequent colonization, since their surfaces and polysaccharides are proadhesive for other bacteria.[29]

Implant surface environment can be maintained in a state resistant to bacterial colonization and favorable for tissue cells by sterility, antibiotics, and specific bacterial blocking agents or by precolonization with eukaryotic cells (Fig. 3–4). After colonization by tissue cells has occurred, the new surface presented to infecting prokaryocytes is the healthy, resistant, polysaccharide (the glycocalyx of mammalian cells) outer layer of the eukaryocyte. There are indications that an intact, fully developed endothelial glycocalyx is resistant to microbial adhesion.[8, 14, 29–32]

Therefore, a biomaterial or biometal surface that is adhesive for appropriate tissue cells and encourages rapid eukaryocytic colonization or integration may be the best strategy for decreasing bacterial colonization. During the initially vulnerable period when random colonization by bacteria of an adhesive surface might occur, antibiotics could be used protectively. Much more study is required of the direct molecular interactions between substrata

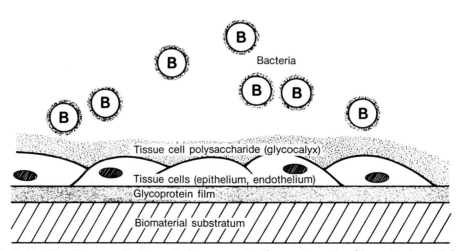

FIGURE 3–4. Healthy tissue cells have their own protective polysaccharide outer layer (glycocalyx), which is resistant to bacterial adhesion.

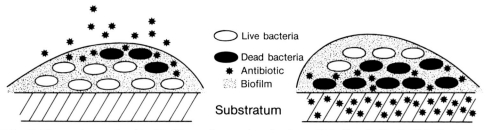

FIGURE 3-5. The polysaccharide biofilm acts as a barrier to antibiotics (left). Antibiotic impregnation into biomaterials may help prevent and treat infection, since a high concentration will be present at the site of bacterial colonization.

surfaces, bacteria, and tissue cells before perfect biomaterials for specific tasks can be designed.

Other Strategies

Antibiotics impregnated into biomaterials provide a logical, though somewhat primitive, method for preventing and treating infection because they are at the site of adhesion in high concentration within the bacterial envelope of initial colonizers (Fig. 3-5). Antibiotics are probably most effective against free-floating or newly attached organisms, not those well shielded by biofilm, hence the efficacy of prophylactic antibiotics. Combined antibiotic therapy may be indicated for polymicrobial or established infections. Antibiotics that penetrate the biofilm or prevent its synthesis should be studied.

Characterization of adhesins and receptors on bacteria, tissues, biomaterials, and conditioning films is required so that saturating or blocking analogs may be developed.

Surgeons should minimize tissue destruction and cleanse the operative site of potential biomaterial or tissue foreign bodies.

The relevance of surface area of biomaterials should be defined.

Biomaterials should be investigated for qualities that enhance, not blunt, host defense mechanisms and that are antagonistic to bacteria but not to eukaryocytes.

The inorganic-biotissue interface should be studied at a molecular level.

In conclusion, bacteria are ancient and highly adaptive organisms. Biomaterials are new but imitate basic compounds and substrata for which bacteria have already evolved colonization and survival strategies. *Man is now in the "race for the surface."*

References

1. Mears DC: Materials and Orthopedic Surgery. Baltimore, Williams & Wilkins, 1979.
2. Dougherty SH, Simmons RL: Infections in bionic man: the pathobiology of infection in prosthetic devices, part 1. Curr Probl Surg 19:221-264, 1982.
3. Dougherty SH, Simmons RL: Infections in bionic man: the pathobiology of infections in prosthetic devices, part 2. Curr Probl Surg 19:269-318, 1982.
4. Kasemo B: Biocompatibility of titanium implants: surface science aspects. J Prosthet Dent 49:832-837, 1983.
5. Absalom DR, Lamberti FV, Policova Z, Zingg W, van Oss CJ, Neuman AW: Surface thermodynamics of bacterial adhesion. Appl Environ Microbiol 46:90-97, 1983.
6. Barth E, Ronningen H, Salheim LF: Comparison of ceramic and titanium implants in cats. Acta Orthop Scand 56:491-495, 1985.
7. Baier RE, Meyer AE, Natiella JR, Natiella RR, Carter JM: Surface properties determine bioadhesive outcomes: methods and results. J Biomed Mater Res 18:337-355, 1984.
8. Webb LX, Gristina AG, Myers RT, Cordell AR, Hobgood CD, Costerton JW: Inhibition of bacterial adherence by antibacterial surface pretreatment of vascular prostheses. J Vasc Surg 4:16-21, 1986.
9. Paerls HW: Influence of attachment on microbial metabolism and growth in aquatic ecosystems. In Savage DC, Fletcher M, eds: Bacterial Adhesion. New York, Plenum Press, 1985, pp 363-400.
10. Albrektsson T, Arnebrandt T, Larsson K, Nylander T, Sennerby L: The effect of a glycoprotein monolayer on the integration of titanium implants. In Williams DF, ed: Transcripts of the Fifth European Conference on Biomaterials. Amsterdam, Elsevier, 1985, p 151.
11. Brown MRW, Williams P: The influence of environment on envelope properties affecting survival of bacteria in infections. Ann Rev Microbiol 39:527-556, 1985.
12. Robb ID: Stereo-biochemistry and function in polymers. In Marshall KC, ed: Microbial Adhesion and Aggregation. Berlin, Springer-Verlag, 1984, pp 39-49.
13. Rutter PR, Vincent B: Physiochemical interactions of the substratum, microorganisms, and the fluid phase. In Marshall KC, ed: Microbial Adhesion and Aggregation. Berlin, Springer-Verlag, 1984, pp 21-38.

14. Gristina AG, Hobgood CD, Barth E: Biomaterial Specificity, Molecular Mechanisms and Clinical Relevance of *S. epidermidis* and *S. aureus* Infections in Surgery. Stuttgart, Gustav Fisher–Verlag, 1987.

15. Gristina AG, Rovere GD, Shoji H, Nicastro JD: An *in vitro* study of bacterial response to inert and reactive metals and to methylmethacrylate. J Biomed Mater Res 10:273–281, 1976.

16. Merritt K, Rickman JD, Crowe TD: Infections of open fractures with *Staphylococcus epidermidis* and *Proteus mirabilis.* Abstract of the 32nd Annual Meeting of the Orthopaedic Research Society. New Orleans, February 17–20, 1986.

17. Ludwicka A, Locci R, Jansen B, Peters G, Pulverer G: Microbial colonization of prosthetic devices in attachment of coagulase-negative staphylococci and "slime" production on chemically pure synthetic polymers. Zbl Bakt Hyg I Abt Orig B 177:527–532, 1983.

18. Gomer R: Surface diffusion. Sci Am 247:98–109, 1982.

19. Brånemark PI, Hansson BO, Adell R, Breine U, Lindström J, Hallén O, Ohman A: Osseointegrated implants in the treatment of the edentulous jaw. Scand J Plast Reconstr Surg (16):1–132, 1977.

20. Petty W, Spanier S, Shuster JJ, Silverthorne C: The influence of skeletal implants on the incidence of infection. J Bone Joint Surg 67A:1236–1244, 1985.

21. Blencke BA, Bromer H, Deubaker KK: Compatibility and long-term stability of glass-ceramic implants. J Biomed Mater Res 12:307–316, 1978.

22. Alberts B, Bray D, Lewis J, Raff M, Roberts K, Watson JD: Molecular Biology of the Cell. New York, Garland Publishing, 1983, pp 93, 113.

23. Merritt K, Turner GE: Adherence of bacteria to biomaterials. Abstract of the 11th Annual Meeting of the Society for Biomaterials. San Diego, 1985.

24. Sutow EJ, Jones DW, Milne EL: *In vitro* crevice corrosion behavior of implant materials. J Dent Res 64:842–847, 1985.

25. Summers AO: Microbial transformation of metals. Ann Rev Microbiol 32:637–672, 1978.

26. Brierly CL: Microbiological mining. Sci Am 247:44–53, 1982.

27. Baier RE: Surface chemical factors presaging bioadhesive events. Ann NY Acad Sci 416:34–57, 1983.

28. Vercellotti GM, McCarthy JB, Lindholm P, Peterson PK, Jacob HS, Furcht LT: Extracellular matrix proteins (fibronectin, laminin and Type IV collagen) bind and aggregate bacteria. Am J Pathol 120:13–21, 1985.

29. Gristina AG, Oga M, Webb LX, Hobgood CD: Adherent bacterial colonization in the pathogenesis of osteomyelitis. Science 228:990–993, 1985.

30. Christensen GD, Simpson WA, Beachey EH: Adhesion of bacteria to animal tissues: complex mechanisms. In Savage DC, Fletcher M, eds: Bacterial Adhesion. New York, Plenum Press, 1985, pp 279–305.

31. Stern GA, Lubniewski A, Allen C: The interaction between *Pseudomonas aeruginosa* and the corneal epithelium. Arch Ophthalmol 103:1221–1225, 1985.

32. Ryan US, Ryan JW, Crutchley DJ: The pulmonary endothelial surface. Fed Proc 44:0013–0019, 1985.

Quentin Anderson, M.D.

4

Radiographic Evaluation of Inflammatory Bone Disease

INTRODUCTION

Early diagnosis of osteomyelitis is mandatory for initiation of antibiotic therapy circumventing potential crippling effects.[1] Plain film radiographic changes do occur in soft tissues and bone, but are often subtle or significantly delayed in onset. Soft tissue swelling adjacent to bony involvement can occur as early as 2 to 3 days. This progresses to displacement or obliteration of muscle planes and fat lines. Bone destruction cannot be detected with less than 30 to 50 percent loss of bone. Typically, bone involvement appears 10 to 14 days after onset and shows a variable pattern.

In our experience, radionuclide imaging (Table 4–1) has been very helpful in early detection of osteomyelitis, whether it be acute hematogenous infection (Fig. 4–1), contiguous soft tissue infection, or a result of penetrating trauma or postsurgical complication. Recent advances made with the introduction of various technetium 99m (^{99m}Tc) phosphate compounds, gallium 67 (^{67}Ga) citrate, and in vitro labeling of leukocytes with indium 111 (^{111}In) oxine offer potential for early and accurate diagnosis of osteomyelitis. This chapter addresses the appropriateness and sequential use of these radiopharmaceuticals.

TECHNETIUM 99m PHOSPHATE

Technetium 99m, with its excellent physical characteristics and easy availability from on-site generator systems, has become the most important radionuclide in bone imaging. After intravenous injection of a technetium phosphate compound, the radiopharmaceutical is rapidly distributed throughout the extracellular fluid compartment. Bone uptake is rapid, with greater than 50 percent of the administered dose delivered to bone within 1 hour.[2] The remainder is excreted by the kidneys into the urine.

The mechanisms and sites of bone localization have not been completely established. Whether it be by diffusion to the bony site with a small amount of absorption onto the surface of the hydroxyapatite crystal or actual binding to the organic matrix, especially immature cartilage, are two postulations. The relative amount of isotope for bone imaging is affected by blood flow and background concentration of radiopharmaceutical throughout the extracellular fluid compartment.

This has led most investigators to utilize the methylene diphosphonate compounds, which tend to clear more rapidly from blood and exhibit a somewhat greater deposition of radioactivity in bone.[3] A 2-hour interval between injection and imaging allows satisfactory clearance of extracellular technetium and improves the target to nontarget ratio of isotope concentration.

Technetium compounds tend to localize in stress with increased blood flow and in those areas where there is increased osteoblastic activity. Two standard techniques are post-clearance 2-hour film studies or more rapid three-phase bone scans.[2] That is, image the area in question during the time of isotope injection followed by immediate blood pool image, plus routine delayed 2-hour film study. By preference, we find that the three-phase study gives us additional information that may be useful for evaluating findings on the 2-hour static images relative to soft tissue versus bony uptake, as one might see with cellulitis or synovitis.

From the Department of Radiology, Hennepin County Medical Center, Minneapolis, Minnesota.

TABLE 4–1. Radionuclide Imaging Studies

Radio-pharmaceutical	Method of Administration	Normal Adult Dose	Injection to Imaging Time	Patient Preparation	Conflicting Examinations/ Medications
Technetium 99m	Intravenous injection	20 mCi	20–25 minutes	1. Hydrate patient to reduce radiation dose to bladder 2. Have patient void prior to imaging	None
Gallium 67	Intravenous injection	5 mCi	6 and 24 hours for soft tissue inflammatory disease; delayed 24 hour images as clinically needed for detection of inflammatory lesion Procedure imaging time: 45 minutes	Bowel preparation after initial images to remove residual isotope from GI tract	Barium studies with residual barium in GI tract
Indium 111	Blood is withdrawn from the patient for initiation of white blood cell labeling; this process takes approximately 2 hours; labeled cells are then reinjected	400–500 mCi Indium 111 oxide	24 hours; earlier imaging studies can be utilized as clinically indicated Procedure imaging time: 30–45 minutes	None	Adequate white blood cell volume for labeling or compatible labeled donor cells

In that there are two major mechanisms for isotope to be distributed to the bony skeleton —blood flow and bone uptake—there are occasions in which technetium phosphate does not give a "hot spot" positive image relative to known pathology but, rather, results in a "cold" nonradioactive lesion.[4] If the inflammatory process has compromised the blood supply, there will be relatively little isotope available for uptake, with a resultant nonradioactive "cold" spot image. A "cold" lesion may also occur when an extremely aggressive neoplasm overcomes any attempt at an osteoblastic response.

The other difficulty with technetium compounds is their sensitivity, for they will be attracted to any area of increased osteoblastic activity. Non-inflammatory entities, such as tumor process, benign bone disease, post-fracture uptake, and previous surgical procedures, must be considered. This points out the importance of clinical as well as plain film radiographic correlation with bone scan findings. Diagnostic accuracy definitely increases by correlating all available imaging studies.

In closing, it should be pointed out that ^{99m}Tc phosphate compounds should be the first choice to diagnose inflammatory bone disease. These compounds are readily available in any radiology department. There are few, if any, contraindications to utilize the isotope.

The isotope is relatively inexpensive and cost-effective. Bone scan studies can be obtained within 2 hours of injection, and the radioisotope is rapidly cleared; consequently, there is a very low radiation hazard to the patient. The isotope has very high detection efficiency and does not interfere with follow-up second stage radionuclide studies such as ^{67}Ga citrate– and ^{111}In–labeled white blood cells.

GALLIUM 67 CITRATE

If the inflammatory lesion has not been adequately documented or detected with a Tc phosphate scan, then it may be necessary to utilize second stage radionuclides such as ^{67}Ga citrate.[5] The potential for localizing inflam-

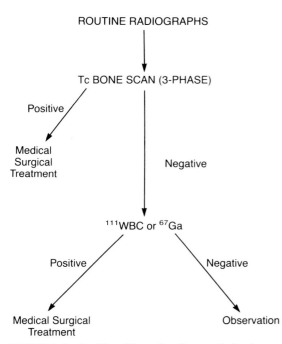

FIGURE 4-1. Algorithm for the radiologic assessment of suspected acute osteomyelitis.

matory disease with ^{67}Ga has survived as a valuable agent in tumor and inflammatory imaging.

Physiologically, intravenous ^{67}Ga is immediately bound to plasma proteins, primarily transferrin.[6] In the first 24 hours, 20 to 30 percent of the administered dose is excreted through the kidneys. After that time, the intestinal mucosa becomes the major route of clearance, along with small amounts excreted via the liver and biliary tract. These modes of excretion account for approximately one third of the administered dose; the remaining two thirds is retained in the body for a prolonged period of time. In addition to activity within the axial skeleton, the liver, spleen, and bowel and, to some degree, salivary glands and breast tissue will retain isotopic activity. If imaging is performed in the first 24 hours, there will be activity within the kidney and bladder.

The mechanism of ^{67}Ga citrate localization in inflammatory disease is complex. Basically, transport of ^{67}Ga citrate is mediated by the gallium transferrin complex with deposition in the inflammatory site. A second mechanism is migration of ^{67}Ga citrate–labeled white blood cells to the inflamed area.

After intravenous administration of ^{67}Ga, scans can be obtained in as short a time as 4 to 6 hours, with follow-up interval 24-hour imaging as needed to detect and differentiate abnormal areas of uptake from normal areas of uptake from normal physiologic clearance. As mentioned, clearance is quite delayed and will preclude utilizing other radionuclides that have similar gamma energies such as ^{99m}Tc– or ^{111}In–labeled white blood cells. The utility of ^{67}Ga in the detection of inflammatory bone disease is for those cases where there is still strong clinical indication or an inflammatory lesion, i.e., a "cold" lesion on Tc phosphate scanning, and when there is a positive phosphate scan but specificity of the uptake can be improved using correlative ^{67}Ga scans.[6, 7]

Gallium 67 uptake relative to ^{99m}Tc scanning has many specific patterns, the greater asset being the relative intensity of uptake of gallium greater than Tc phosphate uptake.[8, 9] Other patterns need to be correlated with specific clinical and plain film radiographic findings.[10]

Overall, there is still a slight possibility that gallium may not detect every inflammatory bone lesion; this has led some investigators to utilize radioactive labeled white blood cells.

RADIOACTIVE LABELED WHITE BLOOD CELLS

Several radionuclides have been successfully labeled with leukocytes and used in the detection of occult inflammatory disease. Currently, the majority of white blood cell–labeled studies are done with ^{111}In oxine. Indium 111 has a relatively short half-life and has many desirable radiobiologic characteristics for detection by available gamma cameras. The labeling process requires some degree of laboratory experience and sophistication utilizing the patient's whole blood or donor-labeled white blood cells.

Technetium localizes as a result of blood flow and interaction with bone metabolism; gallium uptake is mediated by transferrin plasma proteins and in vivo labeling of leukocytes or serum proteins excreted in the inflammatory exudate. Indium-labeled white blood cells will simply be transported by the blood stream and presumably reflect inflammatory activity within the bony skeleton. Several clinical and animal models have alluded to earlier detection by utilizing indium-labeled white blood cells in deference to Tc phosphate scanning.[11]

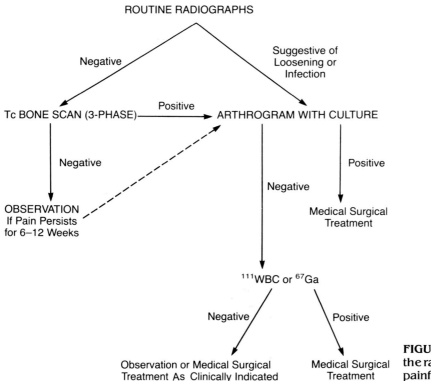

FIGURE 4–2. Algorithm for the radiologic assessment of a painful prosthetic joint.

In most hospital centers, cost and technical demands to label white blood cells limit availability as an imaging technique.[12] These constraints are real, but should not preclude recent advancements in diagnosing acute and low-grade musculoskeletal infections.[13] Overall accuracy appears to be as great as or greater than other imaging techniques, yet warrants strong consideration as a second-stage radionuclide.

SUMMARY

In all infections, except some cases of hematogenous osteomyelitis, technetium phosphate bone scanning is a very sensitive test. Technetium scans do lack specificity, which can be improved by using the three-phase bone scan. ^{67}Ga citrate and ^{111}In labeled white blood cells are useful in diagnosing "cold" lesions as well as useful in diagnosing infection that has been superimposed on damaged bone or postsurgical cases including joint prostheses (Fig. 4–2). The algorithms presented in this chapter outline recommended sequencing of radionuclide scan studies as well as important radiobiologic

and physical characteristics of each radioisotope.

References

1. Duszyndski DO, Kuhn JP, Afshani E, Riddlesberger M Jr: Early radionuclide diagnosis of acute osteomyelitis. Radiology 117:337–340, 1975.
2. Gilday DL, Eng B, Paul DJ, Paterson J: Diagnosis of osteomyelitis in children by combined blood pool and bone imaging. Radiology 117:331–335, 1975.
3. Sullivan DC, Rosenfield NS, Ogden J, Gottschalk A: Problems in the scintigraphic detection of osteomyelitis in children. Radiology 125:731–736, 1980.
4. Berkowitz ID, Wenzel W: "Normal" technetium bone scans in patients with acute osteomyelitis. Am J Dis Child 134:828–830, 1980.
5. Lisbona R, Rossenthall L: Observations on the sequential use of ^{99m}Tc phosphate complex and ^{67}Ga imaging in osteomyelitis, cellulitis and septic arthritis. Radiology 123:123–129, 1977.
6. Graham G, Lundy MM, Frederick RJ, Hartshorne MF, Berger DE: Scintigraphic detection of osteomyelitis with Tc-99m MDP and Ga-67 citrate: concise communication. J Nucl Med 24:1019–1022, 1983.
7. Handmaker H, Giammona ST: Improved early diagnosis of acute inflammatory skeletal-articular diseases in children: a two-radiopharmaceutical approach. Pediatrics 73:661–669, 1984.
8. Tumeh S, Aliabadi P, Weissman BN, McNeil BJ: Chronic osteomyelitis: bone and gallium scan patterns

associated with active disease. Radiology 158:685–688, 1986.

9. LaManna MM, Garbarino JL, German AT, Brady IW: An assessment of technetium and gallium scanning in the patient with painful total joint arthroplasty. Orthopedics 6:580–582, 1983.

10. Graham GD, Lundy MM, Frederick RJ, Berger DE, O'Brien AW, Brown TJ: Predicting the cure of osteomyelitis under treatment: concise communication. J Nucl Med 24:110–113, 1983.

11. Raptopoulos V, Doherty PW, King MA, Johnson K, Gantz NM: Acute osteomyelitis: Advantage of white cell scans in early detection. AJR 139:1077–1082, 1982.

12. Fernandez-Ulloa J, Hughes JA, Krugh KB, Chin D: Bone imaging in infections: Artifacts from spectral overlap between a Tc-99m tracer and In-111 leukocytes. J Nucl Med 24:589–592, 1983.

13. Pring DJ, Henderson RG, Keshavarzian A, Rivett AG, Krausz T, Coombs RRH, Lavender JP: Indium-granulocyte scanning in the painful prosthetic joint. AJR 146:167–172, 1986.

Robert P. Gruninger, M.D.

5

Diagnostic Microbiology in Bone and Joint Infections

. . . relevance depends on the clinical situation of the patient.

A. BALLOWS[1]

PURPOSE AND FUNCTION OF THE MICROBIOLOGY LABORATORY

What the Clinician Should Expect

The purpose of the microbiology laboratory is to aid in the diagnosis, management, and prevention of infectious diseases.[2-5] In contrast to other disciplines in the laboratory, microbiology is more involved in *qualitative* rather than *quantitative* analysis.[6] Thus, the detection of a pathogen in a patient in contrast to a contaminating or colonizing microorganism is a major goal.[5] Further, it is important to obtain this information rapidly in order to aid in patient management and antimicrobial therapy.[7]

Although considerable progress has been made, most of the effort in microbiology involves the traditional time-consuming procedures of isolation, identification, and determination of the antimicrobial susceptibility patterns. Although these operative disciplines remain, changes that have occurred in orthopedic infections have had major impact on the services of the microbiology laboratory. Most important has been the observed increase in spectrum of bacteria or "new pathogens" that cause infections.[2, 8-13] Simultaneously, there has been an increase in the number of available antibiotics. Added to this is the emphasis on cost containment,[14] which has prompted a crit-

ical review of all aspects of diagnostic microbiology, including the appropriateness of a culture.[15] Finally, there has been increased involvement of the microbiology laboratory in infection control, which is particularly important in orthopedics.[4, 16] All of these challenges, both the old as well as new, argue for more physician and microbiologist communication.

Interaction with the Orthopedic Surgeon

Clinical microbiology is challenged by the complex problems related to each patient, procedure, and wound; thus, a culture necessitates individual attention. There is a risk in the laboratory of providing insufficient or excessive information in a culture report.[17-19] Either may be misleading. Early and *direct communication* with a microbiology laboratorian about patient risk factors, antibiotic therapy, precise culture site and what possible microorganisms are being sought will aid in directing the appropriate workup in the laboratory.[7, 17, 20, 21] This in turn will enable a more meaningful microbiology report.[20]

Microbiology Studies and Cost Containment

In contrast to many laboratory tests, the isolation of a single microorganism can result in a cascade of additional testing that might defy the average clinician's imagination. Thus, from the simple Gram stain to the most sophisticated nucleic acid and virulence studies, enormous amounts of time and materials can be consumed. However desirable this is, the advent of cost containment regulation in 1984 has precluded such practices as rou-

From the Department of Laboratory Medicine, Pathology, and Internal Medicine, Hennepin County Medical Center, and The Musculoskeletal Infectious Disease Unit, Metropolitan Medical Center, Minneapolis, Minnesota.

tine.[4, 14, 20, 22] To that extent, inappropriate specimens increasingly will be rejected in the microbiology laboratory.[4] In turn, physician education will become a part of that process.[5] Although the results of a rapid test may preclude the need for culture or require only minimal additional identification and thereby reduce costs, few such tests exist.[2, 3] Conversely, in the control of nosocomial infections, thorough work-up of isolated bacteria may necessitate detailed identification and repeated antibiotic susceptibility testing to detect unusually resistant or "hospital strains."

Nosocomial Infections

The control of nosocomial infections is of particular importance in orthopedics.[16] Wound infections are the second most common nosocomial infection.[23] Major contributing factors to acquiring a nosocomial infection include longer hospitalization, open wounds, central intravenous lines, and antibiotics.[23] All of these risk factors occur in many orthopedic patients in whom a significant number of infections occur even with clean surgery.[16] Therefore, it is important to establish a close working relation between the microbiology laboratory, the orthopedic nursing service, and the hospital epidemiologist in order to expeditiously recognize the clustering of unusual or highly resistant bacteria. In turn, appropriate isolation and preventive measures can be implemented.[16, 23] Measures that reduce transmission of microorganisms from one patient to another, such as hand washing, wound precautions, and isolation of patients with draining wounds containing multiply resistant organism, are fundamental to a successful orthopedic service.

APPROACH TO CLINICAL SPECIMENS

Selection, Collection, Transport, and Rejection

The selection of when and which site to culture in an orthopedic infection is critical. Accurate definition of the type of tissue cultured and collection of the specimen by the most qualified clinician is important.[15] Orthopedic infections, by their very nature, are deepseated.[24, 25] In spite of this, culture should be obtained prior to initiation of antibiotic therapy whenever possible. This is particularly true in acute osteomyelitis, septic arthritis, and preoperatively in previously infected or probably infected patients. In contrast, cultures of superficial wounds or the operative site at the time of extensive debridement in Type III open fractures, although controversial,[26, 27] should not be done routinely because they are not reliable predictors of existing or subsequent bone infection.[28] Even a swab culture of a sinus tract may give misleading results[29] unless Staphylococcus aureus (coagulase-positive) is the predominant isolate or a single species is isolated in pure culture.[18, 29, 30] Deep wound biopsy is recommended. Alternatively, a curetted specimen after cleaning the wound is acceptable.[29, 31] Intraoperative cultures should be taken in all suspected infections even if the patient is receiving antibiotics.[10, 21, 25] The intraoperative site to culture must be individualized according to the patient, the probable pathogen, and the extent of disease. Postoperative wound cultures are not indicated routinely. They may be used to detect a clinical relapse, particularly if a necrotizing or spreading cellulitis is suspected.[32] An occasional exception to this is wound culture for the purpose of infection control.

The preferred type of specimen in most bacterial and yeast infections is aspirated fluid (joint) or pus (wound). In fungal[33] and selected bacterial infections (e.g., anaerobic [Actinomyces] and granulomatous [Mycobacteria]), tissue biopsy from the edge of the wound is preferable. In many situations, both an aspirate of fluid or pus and a biopsy of tissue are appropriate.[9, 18, 34] An aerobic or anaerobic swab, although more commonly used, is appropriate only when neither an aspirate nor a biopsy is obtainable. Aspirates should be collected in a syringe that is made as air-free as possible. Tissue specimens should be placed in a small CO_2-filled container to reduce exposure to air. Bone[35] and tissue biopsy[9, 18] cultures are preferable to swab in assessing infections in pressure sores and prosthetic joints.

It is axiomatic that any specimen for culture should be transported promptly to the microbiology laboratory.[2, 3, 10] Adherence to this recommendation will enhance recovery of important fastidious organisms.[8] In contrast, departure from this or any of the above suggested approaches to specimen collection in orthopedic infections may result in meaningless reports, such as "no pathogen found," "mixed flora," or "normal flora with no predominant isolate found."[20]

Rapid Procedures

Ideally, in order to guide initial antibiotic therapy a rapid test result should be available in 1 to 2 hours.[7, 36] In order to influence decisions during surgery, a rapid test should be available in a matter of minutes. Any one or more of the procedures listed in Table 5–1 may provide meaningful information in the above circumstances. It is important to appreciate that most rapid microbiology tests are *qualitative* in nature and therefore dependent upon the knowledge and experience of the technologist doing the test.

The *direct microscopic examination* of a surgical specimen still is the most rapid diagnostic procedure. It aids in detection of microorganisms and inflammation.[37–39] Characteristic morphology and staining properties of bacteria, yeast, or fungi[33] as well as the nature of an inflammatory response may be observed. This may be helpful in directing both the clinician's early therapy and the microbiologist's culture work-up strategy.

A differential Gram stain should be performed on all specimens.[2, 39, 40] It provides good gram-negative versus gram-positive bacterial morphologic data as well as some measure of inflammation. It is of particular benefit in mixed bacterial infections and septic arthritis. Occasionally the Gram stain is sufficient in some wounds to obviate culture (e.g., *Pasteur-*

ella multocida, group A streptococcal pyoderma). It is critical in necrotizing fasciitis, along with the histopathology of a frozen section, in detecting anaerobic gram-negative rods[32, 41] in deep burn wound sepsis[42] and in detecting clostridial myonecrosis. If the Gram stain is negative and infection is strongly suspected (i.e., many acute inflammatory cells), an *acridine orange stain* (necessitating fluorescent microscope) may aid in detecting gram-negative bacteria. In suspected fungal infections, direct examination of a *10 percent potassium hydroxide (KOH) wet mount* preparation (preferably using a phase microscope) or a *fluorescein calcofluor white stain*[43] will aid in detecting characteristic fungal morphology.[44] Direct microscopy using special stains (e.g., acid-fast, rhodamine-auramine, or a fluorescein-tagged antibody stain) may help make a rapid diagnosis. These procedures should be done only after discussion with the patient's physician.[39]

The development of monoclonal antibodies to specific bacterial antigens has had a major impact in the laboratory. However, with the possible exception of detection of bacterial antigen (e.g., *Haemophilus influenzae*, *Neisseria meningococcus*, *Streptococcus pneumoniae* in synovial fluid),[45–47] these new tests are useful only in the rapid identification of isolated bacteria and *not* for detecting specific bacteria in the clinical specimen.

TABLE 5–1. Rapid Diagnostic Procedures in Microbiology by Direct Microscopic Visualization

Aspirated Fluid/Pus, Swab, or Ground Tissue
Gram stain
  Gram-positive versus gram-negative morphology; inflammatory response
Acridine orange stain*
  If Gram stain is "negative" may aid detection of gram-negative bacteria
Potassium hydroxide (10% KOH) wet preparation†
  Detect fungal morphology; may be diagnostic
Calcofluor white wet preparation*
  Detect fungal morphology; may be diagnostic but also stains collagen and elastin
Ziehl-Neelsen acid-fast stain
  Mycobacteria, Nocardia, Streptomyces

Tissue Imprint (Touch Prep)
Gram stain
  As above
PAS or Wright/Giemsa or methylene blue
  Fungal and fungal-like organisms

---

 * Ultraviolet darkfield or mercury vapor lamp light source microscope.
 † Phase-contrast microscope is better.

Routine Isolation and Identification of Microorganisms

The selection of procedures for the isolation and identification of microorganisms is largely the responsibility of a microbiologist. If the clinician indicates the exact anatomical site of the specimen and which organisms are suspected, the most appropriate direction and extent of work-up in the laboratory will result.[2, 3, 15, 33] In this way, critical, rather than the often occurring uncritical only descriptive microbiologic results can be avoided. Simply indicating whether the specimen is the initial or a follow-up culture can more effectively direct the work-up in the laboratory. Thus, the initial culture of all wounds or abscesses should be thoroughly evaluated; for follow-up specimens from a wound, only a Gram stain may be necessary. Exceptions to this (when a culture should be included in wound follow-up) are suspected cellulitis, wounds contiguous to mucosal surfaces, or wounds in an immunocompromised host or in preparation of skin graft site. In the last situation, it is important to be sure the graft site is free of *S. aureus* (coagulase-positive) or *Streptococcus pyogenes*.

The variety of media available to the microbiologist for isolation and identification of the numerous microorganisms found in orthopedic infections is endless.[2, 3] It would serve little purpose to describe them here. However, as a rule, all primary wound specimens should be cultured initially for *aerobic, facultative anaerobic,* and *strictly anaerobic organisms.* Media for these purposes should include blood agar, chocolate agar *(H. influenzae, Neisseria gonococcus),* and an nutrient-enriched broth for many fastidious microorganisms. Selective media should be used when fungi or acid-fast bacteria (e.g., *Mycobacteria, Nocardia*) and unusual organisms such as L-form bacteria[21] are suspected. In these latter situations, it is important to alert the microbiologist for unusual pathogens in order to ensure that appropriate culture media can be used. Final reports of identification for most organisms should be available in 24 to 48 hours; however, some isolates may take several days to a few weeks for identification (anaerobes) or even several weeks (fungi and mycobacteria). Fortunately, in vitro antibiotic sensitivity studies are often available before complete identification is made.

Testing for Antimicrobial Effectiveness (Table 5–2)

The three major ways to measure antimicrobial effectiveness in vitro are (1) in vitro susceptibility testing of a bacterial isolate; (2) measurement of the patient's inhibitory or

bactericidal serum level against his or her own infectious bacteria; and (3) measurement of the actual serum concentration of the antibiotic the patient is receiving.[2, 3] In vitro antimicrobial susceptibility testing of the clinically significant isolate(s) is the most important and commonly done of these tests.

IN VITRO ANTIMICROBIAL SUSCEPTIBILITY TESTING

In vitro antimicrobial susceptibility testing is a major challenge.[48] In the early years of antibiotics, it was a simple matter to test all available antibiotics, albeit testing was not standardized from one laboratory to the next. Today, in direct contrast, the tests most commonly used are standardized, but there are too many antibiotics available to test all of them against an appropriate isolate.[49] The National Committee for Clinical Laboratory Standards (NCCLS) provides recommendations for standardized tests and suggests the prototype generic antibiotic that can be tested to represent each class of antibiotics.[2] In most clinical laboratories, these recommendations are sufficient. However, when possible, the panel of antibiotics selected for testing in each laboratory should be made in cooperation with clinicians (e.g., infectious disease specialists, surgeons, pediatricians) and should reflect the antibiotics available in the hospital pharmacy.

All in vitro susceptibility studies are based upon:

1. Serial dilutions of the test antibiotic in broth *(broth dilution)* or a solid agar medium *(agar dilution).*

2. Antibiotic diffusion from a paper disc (6 mm) into a solid agar medium *(disc diffusion).*

3. Antibiotic elution from a paper disc into broth *(broth-disc elution).*

GUIDELINES FOR USING IN VITRO SUSCEPTIBILITY TESTS

Broth/Agar Dilution. In the broth/agar dilution methods, the lowest concentration of an antibiotic that inhibits growth of the patient's isolate is designated the MIC (minimal inhibitory concentration).[2, 3] If the MIC level of the antimicrobial can be achieved readily in the patient's serum using normal dosage and route of administration, the organism is said to be *susceptible* or *sensitive* (S) to that antimicrobial. Upon subculture of the MIC broth an MBC (minimal bacteriocidal concentration) can be obtained. This is the lowest concentra-

---

TABLE 5–2. Tests for Antimicrobial Effectiveness

In vitro Bacterial Antimicrobial Susceptibility Test
Broth dilution (MIC, MBC)
Agar dilution (MIC)
Disc diffusion (S, I, R, and an extrapolated MIC)
Broth disc elution (anaerobes)

Serum Bacteriocidal Level
Inhibitory level, 18–24 hours; bactericidal level, 48 hours

Antibiotic Serum Level
Aminoglycosides, vancomycin, chloramphenicol

Abbreviations: MIC = Minimal inhibitory concentration; MBC = minimal bactericidal concentration; S = sensitive; I = intermediate; R = resistant.

tion of antimicrobial agent that allowed less than 0.1 percent of the original culture inoculum to survive.

Disc Diffusion. In the disc diffusion method, the zone of inhibited growth about an antibiotic impregnated disc is measured and compared to a standard test bacterium.[2, 3] In turn, the size of the zone of inhibited growth determines whether the isolate is sensitive (S, large zone); intermediate (I); or resistant (R, small or no zone). Standardization of this qualitative test yields results that correlate well with the quantitative results obtained by the MIC test. It should be apparent that as important as this information is, the interpretation does not take into account variables such as antibiotic distribution into various body sites, antibiotic concentration at the infected site relative to serum concentration, influence of bony sequestrations or foreign bodies or any other local conditions. Most clinicians try to achieve a concentration of antimicrobial agent at the site of infection that is four times or greater than the in vitro MIC.[2, 3, 50] Regardless of the method used most laboratories report results as *S, I,* or *R*.

The disc diffusion method is used in most laboratories and is the most practical method. Its advantages include flexibility in antibiotic selection, reproducibility, and availability of an extrapolated MIC. The disc diffusion method is the most reliable way to detect the methicillin resistant staphylococcus.

Broth Disc Elution. In this method, used almost exclusively for anaerobic bacteria, an antibiotic-impregnated paper disc is placed in an anaerobic broth along with the bacteria to be tested and incubated. Visual results are determined as "no growth" (sensitive) or "growth" (resistant). The test is used for anaerobic bacteria[2, 3] and has limited value in most clinical settings. However, in well-defined anaerobic orthopedic infections (i.e., appropriate and properly collected specimens), the test may be indicated, especially if previous antibiotic failure occurs. In contrast to broth dilution and disc diffusion susceptibility, testing by the NCCLS has not finalized recommendations for test standards. The decision as to which isolates should be tested in vitro and how often the same species from the same site on follow-up culture should be tested is largely the clinician's responsibility. Initially, a pure culture of a gram-negative bacilli or *S. aureus* from a primary wound infection should always be tested. Once done, repeating this is indicated only in clinical relapse or to detect a

multiple antibiotic resistant organism that is important for infection control. Conversely, most streptococci (except group D enterococci) and anaerobes should not be tested routinely for in vitro antimicrobial susceptibility.

Anaerobes seldom need to be tested. Antibiotic sensitivity for most anaerobic isolates is predictable. Susceptibility test results usually are delayed several days so as to make this testing impractical as a matter of routine. Decisions regarding sensitivity studies on bacteria from mixed cultures, on repeat cultures, and on scant growth of common contaminants, such as *Corynebacterium* species, *Bacillus* species, and *Staphylococcus epidermidis* (coagulase-negative), should be discussed with the clinician beforehand. If any of these bacteria were seen on direct smear and cultured from an aspirate or tissue culture, in vitro antimicrobial susceptibility testing may be appropriate.

RAPID TESTS FOR ANTIMICROBIAL SUSCEPTIBILITY

There are a few rapid tests for antimicrobial susceptibility that selectively will be helpful. Several bacteria produce a beta-lactamase, an enzyme that binds to the beta-lactam ring in penicillin, cephalothin, and their cogeners. If the enzyme breaks the ring, the antibiotic becomes inactive. Several methods for direct testing of a pure isolate for beta-lactamase are available. The test is useful in testing isolates of *N. gonococcus*, *Haemophilus* species, and *Bacteroides* species. Some isolates may have a non–beta-lactamase mechanism of beta-lactam antibiotic resistance; thus, a negative beta-lactamase test may require follow-up antimicrobial susceptibility testing (e.g., *Staphylococcus*, *Bacteroides gracilis*, *B. distasonis*). It is possible in some laboratories to have preliminary susceptibility results in 4 to 5 hours if the laboratory has committed automated equipment. For the most part, other than the beta-lactamase test, antimicrobial susceptibility test results are available at 18 to 48 hours and should suffice.

SERUM BACTERICIDAL LEVEL

Determining the serum bactericidal level (SBL), a method introduced decades ago, is another way of measuring antimicrobial effectiveness.[2, 3] This test measures the activity of the patient's own serum against the infecting organism. The lowest dilution of the patient's serum that kills 99.9 percent of a standard inoculum of this organism is called the SBL. Technically, this test is similar to the broth dilution test. It does require close cooperation with the laboratory because the patient's serum must be obtained at precise times of expected *peak* and *trough concentrations* relative to antibiotic administration. The test has had limited use in orthopedics.[51] It has been used in pediatric patients with septic arthritis or acute osteomyelitis to test the adequacy of oral therapy.[51-54] Oral doses are adjusted so that a peak SBL of 1 : 8 or 1 : 16 or more and a trough of 1 : 2 or higher is obtained.[51, 53, 54] Less commonly, the SBL has been used in adults with septic arthritis[55] and osteomyelitis.[56]

ACTUAL SERUM CONCENTRATION

Originally the measurement of the *antimicrobial agent concentration in serum* or other body fluid was done by bioassay methods in the microbiology laboratory. Today, newer, more rapid and reliable methods are available, and usually the test is not performed in the microbiology laboratory. Two reasons for determining these levels are to learn whether an effective therapeutic level is achieved and to guide antibiotic dosage so as to avoid toxic side effects. Assays of the following antibiotic are available in most laboratories: aminoglycosides (amikacin, gentamicin, netilmicin, tobramycin), vancomycin, and chloramphenicol. Assays for other groups of antibiotics used in orthopedic infections (penicillins, cephalosporins, macrolides) either are not available or require special arrangement with reference laboratories that have committed procedures or equipment. Results of aminoglycoside, vancomycin, and chloramphenicol determinations can generally be obtained within the same day, whereas the results of penicillins and cephalosporin may not be available for one or more days. The latter levels are rarely, if ever, indicated.

Special Tests

Special tests are those that necessitate prior arrangement with the laboratory, are used for specific and limited needs, require special handling, and are not considered part of routine microbiologic procedures. Two such tests include the *quantitative tissue culture* and *in vitro antibiotic synergism versus antagonism susceptibility* testing (Table 5–3).

TABLE 5–3. Special Microbiology Tests and Controversies in Infections of Joints and Bones

Special Tests
Quantitative tissue cultures
  $\geq$ than 10^5/gm may be helpful in burn/skin graft patients
In vitro bacterial antimicrobial testing for synergy
  Clinical relevance not established in orthopedic infections

Controversies
Clinical relevance of positive broth culture only
  Particularly *Staphylococcus epidermidis*, other coagulase-negative)
Qualitative/quantitative measurement of biofilm production of isolated microorganisms
  Usually present on any prosthetic indwelling material

Quantitative tissue cultures may fulfill a specific need in burn wound infections and in skin grafting.[42, 57, 58] Simply, this procedure involves obtaining a tissue specimen approximately 1 cm² or 1 gm in weight that is accurately weighed, ground, and suspended in a known volume of broth. This is followed by a Gram stain to estimate the number of bacteria per milliliter and usually by four to five serial dilutions so that inoculum onto an agar plate will facilitate an accurate colony count. The actual number of bacteria per gram of tissue can be calculated from these data. In burns or skin grafts, $\geq 10^5$/gm tissue are considered significant. On the other hand, such cultures at the time of thorough debridement in Type II open fractures have not been predictive of subsequent infection.[28] Other uses of quantitative tissue cultures in orthopedic infections are unclear or controversial.[42, 57]

In vitro antimicrobial testing for *synergism* and *antagonism* is rarely indicated in orthopedic infections. This test measures the sum effect in vitro when two antibiotics are used in combination against a pathogen. If inhibitory effect is greater than the total additive effect of the combined antibiotics, it is considered *synergistic*.[2, 3] Conversely, if one antibiotic diminishes the activity of the other, it is considered *antagonistic*. Several methods are available in the laboratory for this test. The test has had its greatest use in evaluation of combined antibiotic therapy in infectious endocarditis, particularly when the infection is due to *Enterococcus*.[2] Although combinations of antibiotics are frequently used in orthopedic infections, there are no well-documented in vitro synergy or antagonism studies to correlate treatment efficacy in patients. It is a test to consider in a persistent infection caused by the same pathogen that appears refractory to antibiotic treatment.

Laboratory Controversies in Orthopedic Infections

There are many controversies in clinical microbiology that relate to orthopedic infections. Some of these have been referred to above, such as serum bactericidal levels, quantitative tissue cultures, extent of descriptive microbiology with each isolate particularly in mixed bacterial infections, the frequency of repeat cultures from a wound site, frequency of antibiotic susceptibility testing of a previously isolated pathogen from the same site, and the value of superficial wound cultures in deep-seated infections (see the next section, Microorganisms Encountered in Orthopedic Infections). Two additional controversies should be mentioned.

One relates to the interpretation of a positive back-up broth culture from a surgical wound site, particularly when the isolate is *Staphylococcus* (coagulase-negative) that was not seen in the direct Gram stain or on the primary culture plates. In the absence of bone cement or a prosthesis, this in all probability is a true contaminant and at worst is of little consequence to the otherwise normal patient. On the other hand, it is well known that this organism is an important pathogen with orthopedic prostheses,[25] albeit it often produces an indolent illness with little inflammation. To further complicate matters, this organism, as with many bacteria, can remain as a latent (dormant in situ) infection, only to appear much later as active and clinically important infection.[25] Most microbiologists believe it is important to place part of a wound or abscess specimen into enriched broth media as part of the primary culture. Often this broth aids in the isolation of fastidious bacteria, anaerobes, and so on. However, the interpretation of "broth-only positive" culture of normal flora most often is arbitrary. The tendency is to disregard the isolate as a contaminant in an otherwise uncomplicated case.[31, 38]

The second controversy relates to the role of *slime* or *glycocalyx* biofilm that is produced by bacteria on synthetic materials used in orthopedic surgery.[58] The question for the microbiology laboratory is whether to test bacteria for slime production. Certainly, if this is a virulence factor of certain bacteria, it should be determined. If, however, there is no correlation with active infection or mechanical disruption of orthopedic prostheses, slime detection has no applied clinical value. Until this question is more clearly resolved, it seems inappropriate to test for this bacterial property (Gristina AG, personal communication).

MICROORGANISMS ENCOUNTERED IN ORTHOPEDIC INFECTIONS

Joints

The etiologic agents of infectious arthritis (see Chapters 20, 21, 26, 28) include the four major categories of microorganisms (bacteria, fungi, viruses, and parasites).[2] In this section, emphasis is on bacterial arthritis. Fungal arthritis is uncommon (see Chapter 21), and infectious arthritis is not a feature of any of the common parasitic infections. Some of the more commonly encountered agents in *natural infections* of joints are listed in Table 5–4.[2, 59] *Staphylococcus aureus* is the most frequently isolated etiologic agent in all infectious arthritis. However, the frequency of isolation of other etiologic agent varies considerably, based upon age and various epidemiologic factors. Thus *N. gonorrhoeae* is more common in adults younger than 30 years of age and *H. influenzae*, Type b, is more common in children under 2 years old.[59] These three bacteria, along with the various *Streptococcus* species, comprise well over a majority of known isolates in joint infections. These bacteria usually can be recovered in the laboratory if attention is given to careful collection of joint fluid in a sterile syringe and use of appropriate primary isolation media. An enriched broth is particularly important for recovery of anaerobes,[2, 3, 8] which uncommonly have caused septic arthritis.[8] In contrast, *prosthetic joint infections* are most often associated with skin flora.[10, 25] *Staphylococcus epidermidis;* other coagulase-negative staphylococci; *Corynebacterium* species; *Propionibacterium,*[60] which are indigenous to the skin; and gram-negative bacilli, which are transient skin colonizers, are the most common isolates. Often these infections occur late after surgery,[61] produce little inflammatory response, and yield negative Gram stains and scant growth on culture. At times it is difficult to interpret the laboratory results (see the previous section on laboratory controversies). Other etiologic microorganisms in septic arthritis include viruses (e.g., coxsackievirus,

TABLE 5–4. More Common Bacteria Encountered in Orthopedic Infections

Infectious Arthritis		Osteomyelitis
Most common	Staphylococcus aureus (coagulase-positive)	Most common
Common in infants	Haemophilus influenzae	Rare
+	Haemophilus sp (other)	+
+	Beta-hemolytic streptococcus (group A or B)	+
+	Streptococci (other) (Streptococcus pneumoniae)	
Common in young adults	Neisseria gonorrhoeae	
+	Salmonella	Sickle cell disease
+	Pseudomonas	Sneakers, water
Cat or dog bite	Pasteurella multocida	Same
Prosthetic	Enterobacteriaceae*	Trauma, reparative materials in fractures
Human bite	Fusobacterium sp.	Human bite, oral disease
Drug addicts	Eikenella corrodens	Drug addicts
Human bites	Bacteroides sp.	Human bite, oral disease
+	Peptostreptococcus sp.	+
Seen, +/– culture	Borrelia burgdorferi	
Prosthesis	Staphylococcus epidermidis (other coagulase-negative staphylococcus)	Reparative materials in fractures
Prosthesis	Corynebacterium sp.	
+	Propionibacterium sp.	
+	Actinomyces sp.	Jaw
+	Mycoplasma sp.	
+	Mycobacteria sp.	+

* Enterobacteriaceae include several gram-negative bacilli (e.g., Escherichia coli, Enterobacter, Klebsiella sp., etc.).
Plus signs = positive, or occurs.
Blank spaces = not described, or does not occur.

echovirus), *Mycobacterium, Mycoplasma* (?), spirochetes *(Borrelia burgdorferi),* and *Actinomyces* species. Attempts to recover any of these should be done only after consulting with the microbiologist.

Bones

The etiologic agents of bone infections (i.e., osteomyelitis), excluding primary infectious involvement of bone marrow with contiguous connective tissue, include only two of the four categories of microorganisms.[2] They are fungi (see Chapter 21) and bacteria. *Staphylococcus aureus* is clearly the most frequent isolate from all osteomyelitis.[3, 13, 25, 61] The order of frequency of other bacteria (Table 5–4), as with septic arthritis, varies considerably, depending upon age and epidemiologic factors and whether the osteomyelitis is acute, subacute, or chronic hematogenous; post-traumatic[12]; or without orthopedic hardware.[11, 25, 59, 61] Appropriate specimens for each of these clinical conditions vary. In general, the following is appropriate. Acute hematogenous osteomyelitis should include a blood culture in the early febrile period and preferably an aspirate from the metaphysis or point of maximal periosteal

tenderness. Both specimens should be obtained before empiric antibiotic therapy. In the other forms of osteomyelitis, the preferred specimen should be obtained intraoperatively and should include any bony sequestration, bone biopsy, or scraping from the infected site.[2, 9] An aspirate of purulent material should be included. If neither type of specimen is obtainable, a swab may suffice. In the event of a therapeutic amputation, a culture of the removed tissue should not be taken routinely unless the patient is acutely ill or there are medical legal issues or epidemiologic concerns. All specimens should be processed as with joint fluid, with the additional step of grinding all tissue or bone specimen prior to inoculating culture media.

SUMMARY

The clinical microbiology laboratory is increasingly challenged by the spectrum of orthopedic infections. Advances in reparative and reconstructive surgery, for example, have brought new "pathogens" to the foreground. Newer antibiotics have created new in vitro antimicrobial susceptibility testing. Concern for nosocomial infection justifiably has increased. All of this in the face of cost containment attests to the challenges in clinical microbiology. Critical to meeting these challenges will be close communication between the orthopedic physicians and the clinical microbiologist.[5]

References

1. Ballows A: Introductory comments: clinical relevance in microbiology. Proceedings of the 1975 Aspen Conference: Clinical Relevance in Microbiology. Chicago, College of American Pathologists, 1977.
2. Finegold SM, Baron EJ: Bailey and Scott's Diagnostic Microbiology, 7th ed. St. Louis, CV Mosby, 1986.
3. Lennette EH, Balows A, Hauser WJ Jr, Shadomy HJ: Manual of Clinical Microbiology, 4th ed. Washington, DC, American Society of Microbiology, 1985.
4. Gavin TL: The laboratory microbiologist in clinical medicine. Ann Intern Med 89:789–790, 1978.
5. Neu HC: What should the physician expect from the microbiology laboratory? Ann Intern Med 89:781–784, 1978.
6. Sonnenwirth AC: Constraints under which the microbiology laboratory functions. Ann Intern Med 89:785–788, 1978.
7. Ellner PD: The clinician-microbiologist interaction: continuing indications for an essential dialog (editorial). Clin Micro Newsletter 8:177–178, 1986.
8. Sim FH: Anaerobic infections. Orthop Clin North Am 6:1049–1056, 1975.
9. Stratton IB: Deep implant infection in orthopedics (abstract) J Bone Joint Surg 57-B:249, 1975.
10. Gristina AG, Kolkin J: Total joint replacement and sepsis. J Bone Joint Surg 65-A:128–134, 1983.
11. Inman RD, Gallegos KV, Brause BD, Redecha PB, Christian CL: Clinical and microbial features of prosthetic joint infection. Am J Med 77:53, 1984.
12. Meyers BR, Berson BL, Gilbert M, Hirschman SZ: Clinical patterns of osteomyelitis due to gram-negative bacteria. Arch Intern Med 131:228–233, 1973.
13. Pichichero ME, Friesen HA: Polymicrobial osteomyelitis: report of three cases and a review of the literature. Rev Infect Dis 4:86–96, 1982.
14. Bartlett RC: Effect of DRGs on utilization of the microbiology laboratory. Infect Control 6:323–325, 1985.
15. Westerman EL: Clinical aspects of wound and anaerobic infections: medical perspective. In Smith JW, ed: The Role of Clinical Microbiology in Cost-Effective Health Care. Skokie, Ill, College of American Pathologists, 1985, pp 325–332.
16. O'Riordan C, Adler JL, Banks HH, Finland M: Wound infections on an orthopedic service: a prospective study. Am J Epidemiol 95:442–450, 1972.
17. Griner PF, Glaser RJ: Misuse of laboratory tests and diagnostic procedures. N Engl J Med 307:1336–1339, 1982.
18. Robson M, Heggers JP: Surgical infection. I. Single bacterial species or polymicrobic in origin. Surgery 65:608–610, 1969.
19. Lipsky BA, Plorde JJ: Bacterial culture specimens: categories, collection and interpretation. Postgrad Med 64:80–83, 86–87, 90–92, 1978.
20. MacLowry JD: General laboratory aspects of wound infections. In Smith JW, ed: The Role of Clinical Microbiology in Cost-Effective Health Care. Skokie, Ill, College of American Pathologists, 1985, pp 341–348.
21. Gordon SL, Greer RB, Craig CP: Recurrent osteomyelitis: report of four cases culturing L-form variants of staphylococci. J Bone Joint Surg 53-A:1150–1156, 1971.
22. Bartlett RC: Cost containment in microbiology. Clin Lab Med 5:761–791, 1985.
23. Aber RC, Garner JS: Postoperative wound infections. In Wenzel RP, ed: Handbook of Hospital Acquired Infections. Boca Raton, Fla, CRC Press, 1981, pp 303–316.
24. Shannon JG, Woolhouse FM, Eisinger PJ: The treatment of chronic osteomyelitis by saucerization and immediate skin grafting. Clin Orthop 96:98–107, 1973.
25. Fitzgerald RH, Nolan DR, Ilstrup DM, Van Scoy RE, Washington JA: Deep wound sepsis following total arthroplasty. J Bone Joint Surg 59-A:847–855, 1977.
26. Patzakis MJ, Harvey JP, Ivler D: The role of antibiotics in the management of open fractures. J Bone Joint Surg 56-A:532–541, 1974.
27. Lawrence RM, Hoeprich PD, Huston AC: Quantitative microbiology of traumatic orthopedic wounds. J Clin Microbiol 8:673–675, 1978.
28. Gruninger RP, Kennedy K, Klicker RE, Gustilo RB: Quantitative Tissue and Swab Culture at Wound Debridement in Type III Open Fracture (abstract). 85th Annual Meeting of the American Society for Microbiology, Las Vegas, Nevada, March 3–7, 1985 (No. C 195, p 332).
29. Sapico FL, Canawati HN, Witte JL: Quantitative aerobic and anaerobic bacteriology of infected diabetic feet. J Clin Microbiol 12:413–420, 1980.
30. Mackowiak PA, Jones SR, Smith JW: Diagnostic value of sinus-tract cultures in chronic osteomyelitis. JAMA 239:2772–2775, 1978.
31. Louie TJ, Bartlett JG, Tally FP, Gorbach SL: Aerobic and anaerobic bacteria in diabetic foot ulcers. Ann Intern Med 85:461–463, 1976.
32. Janevicius I, Hann SE, Batt MD: Necrotizing fasciitis. Surg Gynecol Obstet 154:97–102, 1982.
33. Ajello L: Problems in the laboratory diagnosis of opportunistic fungus disease. In Chick EW, Balows A, Furcolow ML, eds: Opportunistic Fungal Infections. Springfield, Ill, Charles C Thomas, 1975, pp 31–35.
34. Ziment I, Miller LG, Finegold SM: Nonsporulating anaerobic bacteria in osteomyelitis. Antimicrob Agents Chemother 7:77–85, 1967.
35. Sugarman B, Hawes S, Musher DM, Kilma M, Young EJ, Pircher F: Osteomyelitis beneath pressure sores. Arch Intern Med 143:683–688, 1983.
36. Jorgensen JH: Clinical situations in which rapid methods may be applied. Diagn Microbiol Infect Dis 3:3S–7S, 1985.
37. Grobbelar CJ: Hip replacement: frozen section as an additional method of detecting latent infection. J Bone Joint Surg 57-B:259, 1975.
38. Wilson PD. Joint replacement. South Med J 70:55–60, 1977.
39. Murray PR: The role of microscopy in the microbiology laboratory. Clin Micro Newsletter 6:89–91, 1984.

40. Ellner PD: Microbiology and laboratory procedures. In Eftekhar NS, ed: Infection in Joint Replacement Surgery. St. Louis, CV Mosby, 1984, pp. 3–25.

41. Stameenkovic I, Lew PD: Early recognition of potentially fatal necrotizing fasciitis. N Engl J Med 310:1659–1693, 1984.

42. Krizek TJ, Robson MC: Evolution of quantitative bacteriology in wound management. Am J Surg 130:579–584, 1975.

43. Elder BL, Roberts GD: Rapid methods for the diagnosis of fungal infections. Lab Med 17:591–596, 1986.

44. O'Hara M: Histopathologic diagnosis of fungal diseases. Infect Control 7:78–84, 1986.

45. Feldman SA, DuClos T: Diagnosis of meningococcal arthritis by immunoelectrophoresis of synovial fluid. Appl Microbiol 25:1006–1007, 1973.

46. DeLuca PA, Gutman LT, Ruderman RJ: Counterimmunoelectrophoresis of synovial fluid in the diagnosis of septic arthritis. J Pediatr Orthop 5:167–170, 1985.

47. Dorff RJ, Ziolkowski JS, Rytel MW: Detection by counterimmunoelectrophoresis of pneumococcal antigen in synovial fluid from septic arthritis. Arthritis Rheum 18:613–615, 1975.

48. Loveless MO: The role of susceptibility testing in appropriate selection of antibiotics. Lab Med 17:75–77, 1986.

49. Hindler JA, Kelley SG: Reference chart for commonly used antibacterial agents. Lab Med 17:476–479, 1986.

50. Ellner PD, Neu HC, Fink DJ: The inhibitory quotient: a method for interpreting minimum inhibitory concentration data. JAMA 246:1575–1578, 1981.

51. Prober CG, Yeager AS: Use of serum bactericidal titer to assess the adequacy of oral antibiotic therapy in the treatment of acute hematogenous osteomyelitis. J Pediatr 95:131–135, 1979.

52. Stratton CW: The usefulness of the serum bactericidal test in orthopedic infections. Orthopedics 7:1579–1580, 1984.

53. Tetzlaff TR, McCracken GH, Nelson JD: Oral antibiotic therapy for skeletal infections in children. II. Therapy of osteomyelitis and suppurative arthritis. J Pediatr 92:485–490, 1978.

54. Kolyvas E, Ahronheim G, Marks MI, Gledhill R, Owen H, Rosenthal L: Oral antibiotic therapy of skeletal infections in children. Pediatrics 65:867–871, 1980.

55. Parker, RH, Schmid FR: Antibacterial activity of synovial fluid during therapy of septic arthritis. Rheumatology 14:96–104, 1971.

56. Jordan GW, Kawachi MM: Analysis of serum bactericidal activity in endocarditis, osteomyelitis and other bacterial infections. Medicine 60:49–61, 1981.

57. Marshall KA, Edgerton MT, Rodeheaver GT, Magee CM, Edlich RF: Quantitative microbiology: its application to hand injuries. Am J Surg 131:730–733, 1976.

58. Gristina AG, Costerton JW: Bacterial aherence to biomaterials and tissue. J Bone Joint Surg 67-A:264–273, 1985.

59. Gutman LT: Acute, subacute, and chronic osteomyelitis and pyogenic arthritis in children. Curr Prob Pediatr 15:1–56, 1985.

60. Launder WJ, Hungerford DS: Late infection of total hip arthroplasty with *Propionibacterium acnes:* a case and review of the literature. Clin Orthop 157:170–177, 1981.

61. Mitchell C, Ehrlich MG, Siffert RS: Comparative bacteriology of early and late orthopedic infections. Clin Orthop 96:277–287, 1973.

David N. Williams, M.D.

CHAPTER

6

Antibiotic Penetration into Bones and Joints

INTRODUCTION

Antibiotics are used prophylactically in orthopedic surgery, primarily at the time of major reconstructive surgery, and therapeutically in osteomyelitis, septic arthritis, open fractures, and soft tissue infections. The appropriate use of antibiotics in these situations requires a knowledge of the antimicrobial spectrum, pharmacokinetics, safety profile, and (increasingly) cost. This chapter focuses on one aspect of antibiotic pharmacokinetics, namely, antibiotic penetration into bones, synovial tissue, and synovial fluid.

ASSAY OF ANTIBIOTIC LEVELS

General Considerations

BONE

The lack of widely accepted standard assay methods results in special problems in interpreting bone antibiotic levels reported in the literature. There are several technical problems still to be solved, such as the optimum antibiotic extraction procedure and the contribution of blood or serum to the "bone" antibiotic level, particularly in highly vascularized fragments. Thus, comparisons between published bone antibiotic levels must take into account such diverse factors as route (oral, intramuscular, intravenous) and timing of antibiotic administration, anatomic site (knee, hip), type of bone (cortical, cancellous), origin (human, nonhuman), bone status (infected or inflamed versus noninflamed), timing of bone

From Park Nicollet Medical Center, St. Louis Park, Minnesota.

sampling, and size and preparation of bone fragments to be analyzed as well as details of the bioassay and standards used to determine bone antibiotic concentrations.

The methods employed to assay bone antibiotic levels vary, but usually an agar diffusion method is used. This method is a bioassay and employs a very sensitive indicator organism seeded into an agar gel upon which paper discs containing antibiotic are placed. In the case of bone and synovial fluid tissue, buffered homogenates are prepared and placed in cylinders or into wells that have been cut into the agar. The antibiotic in the sample then diffuses into the agar and inhibits growth of the indicator organism. The diameter of the zone of inhibition is proportional to the concentration of antibiotic in the sample. Standards, containing known quantities of antibiotic, are prepared and assayed in the same way as the test sample, and standard curves are constructed.

Bone assay methods can be broadly divided into two major categories:

1. The elution of the antibiotic from bone fragments placed in a buffer (usually phosphate) solution. The bone is first washed, mechanically crushed, and then suspended in the buffer for assay, as noted above.

2. Direct placement of an antibiotic-containing bone fragment onto the assay plate. While the size of the bone fragment is being standardized, no other preparation is undertaken.

In each case, appropriate standards are assayed concomitantly, and because of the difficulties intrinsic in such assays, they are invariably done in triplicate. The bone antibiotic concentration must be reviewed in light of many factors, including the sensitivity of the actual or likely infecting organism and the complex issue of protein binding.

SYNOVIAL TISSUE

Assay of synovial tissue antibiotic levels poses some of the same technical problems as those seen in assay of bone antibiotic levels, although not to the same degree. The chief concerns are blood contamination of the tissue (falsely elevating the levels) and extraction procedures. The methodology is similar to that described for assay of bone antibiotic levels.

SYNOVIAL FLUID

Assay methods for synovial fluid antibiotic levels are much more standard and reproducible than those for bone and synovial tissue. The most widely used method is the agar diffusion assay described earlier. Synovial fluid standards are prepared by adding known antibiotic concentrations to pooled human synovial fluid and standard curves formulated by plotting the zones of inhibition on semi-logarithmic paper. As in the case of most assays, variables do exist, the chief of which is whether the synovial fluid levels were obtained from an inflamed versus a noninflamed joint.

The ability of an antibiotic to penetrate the membranous barriers between the blood and synovial fluid compartments is solute- and size-dependent, whereas the permeability of these membranes is inflammation-dependent. Capillary pore size increases with inflammation, permitting entrance of more antibiotic into the synovial compartment. The penetrance of antibiotics into synovial fluid is also related to the white blood cell count and the protein (albumin) concentration. Therefore, the greater the degree of inflammation, the greater the protein concentration and white blood cell accumulation into the synovial fluid space. It is for these reasons that nearly all antibiotics achieve satisfactory synovial fluid levels in the presence of inflammation. The analysis of antibiotic penetration into the synovial fluid of patients suffering acute exacerbations of rheumatoid arthritis provides a useful model for the study of septic arthritis, since the joint is acutely inflamed with polymorphonuclear leukocyte infiltration but no bacteria are present.[1]

Additional Considerations

MICROBIOLOGY

The importance of relating the bone antibiotic concentration to the sensitivity of the likely infecting organism was referred to earlier. For example, cephalothin administration results in rather unimpressive bone concentrations but the drug remains useful by virtue of its greater activity versus *Staphylococcus aureus.* There are major differences in the activity of cefamandole, cefoxitin, and ceforanide with respect to, for example, *S. aureus;* the MIC-90 (antibiotic concentration required to inhibit 90 percent of a standard bacterial inoculum) is 1, 4, and 8 $\mu g/ml$, respectively. Other authorities have advocated relating antibiotic activity to some form of "kill ratio" (ratio of mean minimum inhibitory concentration [MIC] of the organism to the antibiotic tissue level). Drugs with the greatest degree of antimicrobial activity and the best tissue penetration will have the highest "kill ratios." It is thought that a "kill ratio" of greater or equal to four to one (4:1) is optimal for predicting clinical response. What is, however, mandatory is that tissue antibiotic levels exceed the MIC of the infecting organism.

METHOD OF ANTIBIOTIC ADMINISTRATION

Antibiotics may be administered orally, intramuscularly, or intravenously. Usually, intravenous antibiotics are given in "pulse" doses but there are reports[2] describing higher bone antibiotic concentrations when the antibiotic was administered by constant intravenous infusion. In the study by Williams and co-workers[3] of bone and serum concentrations of five cephalosporin drugs, although there was no clear-cut relationship between serum and bone antibiotic concentrations, the antibiotics with the highest serum levels and longest half-lives usually were found to have the highest bone concentrations.

There is now an increasing body of information showing that adequate bone levels can be achieved with orally administered antistaphylococcal drugs (Table 6–1).

TIMING

Williams and co-workers[3] demonstrated, in graphic fashion, the fact that for five cephalosporins, higher bone antibiotic concentrations occurred at 50 to 70 minutes after infusion than at 100 to 150 minutes following drug administration (Table 6–2). Their data emphasized the fact that maximal bone antibiotic concentrations occurred within the first 60 minutes of drug administration.

TABLE 6–1. Concomitant Bone and Serum Antibiotic Concentrations in Patients Undergoing Simultaneous Bilateral Joint Arthroplasties

Antibiotic/Dose	Joint Studied	First Operation[†]		Second Operation		Time[‡] (Minutes)
		Bone	Serum	Bone	Serum	
Cefoxitin, 2 gm	Knee	11.0	78.0			55
				1.9	49.0	90
Cefoxitin, 1 gm	Knee	1.6	15.4			60
				1.1	5.6	138
Cephalothin, 1 gm	Knee	0.6	2.9			80
				0.3	1.4	145
Cephalothin, 1 gm	Knee	0.3	2.0			115
				0.3	1.6	140
Cephalothin, 2 gm	Knee	1.3	60.0			60
				0.6	30.0	125
Ceforanide, 2 gm	Knee	30.4	162.0			50
				11.2	132.0	90
Ceforanide, 2 gm	Knee	17.7	197.0			65
				5.7	131.0	133
Cefamandole, 2 gm	Knee	3.4	44.0			66
				2.1	26.0	106
Cefazolin, 1 gm	Hip	8.6	70.8			60
				5.2	30.0	150
Cefazolin, 1 gm	Knee	3.5	49.0			76
				1.7	39.0	149

* Modified from Williams DN, Gustilo RB, Beverley R, Kind AC: Clin Orthop 179:254–265, 1983.

† First and second operation indicate the sequence of surgery, which was usually left followed by right.

‡ Time represents the number of minutes from the initial antibiotic administration to the subsequent removal of the bone specimen.

ANATOMIC SITE

A tendency for decreased bone antibiotic concentrations in patients undergoing knee surgery compared with those undergoing hip surgery was first noted by Schurman and colleagues.[4] However, these differences were not statistically significant. Williams and associates[3] confirmed this trend and documented a statistically significant difference with regard to cefazolin administered in a 1-gm dose. These observations were subsequently confirmed by Cunha and others.[5] They demonstrated different penetration characteristics of cefazolin and cephradine in patients undergoing total knee as opposed to total hip arthroplasty. Peak bone levels of these two cephalosporins in total knee replacement patients were significantly lower than the bone levels in total hip replacement patients. The reduction in peak bone levels was associated with a prolonged bone half-life of the cephalosporins. These differences are presumed to be related to the use of the tourniquet in knee surgery, despite the fact that antibiotics are invariably infused before application of the tourniquet. These data underscore the importance of giving a 2-gm dose of antibiotic prior to prosthetic knee arthroplasty, so as to ensure adequate antibiotic tissue levels before potential contamination. It should also be noted that for most antibiotics studied, cancellous bone levels are higher than the denser cortical levels. Finally, it must be emphasized that antibiotic concentrations have been derived at the time of elective prosthetic joint arthroplasty. In these circumstances, the bone is invariably noninflamed and the bone sample usually obtained after a single parenteral dose of antibiotic.

Protein Binding

The principles involved in antibiotic tissue penetration have recently been reviewed.[6] The importance of serum protein binding, and specifically the fact that the free or non–protein-bound drug has the most biological activity, needs to be emphasized. These authors[6] also underscore the fact that multiple doses of an antibiotic agent are required before equilibrium is achieved between the intravascular and extravascular spaces. As previously indicated, most bone antibiotic levels have been derived from single-antibiotic dose administration in noninflamed bone.

TABLE 6-2. Antibiotic Concentrations in Bone*

Reference	Drug	Method of Administration	Dose S/M	No. of Patients	T½ Serum (Hrs)	Serum Concentration (μg/ml) (Range)	Bone Concentration (μg/G) (Range)	Time Specimens Obtained After Antibiotic Dose (Hrs)	Ratio (%)	Notes
11	Gentamicin	IM	1.7 mg/kg (M)	3	2.0	5.2 (3.7-7.1)	1.22 (<2-3.6)	1-2	30	U
12	Cefadroxil	Oral	1.0 (M)	14	1.3	21.5 (±2.3)	5.0 (±0.9)	2	23	U, CO
13	Cefadroxil	Oral	0.5 (S)	6	1.3	6.33	0.4	4	6.3	U, CA
							0.9	4	14.2	U, C
14	Cephalothin	IV	1.0 (S)	21	0.5	23.0	2.8	0.67	12.0	U
15	Cephalothin	IV	2.0 (S)	28	0.5	41.6 (±3.8)	2.5 ± 0.4	0.87	6.0	U, CA
3	Cephalothin	IV	1.0 (S)	14	0.5	5.3	0.5	1.52	9.4	U, CA
3	Cephalothin	IV	2.0 (S)	24	0.5	31.5	0.9	1.05	2.9	U, C
14	Cefazolin	IV	1.0 (S)	31	2.0	80.0	30.0	0.67	37.5	U, CA
3	Cefazolin	IV	1.0 (S)	17	2.0	51.7	5.9	1.15	11.4	U, CA
3	Cefazolin	IV	2.0 (S)	6	2.0	98.3	14.9	0.85	15.2	U, CA
3	Cefoxitin	IV	1.0 (S)	17	0.8	17.5	3.6	1.23	20.6	U, CA
3	Cefoxitin	IV	2.0 (S)	20	0.8	39.0	6.3	1.15	16.2	U, C
16	Cefotaxime	IV	2.0 (S)	19	1.2	61.0	5.4	0.5-1.0	8.8	U
17	Ceftazidime	IV	2.0 (S)	12	2.85	7.14	28.6 ± 1.3	1.0	40.0	U, CO, MC
18	Cloxacillin	Oral	1.0 (S)	5	0.5	17.7 (±2.4)	1.7 (±0.9)	2	9.6	U
9	Oxacillin	IV	1.0 (S)	22	0.5	18.9 (5.0-33.0)	2.1 (0.3-14.5)	1	11.0	U
19	Oxacillin	IV	1.0 (S)	16	0.5	26.4 (11.0-55.0)	3.60	0.92	13.7	U
11	Penicillin G	IV	2 million (M)	3	0.5	5.0 (0.5-9.4)	<1	0.5-1.0	<20	U
20	Doxycycline	Oral	0.2 (S)	6	20	3.6 (±0.8)	2.6 (±2.0)	3	72	U
20	Clindamycin	Oral	0.3 (S)	6	2.0	2.8 (±1.2)	0.6 (±0.4)	1.5	21.4	U
21	Clindamycin	IV	0.3 (M)	8	2.0	6.5 (1.7-24.0)	1.3 (0.4-4.9)	4.0	29.0	U
14	Erythromycin	Oral	0.5 (S)	6	1.5	1.3 (0.1-2.1)	0.2 (±0.1)	1.5	18.0	U
22	Erythromycin	IV	1.0 (S)	4	1.5	9.8 (7.6-11)	3.8 (1.8-5.5)	1.25-2.5	39	U, CA
							0		0	U, C, CO
23	Rifampin	Oral	0.3 (M)	8	3.0	6.0 (±2.6)	1.2 ± 0.5	3-4	19	U

* Modified and adapted from Gerding DN, Peterson LR, Hughes CE, Bamberger DM: Extravascular antimicrobial distribution in man. In Lorian V, ed: Antibiotics in Laboratory Medicine. Baltimore, Williams & Wilkins, 1985, pp 938-994.

Abbreviations: S = Single dose; M = multiple dose; IM = intramuscular; IV = intravenous; U = uninfected; CA = cancellous bone; CO = cortical bone; C = corrected for blood; MC = blood contamination minimal.

ANTIBIOTIC CONCENTRATIONS

Bone

Data for selected antibiotics are as listed in Table 6 – 1. Much of this information has been modified and adapted from a review by Gerding and associates.[7] Data have been selectively tabulated emphasizing those antibiotics most relevant to clinical orthopedics. For the most part, data have been derived from patients undergoing prosthetic joint arthroplasty wherein a single antibiotic dose has been used prior to bone assay. Very few sources in the literature give information about the vascularity of the bone sampled, which would be another influence on the bone antibiotic concentration.

The choice of antibiotic for surgical prophylaxis and therapy depends on a number of factors, including predictable bone antibiotic concentration, cost, and activity against actual or potential infecting organisms. In prophylaxis for primary prosthetic joint arthroplasty, it is the author's current practice to use cefazolin, 2 gm, prior to surgery, followed by 1 gm intravenously every 8 hours for 24 hours.

The antibiotic choices for established osteomyelitis vary with the actual or likely infecting organisms. The likely infecting organism, in turn, varies with such diverse factors as the patient's age and underlying disease. The semisynthetic penicillins, cephalosporins, clindamycin, and vancomycin are the primary drugs in the treatment of staphylococcal osteomyelitis. In enteric gram-negative bone infection, or where mixed infections occur (as in the diabetic foot), second- and third-generation cephalosporins, alone or in combination with other drugs, have primacy over the aminoglycosides because of their excellent *in vitro* activity and diffusion. Moreover, the prolonged treatment (4 to 6 weeks) required in osteomyelitis and the concern about toxicity make the cephalosporins good choices. When the bacterial pathogen is known, final therapeutic decisions can be made on the basis of *in vitro* antibiotic sensitivities, with particular consideration given to the likely bone antibiotic concentration/MIC ratio. The antibiotic with the highest ratio should give the best result, provided that the drug is not unduly toxic.

Synovial Tissue

Data on synovial tissue are relatively sparse (Table 6 – 3). Concerns about the validity of tissue antibiotic levels are discussed elsewhere. Generally, synovial tissue levels are approximately one third or less of concomitant serum levels, and in many studies are actually lower than the concomitant bone levels.[8, 9] For example, Fitzgerald et al[8] reported mean synovial tissue levels for cephalothin of 2.4 mg/gm compared with bone levels of 3.9 mg/gm and serum levels of 11.9 mg/ml.

Synovial Fluid

As a generalization, synovial fluid antibiotic levels are about 60 to 70 percent of concomitantly drawn serum antibiotic levels. Thus, the previous practice of local instillation of antibiotics into a joint space is unwarranted and indeed contraindicated, since such administration may result in a chemical synovitis. Selected synovial fluid antibiotic levels are as listed (Table 6 – 4). Unlike data for bone antibiotic concentration, many of the studies cited involve patients with infections who have received multiple antibiotic doses. Also included are some data on synovial fluid antibiotic levels following oral drug administration. This is to reflect the current pediatric practice, in treating septic arthritis, of initiating oral antibiotic administration after clinical improvement with parenteral therapy. In a study by Sattar and colleagues,[10] an attempt was made to gather more information about antibiotic pharmacokinetics in synovial fluid by placing an indwelling catheter into the joint and taking multiple synovial fluid samples over time. In general, synovial fluid antibiotic levels peaked slightly later and disappeared more slowly than corresponding serum antibiotic levels. Four different antibiotics were studied in 20 patients with noninfected knee effusions (mainly patients with rheumatoid arthritis). Antibiotic synovial fluid levels of cephradine and flucloxacillin were lower than in similar studies of data generated for sodium fucidate and amoxicillin.

The most frequent joint pathogens are *Neisseria gonorrhoeae, Staphylococcus aureus,* and *Haemophilus influenzae,* but the prevalence of these and other pathogens varies with age. For example, enteric gram-negative organisms are important in neonatal bone infection and, to a lesser extent, in bone infections in the elderly. Similarly, group B *Streptococcus* has become an important pathogen in neonatal bone infection. Penicillins or cephalosporins are the initial drugs of choice in most cases of septic arthritis, and most of the published data on synovial fluid antibiotic levels involve these drugs.

TABLE 6–3. Antibiotic Concentration in Synovial Tissue

Reference	Antibiotic	Route of Administration	Dose	No. of Patients	Serum T½ (Hrs)	Mean Serum Concentration (mg/ml) (Range)	Time of Specimen Collection (Hrs)	Synovial Tissue Concentration (mg/gm)	Bone Concentration (mg/gm)
9	Cephalothin	IV (S)	1 gm	19	0.5	11.9 (6.6–20.5)	1	2.4 (0.9–5.6)	3.9
9	Oxacillin	IV (S)	1 gm	14	0.5	18.9 (5.0–32.8)	1	1.8 (0.3–5.6)	2.1
24	Cefuroxime	IV (S)*	1 gm	7*	—	—	0.25–0.5	36.4 (15–76.2)	8.7
24	Cefuroxime	IV (S)	1 gm	3†	—	—	0.25–0.5	27.3 (5.4–60.0)	10.3
24	Cefuroxime	IV (S)	1.5 gm	5†	—	—	0.25–0.5	28.3 (19.8–34.2)	31.4
24	Cefuroxime	IV (S)	1.5 gm	5†	—	—	0.25–0.5	8.0 (0–21.8)	11.4
8	Clindamycin	IM and IV	0.3 gm 0.3 gm	12	2.0	5.01 (±1.16)	2–3	3.29 (±0.71)	5.01 (±1.16)

* Hip arthroplasty.
† Knee arthroplasty.
Abbreviations: IM = Intramuscular; IV = intravenous.

TABLE 6–4. Antibiotic Concentrations in Joint Fluid*

Reference	Antibiotic	Method of Administration	Dose S/M	No. of Patients	Serum T½ (Hrs)	Mean Serum Concentration (μg/ml) (Range)	Time Specimens Obtained (Hrs)	Mean Joint Fluid Concentration (μg/ml)	Ratio (%) Joint Fluid / Serum
25	Gentamicin	IM	1.0–1.5 mg/kg (S)	6	2.0	4.0 (2.4–6.5)	1.0–3.5	3.2 (2.4–4.4)	80
25	Tobramycin	IM	1.0–1.5 mg/kg (S)	7	2.0	2.7 (1.0–5.6)	1.5–4.0	2.4 (1.3–4.6)	89
13	Cefadroxil	Oral	0.5 gm (S)	5	1.3	7.30	2.0	7.14	98
13	Cefadroxil	Oral	0.5 gm (S)	6	1.3	6.33	4.0	5.35	84
4	Cefazolin	IV	1.0 gm (S)	7	1.8	103.5 (85–122)	0–0.25	17.3 (0.5–30.5)	17
4	Cefazolin	IV	1.0 gm (S)	15	1.8	81.4 (56–135)	0.25–0.5	26.2 (7.1–63)	32
26	Ampicillin†	IV	25–52 mg/kg (M)	4	1.1	7.8 (2.1–15.8)	1.0–5.0	11.6 (1.7–27.0)	149
27	Ampicillin†	Oral	50 mg/kg (M)	5	1.1	9.3 (3.8–20.0)	2.0	11.7 (4.8–20.0)	126
28	Ampicillin	Oral	0.5 gm (S)	4	1.1	2.3 (1.38–3.48)	2.0	1.0 (0.4–2.0)	43
27	Cloxacillin†	Oral	25 mg/kg (M)	7	0.5	7.7 (2.1–19.0)	2.0	5.0 (1.7–11.0)	65
27	Dicloxacillin†	Oral	25 mg/kg (M)	6	0.5	13.6 (9.2–28.0)	2.0	9.5 (3.2–23.0)	70
29	Nafcillin	IM	1.5 gm (S)	20	1.0	15.5 (7.9–26.0)	1.0	2.7 (0.5–7.0)	17
26	Penicillin G†	IV	25 mg/kg (M)	3	0.5	2.60 (0.16–5.1)	1.0–2.0	2.6 (0.08–5.1)	100
30	Vancomycin	IV	500 mg (M)	6	6.0	7.0 (5.2–8.7)	1.0–1.65	5.7 (4.0–6.4)	81

* Modified from Gerding DN, Peterson LR, Hughes CE, Bamberger DM: Extravascular antimicrobial distribution in man. In Lorian V, ed: Antibiotics in Laboratory Medicine. Baltimore, Williams & Wilkins, 1985, pp 938–994.

† Infected joints.

Abbreviations: S = Single dose; M = multiple dose.

One other major consideration in antimicrobial activity is the influence of pH. As a result of the accumulation of inflammatory products, synovial fluid pH levels are invariably lower than septic arthritis. This may make the use of antibiotics such as the aminoglycosides and macrolides, which are less active at an acid pH, less desirable, particularly when good alternate drugs exist.

Finally, it should be noted that in the treatment of septic arthritis, systemic antibiotic treatment should be combined with repeated local aspiration. The only exception is in hip joint infection, if, owing both to the relative inaccessibility of the joint space and the tenuous nature of the blood supply, arthrotomy is advised.

References

1. Morgan JR, Paul LA, O'Sullivan M, Williams BD: The penetration of ceftriaxone into synovial fluid in the inflamed joint. J Antimicrob Chemother 16:367–371, 1985.
2. Patel D, Moellering RC, Thrasher K, Fahmy NR, Harris WH: The effect of hypotensive anesthesia and cephalothin concentrations in bone and muscle of patients undergoing total hip replacement. J Bone Joint Surg 61A:531, 1979.
3. Williams DN, Gustilo RB, Beverley R, Kind AC: Bone and serum concentrations of five cephalosporin drugs: relevance to prophylaxis and treatment in orthopedic surgery. Clin Orthop 179:254–265, 1983.
4. Schurman OJ, Hirshman HP, Kajiyama G, Moser K, Burton DS: Cefazolin concentrations in bone and synovial fluid. J Bone Joint Surg 60A:359–362, 1978.
5. Cunha BA, Gossling HR, Pasternac HS, Nightingale CH, Quintiliana R: Penetration of cephalosporins into bone. Infection 12:80–84, 1984.
6. Peterson LR, Gerding DN: Antibiotic tissue penetration. In Peterson PK, Verhoef J, eds: Antimicrobial Agents Annual, No. 1. New York, Elsevier, 1986, pp 515–525.
7. Gerding DN, Peterson LR, Hughes CE, Bamberger DM: Extravascular antimicrobial distribution in man. In Lorian V, ed: Antibiotics in Laboratory Medicine. Baltimore, Williams and Wilkins, 1985, pp 938–994.
8. Baird P, Hughes S, Sullivan M, Willmoti: Penetration into bone and tissues of clindamycin phosphate. Postgrad Med J 54:65–67, 1978.
9. Fitzgerald RH, Kelly PJ, Synder RJ, Washington JA: Penetration of methicillin, oxacillin, cephalothin, into bone and synovial tissues. Antimicrob Agents Chemother 14:723–726, 1978.
10. Sattar MA, Barrett SB, Cawley MID: Concentrations of some antibiotics in synovial fluid after oral administration, with special reference to antistaphylococcal activity. Ann Rheum Dis 42:67–74, 1983.
11. Smilak JD, Flittie WH, Williams TW: Bone concentrations of antimicrobial agents after parenteral administration. Antimicrob Agents Chemother 9:169–171, 1976.
12. Quintiliani R: A review of the penetration of cefadroxil into human tissue. J Antimicrob Chemother 10(Suppl B):33–38, 1982.
13. Valencia-Chinas A, Galindo-Hernandez F, Reyes-Sanchez J, Flores-Mercado F: Concentrations of cefadoxil in osteoarticular tissues (abstract 338). In Program and Abstracts: The 11th International Congress of Chemotherapy and 19th Interscience Conference on Antimicrobial Agents and Chemotherapy. Washington, DC, American Society for Microbiology, 1979.
14. Cunha BA, Gossling HR, Pasteinak HS, Nightingale CH, Quintiliani R: The penetration characteristics of cefazolin, cephalothin, and cephradine into bone in patients undergoing total hip replacement. J Bone Joint Surg 59A:856–859, 1977.
15. Schurman OJ, Hirshman HP, Burton DS: Cephalothin and cefamandole penetration into bone, synovial fluid, and wound drainage fluid. J Bone Joint Surg 62A:981–985, 1980.
16. Wittman DH, Schassan HH, Freitag V: Pharmacokinetic studies and results of a clinical trial with cefotaxime (HR-756). In Nelson JD, Grassi C, eds: Current Chemotherapy and Infectious Disease: Proceedings. Washington, DC, American Society for Microbiology, 1980, pp. 114–116.
17. Wittman DH, Schassan HH, Kohler E, Seiberg W: Pharmacokinetic studies of ceftazidime in serum, bone, bile, tissue fluid and peritoneal fluid. J Antimicrob Chemother 8 (Suppl B):293–297, 1981.
18. Sinot J, Lopitaux R, Sinot J, Delisle JS, Rampon S, Cluzel R: Diffusion de la cloxacilline dans le tissue osseux human apies administration par voie orale. Pathol Biol 30:332–335, 1982.
19. Kramer J, Weuta H: Untersuchungen uber serumund Knocheuspiegel nach Injektion von oxacillin und carbenicillin. Z Orthop 110:216–223, 1972.
20. Bystedt H, Dahlback A, Dornbusch K, Nord CE: Concentration of azidocillin, erythromycin, doxycycline plus clindamycin in human mandibular bone. Int J Oral Surg 7:442–449, 1978.
21. Dornbusch K, Carlstrom A, Hugo H, Lindstrom A: Antibacterial activity of clindamycin and lincomycin in human bone. J Antimicrob Chemother 3:153–160, 1977.
22. Sorensen TS, Colding H, Schroeder E, Rosdahl VT: The penetration of cefazolin, erythromycin and methicillin into human bone tissue. Acta Orthop Scand 49:549–553, 1978.
23. Sinot J, Drive L, Lopitaux R, Glannder Y: Etude de la diffusion de la rifampicine dans le tissu osseux spongieux et compact au cours de protheses totales de hanches. Pathol Biol 31:438–441, 1983.
24. Hughes SPF, Want S, Darrell JH, Dash CH, Kennedy M: Prophylactic cefuroxime in total joint replacement. Int Orthop 6:155–161, 1982.
25. Dee TH, Kozin F: Gentamicin and tobramycin penetration into synovial fluid. Antimicrob Agents Chemother 12:548–549, 1977.
26. Nelson JD: Antibiotic concentrations in septic joint effusions. N Engl J Med 284:349–353, 1971.
27. Nelson JD, Howard JB, Shelton S: Oral antibiotic therapy for skeletal infections of children. Pediatrics 92:131–134, 1978.
28. Howell A, Sutherland R, Rolinson GN: Effect of protein binding on levels of ampicillin and cloxacillin in synovial fluid. Clin Pharmacol Ther 13:724–732, 1972.
29. Viek P: Concentration of sodium nafcillin in pathological synovial fluid. Antimicrob Agents Chemother 1961:379–383, 1962.
30. Geraci JE, Heilman FR, Nichols DR, Wellman WE, Ross GT: Some laboratory and clinical experiences with a new antibiotic, vancomycin. Proc Staff Mtgs Mayo Clin 31:564–582, 1956.

David N. Williams, M.D.

Antibiotic Prophylaxis in Bone and Joint Surgery

INTRODUCTION

Although the use of prophylactic antibiotics is now accepted practice in patients undergoing prosthetic joint arthroplasty[1-4] and in those who have sustained femoral neck fractures,[5,6] its acceptability in other clean orthopedic surgical procedures remains controversial.[7,8] Infection is an infrequent accompaniment of prosthetic joint arthroplasty (1 to 2 percent),[9] but the consequences are devastating, requiring both prolonged antibiotic therapy and possibly extensive surgical treatment.[10,11] The serious morbidity associated with prosthetic joint infection is the major rationale for antibiotic prophylaxis. Morbidity can be measured not only in economic terms (prolonged hospital stay and the cost of various surgical procedures) but also by the serious physical and psychological consequences that may result.

Currently, one fourth to one half of all antimicrobial usage is for the prevention rather than the treatment of infection.[7] Prophylactic antibiotic use is expensive but may also result in other undesirable sequelae, such as drug-related side effects, and in an unfavorable influence on the microflora of the patient and hospital. These and other concerns have resulted in several changes in the use of prophylactic antibiotics. The importance of instituting antibiotic therapy immediately prior to surgery has been demonstrated in the laboratory[12,13] and by clinical trials,[14] and there is now increasing evidence that prophylactic antibiotic use can be limited to 24 hours following most surgical procedures.[4,15-17] Indeed, there is now newer information indicating that for many procedures, antibiotic use can be limited to a single preoperative dose.

Other more recent changes include the recognition that different antibiotic regimens may be indicated for different types of surgical situations, as in, for example, the regimens used in primary as opposed to revision arthroplasty. There is also an increasing awareness of the need to direct antibiotic prophylaxis against likely pathogens. Thus, in some centers prophylaxis against methicillin-resistant *Staphylococcus epidermidis* may be an issue.

The past decade has also seen advances in other factors that relate to postsurgical infection, such as changes in the operating room design aimed at reducing the possibility of intraoperative implantation of airborne bacteria.[18,19] Antibiotics, therefore, may play a relatively minor role in reducing the infection rate, since other factors, such as surgical skills and new operative techniques,[20] may be of greater import. In some centers, these modalities result in such very low infection rates that the use of prophylactic antibiotics is obviated.

This chapter reviews the use of prophylactic antibiotics in primary prosthetic joint arthroplasty; fractures of the femoral neck; other major orthopedic surgeries, such as the insertion of Harrington rods; and clean orthopedic surgeries. The specific problems of prevention and treatment of infection in revision joint arthroplasty are discussed elsewhere.

The use and rationale of prophylactic antibiotics, the special problems of antibiotic selection in the penicillin-allergic patient, and the prophylactic regimens for invasive procedures in patients with established joint prostheses are discussed.

USE AND RATIONALE OF ANTIBIOTIC PROPHYLAXIS

Bacteriology

The patient's skin remains the major source of orthopedic infections. Although the preva-

From the Department of Medicine, University of Minnesota, and Park Nicollet Medical Center, Minneapolis, Minnesota.

lence of the specific pathogen varies from one center to another, staphylococcal organisms continue to account for over 60 percent of infections. Over the past decade or so, an increased predominance of *S. epidermidis* over *Staphylococcus aureus* as the primary infecting organism has been reported at some centers. This trend may have important consequences in terms of prophylaxis, since many isolates of *S. epidermidis* are multiply antibiotic-resistant. Moreover, this is the organism, *par excellence,* in which routine antibiotic disc diffusion studies may give erroneous sensitivity data. For example, an isolate of *S. epidermidis* that is "methicillin-resistant" will, under appropriate testing conditions, be found to be resistant to all semisynthetic penicillins as well as to the cephalosporins, irrespective of the result of the antibiotic disc diffusion studies.

Aerobic enteric gram-negative rods (such as *Escherichia coli* and *Proteus* species) account for 10 to 20 percent of infections; other relatively nonpathogenic organisms, such as streptococcal and corynebacterial isolates, make up the remainder. The importance of the biofilm (glycocalyx) produced by certain microorganisms and its protective influence from both antibiotic and host defense mechanisms are discussed elsewhere.

Concern regarding the potential for selecting out resistant organisms is exemplified in a study by Burnett and co-workers[6] on antibiotic prophylaxis in femoral neck fractures. Seven (22 percent) of 32 organisms isolated after surgery from the placebo-treated group were found to be resistant to cephalosporins compared with ten (42 percent) of 24 cultures from the cephalothin-treated group; most of the bacteria isolated following surgery were from the urinary tract. Although this difference was not statistically significant, the trend prompted the authors to speculate that a reduction in antibiotic-resistant organisms could result if an abbreviated course of antibiotics was used. There are no data to confirm or refute this speculation.

Patient Characteristics

It is clear that certain patient characteristics predispose to infectious sequelae, and, to the degree possible, patients should be evaluated with these considerations in mind. For the most part, data have been derived from studies of patients undergoing prosthetic joint surgery; however, these characteristics are applicable whenever prophylactic antibiotics are used in orthopedic surgery.

The overall risk of infection depends upon such diverse factors as the patient's host defenses, the nature and virulence of the contaminating organism, previous surgery at the operative site, duration of hospitalization prior to surgery, duration of surgery, and evidence of distant foci of infection (e.g., skin, dental, urinary tract). With regard to host defenses, many papers underscore the fact that patients with rheumatoid arthritis, particularly those taking steroids, are especially vulnerable to both early and late prosthetic joint infections. There are similar data indicating increased risk with extremely advanced age, poor nutrition, and gross obesity. Some of these risks can be diminished by a diligent preoperative evaluation. Theoretically, prosthetic joint and other infections could be the result of an untreated infection elsewhere in the body, perhaps caused by a bacteremia during the procedure itself. Patients, therefore, should be examined and evaluated prior to surgery for both occult and overt forms of infection, which should be treated prior to prosthetic joint implantation.

The incidence of infection following total knee arthroplasty is approximately twice that following hip surgery (2 percent versus 1 percent) and may be related to differences in the prostheses. However, it is more likely a result of anatomic factors, such as the proximity of the skin (and therefore potential pathogens) to the underlying prosthesis. Thus, it has been argued that a wound infection following total knee arthroplasty invariably affects the prosthesis owing to its proximity to the wound.

SYSTEMIC ANTIBIOTICS

In most of the major centers where prophylactic antibiotics are used, cephalosporins are favored as the antibiotics of choice. In several of the early studies, penicillin, cloxacillin, and other semisynthetic penicillins were used; this is still true for some centers in western Europe. In the United States, cephalosporins have been favored for many reasons: they are relatively nontoxic, inexpensive, and effective against most of the potential pathogens important in orthopedic surgery.

The rationale of antibiotic prophylaxis was established by the pioneering work of Burke[12] and Miles and associates[13] in the late 1950s. The critical importance of having antibiotics in the tissue at the time of bacterial contamination was documented, and it was clear that in appropriate situations prophylactic antibiotics had to be administered before surgery because of the possibility of intraoperative contamination. Although this thesis has long been accepted, the results of some surveys on the use of prophylactic antibiotics have been rather disappointing. Crossley and Gardner,[21] in a survey of 27 hospitals in metropolitan Minnesota, found that in 265 orthopedic procedures, antibiotics were given immediately prior to surgery (within 4 hours) in only 49 percent of the cases and were initiated more than 4 hours prior to surgery in 10 percent of the cases. Antibiotics were first administered intraoperatively in 24 percent, and in 17 percent of the cases the first antibiotic dose was administered after surgery. In a much smaller study performed by Fry and colleagues[12] only 59 percent of 29 prosthetic joint surgical cases received antibiotics before surgery.

The duration of prophylactic antibiotic administration after surgery has undergone a major change; in early reports of prosthetic joint surgery,[1, 2] antibiotics were frequently administered for 14 days, often in oral form. In a study of patients following total hip arthroplasty,[4] no difference in infection rates was found between those receiving prophylactic antibiotics for 1 day and those receiving antibiotics for 7 or 10 days after surgery. Similarly, Nelson and co-workers[15] found no difference in infection rates between patients receiving antibiotics for 1 day and those receiving antibiotics for 7 days after surgery. This is in accord with the authors'[23] experience comparing the incidence of infection in 1791 total joint arthroplasties treated over 7 years (Table 7–1). The authors' current practice is to administer a single 2-gram intravenous dose of cefazolin, in the surgical ante-room, immediately prior to surgery and to continue with 1 gm intravenously (IV) every 8 hours for 24 hours after surgery. This ensures appropriate timing of the antibiotic dose before surgery and avoids delays occasioned by orders to give the first dose of antibiotic "on call" to the operating room. In addition, in the unlikely event of an accelerated antibiotic reaction such as anaphylaxis, the patient is in a controlled situation for resuscitation. A couple of studies[24, 25] clearly indicate that antibiotics diffuse rapidly into both the synovial fluid and bone, and in one of the studies[25] peak bone levels of five different cephalosporin drugs invariably occurred within 60 minutes of administration.

Selection of prophylactic antibiotics in orthopedic surgery requires consideration of a number of factors, including bone antibiotic concentrations, sensitivity of the likely infecting organism, and cost. The advantage of administering 2 gm of a chosen drug rather than the usual 1 gm is predicated on the higher bone levels obtained with the 2-gm doses. It would be prudent to provide the highest possible bone antibiotic level when bacterial contamination would be most likely, i.e., at the time of surgery. After the initial antibiotic dose, therapy is continued for a further 24 hours. Data indicate that such a regimen results in adequate antibiotic concentrations in Hemovac wound drainage fluid (Zimmer Co., Edina, Minn.) for several days after surgery (Williams and Gustilo, unpublished observations). Abbreviating the duration of antibiotic therapy may reduce the incidence of antibiotic-associated side effects, including antibiotic-associated colitis and drug fever, and IV-associated phlebitis, as well as reduce the likelihood of selecting out antibiotic-resistant

TABLE 7–1. Infection in Total Joint Arthroplasty (Comparison of 3 Days *versus* 1 Day of Preventive Antibiotic Use)*

| Duration of Postoperative Antibiotic | Hip† | | | Knee† | | | Total | Percent |
	No. of Joints Replaced	No. of Infections‡	Percent	No. of Joints Replaced	No. of Infections‡	Percent		
1975–1979	3 Days	750	4	0.53%	591	4	0.68%	1341	0.6%
1980–1982	1 Day	264	2	0.75%	186	1	0.53%	450	0.67%
1975–1982		1014	6	0.59%	777	5	0.64%		

* From Williams DN, Gustilo RB: The use of preventive antibiotics in orthopaedic surgery. Clin Orthop 190:83, 1984.[23]

† Number of joints replaced.

‡ Deep infections.

organisms. Moreover, abbreviating the duration and the number of antibiotics inevitably reduces cost.

There has been some debate, of late, with regard to the substitution of a second- or even a third-generation cephalosporin for the more traditional first-generation cephalosporin in orthopedic prophylaxis. There are no data to support this, and most authorities would urge continued use of first-generation cephalosporins for most orthopedic prophylaxis. There may be a case for using some of the second-generation cephalosporins, such as cefonicid or ceforanide, which can be administered once or twice a day. As is discussed elsewhere, a different regimen may be indicated in revision arthroplasty.

Topical Antibiotics

Riska[26] compared 362 patients treated with total hip arthroplasty in whom local irrigation of neomycin and bacitracin (1 gm/dl) into the operating field was undertaken with a similar group of 106 patients who had received prophylactic penicillin treatment. The incidence of infection in the group treated with local irrigation was 0.8 percent compared with 2.8 percent in the group treated with penicillin. This author would not advise using penicillin alone for prophylactic treatment. In an article by Roth and associates,[27] the issue of topical antibiotics in orthopedics was reviewed. These authors could find only one published study evaluating the use of antibiotic lavage in orthopedic surgery, and they felt that the methodology and study design precluded an appropriate evaluation of this work. Thus, in contemporary orthopedic practice, topical antibiotics have not found a role.

Antibiotic-Impregnated Cement

Work dealing with antibiotics and cement was pioneered by Buchholz and Engelbrecht[28] and Buchholz and associates,[29] with gentamicin being the most frequently used drug. Most investigators have limited the amount of gentamicin added to the cement to about 2 gm. Other drugs have been used, but there has been concern about possible allergic sequelae. There are data indicating that antibiotics diffuse out of the cement in the first 4 days, that serum levels are detected for the first couple of days, and that thereafter the antibiotic elutes slowly over a matter of months.[30] Lauten-

schlager and colleagues[31] have shown that when antibiotics are added to methylmethacrylate in a water solution, they cause a significant decrease in the mechanical strength of the cement, a weakening not found when the antibiotics are used in powdered form.

Antibiotic-impregnated cement has been used both in prophylaxis and in the treatment of established infection. As far as the prophylactic studies are concerned, the largest was published by Josefsson and others.[32] This was a multicenter study that compared systemic antibiotic prophylaxis with the use of gentamicin-impregnated cement. That study has been critically reviewed by Norden,[33] who points out some inconsistencies in this multicenter trial. However, in sum, the incidence of deep-seated infection in the antibiotic-impregnated cement group, in Josefsson's study,[32] was 0.4 percent compared with 1.6 percent in those receiving systemic antibiotics.

SPECIFIC USES OF PROPHYLACTIC ANTIBIOTICS

Prosthetic Joints

The rationale for the use of prophylactic antibiotics in orthopedic surgery is best validated with prosthetic joints. It has been estimated that approximately 75,000 total hip arthroplasties are performed on 65,000 patients annually in the United States.[34] Several prospective, randomized, double-blind studies of good quality reinforce the fact that prophylactic antibiotic therapy reduces the incidence of deep-seated infection to less than 1 percent compared with approximately 4 percent when a placebo is used. The choice of prophylactic antibiotics is a continuing debate, with the author's bias toward the use of cefazolin because of its good bone penetration and its half-life (approximately 2.5 hours), making 8-hour dosing feasible.

As previously discussed, the author strongly favors administering larger antibiotic doses in the surgical anteroom before surgery as well as advocating shorter courses of antibiotics. It is unnecessary to wait for the removal of all drainage devices prior to the cessation of antibiotic prophylaxis.

Femoral Fractures

Two papers describing prospective, randomized, controlled trials of the use of antibiotics in femoral neck fractures treated by pinning found a reduction in the infection rate from approximately 5 percent in the placebo-treated group to approximately 1 percent in the antibiotic-treated group.[5, 12] We employ the same antibiotic approach as with prosthetic joint patients.

Extensive Orthopedic Surgery (Insertion of Harrington Rods)

Prophylactic antibiotics are widely used in patients treated by spinal fusion with Harrington rods. There is, however, no published trial on their efficacy. However, the same concerns that apply to prosthetic joint patients would logically apply to this procedure, namely, infection in a situation where there is both massive soft tissue reconstruction and the use of prosthetic materials.

Clean Orthopedic Surgery

The lack of an adequate, randomized, double-blind prospective study dealing with clean orthopedic surgery has led to much controversy. In the paper by Pavel and co-authors[8] (the most widely quoted article), the type of surgery is not clearly stated. Thus, the validity of suggesting that all "clean" orthopedic surgery patients should receive preventive antibiotics has been questioned.[7] There may be some decrease in the frequency of wound infections in patients receiving antibiotics in clean orthopedic surgery, such as laminectomy,[35] but the advantages do not appear to justify routine antibiotic administration. However, some orthopedic surgeons routinely administer a single antibiotic dose before surgery in patients undergoing meniscectomy and laminectomy.

SPECIAL CONSIDERATIONS

Penicillin Allergy

The selection of an appropriate antibiotic in a patient with documented penicillin allergy frequently poses a problem. We would urge avoidance of cephalosporins in a patient with a history of an accelerated skin or other reaction within 24 hours of penicillin administration. In that setting, the major choices are either the use of clindamycin or vancomycin, usually in combination with a brief course of gentamicin. Note should be made of the fact that vancomycin should be infused slowly (over 60 minutes)

to avoid the untoward cutaneous reaction referred to as "the red man syndrome."

Antibiotic Prophylaxis in Patients with Prosthetic Joints

Many series indicate that about 20 to 30 percent of prosthetic infections occur after a pain-free interval of several years (late infections). We urge patients to notify their orthopedist in the event of any significant infectious process, since it appears that most late prosthetic joint infections are hematogenously spread. Thus, any significant infection should be promptly and thoroughly treated. There is, however, controversy regarding the use of prophylactic antibiotics for dental and other surgery. In a paper by Stinchfield and colleagues,[36] two of nine patients with late hematogenous infection of a total joint had concomitant oral infections. The fact that more than 50 percent of all prosthetic joint infections have been due to staphylococci, however, raises concerns about overemphasizing the importance of a dental source, since *S. aureus* would be an unlikely oral pathogen. Nonetheless, it is the author's current practice to advise patients with prosthetic joints or who are having dental work, cystoscopy, or other procedures that carry a risk of transient bacteremia to receive preoperative antibiotic prophylaxis in much the same way as patients with cardiac valvular prostheses. In this regard, there have been some recent changes with a less rigorous use of parenteral prophylactic regimens and an abbreviation of the duration of treatment.[37] The author feels that the now long-standing British practice of using a single prophylactic oral dose of amoxicillin (3 gm), prior to "at-risk" procedures, has a great deal of merit.

References

1. Carlsson AS, Lidgren L, Lindberg L: Prophylactic antibiotics against early and late deep infections after total hip replacement. Acta Orthop Scand 48:405, 1977.
2. Ericson C, Lidgren L, Lindberg L: Cloxacillin in the prophylaxis of postoperative infections of the hip. J Bone Joint Surg 55A:808, 1973.
3. Hill C, Mazas F, Flamant R, Evrard J: Prophylactic cephazolin versus placebo in total hip replacement. Lancet 1:795, 1981.
4. Pollard JP, Hughes SPF, Scott JE, Evans MJ, Benson MKD: Antibiotic prophylaxis in total hip replacement. Br Med J 1:707, 1979.
5. Boyd RJ, Burke JF, Colton T: A double blind clinical trial of prophylactic antibiotics in hip fractures. J Bone Joint Surg 55A:1251, 1973.

6. Burnett JW, Gustilo RB, Williams DN, Kind AC: Prophylactic antibiotics in hip fractures. J Bone Joint Surg 62A:457, 1980.
7. Hirschmann JV, Inui TS: Antimicrobial prophylaxis: critique of recent trials. Rev Infect Dis 2:1, 1981.
8. Pavel A, Smith RL, Ballard A, Larsen IJ: Prophylactic antibiotics in clean orthopedic surgery. J Bone Joint Surg 56A:777, 1974.
9. Fitzgerald RH, Nolan DR, Ilstrup DM, Von Scoy RE, Washington JA, Coventry MB: Deep wound sepsis following total hip arthroplasty. J Bone Joint Surg 59A:847, 1977.
10. Nelson JP: Deep infection following total hip arthroplasty. J Bone Joint Surg 59A:1042, 1977.
11. Petty W, Goldsmith S: Resection arthroplasty following infected total hip arthroplasty. J Bone Joint Surg 62A:889, 1980.
12. Burke JF: The effective period of preventative antibiotic action in experimental incisions and dermal lesions. Surgery 50:161, 1961.
13. Miles AA, Miles EM, Burke J: The value and duration of defense reactions of the skin in the primary lodgement of bacteria. Br J Exp Pathol 38:79, 1957.
14. Polk HC, Lopez-Mayor JF: Postoperative wound infection: a prospective study of determinant factors and prevention. Surgery 66:97, 1969.
15. Nelson CL, Green TG, Porter RA, Warren RD: One day versus seven days of preventive antibiotic therapy in orthopedic surgery. Clin Orthop 176:258, 1983.
16. Polk BF, Shapiro M, Goldstein P, Tager IB, Goren-Shite B, Schoenbaum SC: Randomized clinical trial of perioperative cefazolin in preventing infection after hysterectomy. Lancet 1:437, 1980.
17. Strachan CJL, Black J, Powis SJA, Waterworth TA, Wise R, Wilkinsen AR, Burdon DW, Severn M, Mitra B, Norcott H: Prophylactic use of cefazolin against wound sepsis after cholecystectomy. Br Med J 1:1254, 1977.
18. Letts RM, Doermer E: Conversation in the operating theater as a cause of airborne bacterial contamination. J Bone Joint Surg 65A:357, 1983.
19. Moggio M, Goldmer JL, McCollum E, Beissinger SF: Wound infections in patients undergoing total hip arthroplasty. Arch Surg 114:815, 1979.
20. McCue SF, Berg EW, Saunders EA: Efficacy of double gloving as a barrier to microbial contamination during total joint arthroplasty. J Bone Joint Surg 63A:811, 1981.
21. Crossley KB, Gardner LC: Antimicrobial prophylaxis in surgical patients. JAMA 245:722, 1981.
22. Fry DE, Harbrecht PJ, Polk HC Jr: Systemic prophylactic antibiotics. Arch Surg 116:466, 1981.
23. Williams DN, Gustilo RB: The use of preventive antibiotics in orthopaedic surgery. Clin Orthop 190:83, 1984.
24. Schurman DJ, Hirschman HP, Burton DS: Cephalothin and cefamandole penetration into bone, synovial fluid and wound drainage fluid. J Bone Joint Surg 62A:981, 1980.
25. Williams DN, Gustilo RB, Beverly R, Kind AC: Bone and serum concentrations of five cephalosporin drugs: relevance to prophylaxis and treatment in orthopedic surgery. Clin Orthop 179:253, 1983.
26. Riska EB: Are antibiotics necessary in the prevention of infection in total hip replacement? Ann Chir Gynaecol 69:122, 1980.
27. Roth RM, Gleckman RA, Gantz NM, Kelly N: Antibiotics irrigation: a plea for controlled clinical trials. Pharmacotherapy 5:222, 1985.
28. Buchholz HW, Engelbrecht E: Uber die Depotwirkung einiger Antibiotika bei Vermischung mit dem Kunstharz Palacos. Chirurgie 41:511, 1970.
29. Buchholz HW, Engelbrecht E, Rottger J, Seigel A: Erkenntnisse nach Wechsel von uber 400 infizierten Huftendoprothesen. Orthop Praxis 12:1117, 1977.
30. Gristina AG, Kolkin J: Current concepts review: total joint replacement and sepsis. J Bone Joint Surg 65A:128, 1983.
31. Lautenschlager EP, Marshall GW, Marks KE, Schwartz J, Nelson CL: Mechanical strength of acrylic bone cements impregnated with antibiotics. J Biomed Mater Res 10:837, 1976.
32. Josefsson G, Lindberg L, Wiklander B: Systemic antibiotics and gentamicin-containing bone cement in the prophylaxis of postoperative infections in total hip arthroplasty. Clin Orthop 159:194, 1981.
33. Norden CW: A critical review of antibiotic prophylaxis in orthopedic surgery. Rev Infect Dis 5:928, 1983.
34. National Institutes of Health Consensus Development Conference Summary, Vol. 4, No. 4. Total Hip Joint Replacement, 1982.
35. Horwitz NH, Curtin JA: Prophylactic antibiotics and wound infections following laminectomy for lumbar disc herniation. J Neurosurg 43:727, 1975.
36. Stinchfield FE, Bigliani LU, Neu HC, Goss TP, Foster CR: Late hematogenous infection of total joint replacement. J Bone Joint Surg 62A:1345, 1980.
37. Kaye D: Prophylaxis for infective endocarditis: an update. Ann Intern Med 104:419, 1986.

Robert P. Gruninger, M.D.
Dean T. Tsukayama, M.D.
Barbara Wicklund, B.S., MT (ASCP)

CHAPTER

8

Antibiotic-Impregnated PMMA Beads in Bone and Prosthetic Joint Infections

INTRODUCTION

The treatment of orthopedic wounds is a continuous challenge. Not surprisingly, various types of local treatment for persistent wounds date back to the origin of humans, albeit the precise role of infection, particularly that due to bacteria, was not appreciated until the end of the last century.[1-3] Prior to that, it is reasonable to assume that bacteria and fungi were the major cause of these problems, particularly in wounds that did not heal.[3, 4] It can be presumed that treatment was empiric in the various orthopedic injuries. Surely, debridement, excision, and amputation were part of treatment as it exists today. However, the application of various natural or contrived substances and even maggots were tried to help healing.[1, 2] Many times, these efforts were effective, even though infection as we know it today was not recognized. Thus, the belief in "laudable pus" by Greek physicians is the classic example of the historic understanding of wound pathology.[4] In spite of the existence of microbes, as clearly shown by electron microscopy in fossils that predate humans,[5] the sense that another biologic form could exist, much less cause disease, i.e., infection, was not appreciated until "bread mold" was seen in wounds and considered important.[3] Even the major observations of microscopic "animals"

by Van Leeuewenhoeck in the seventeenth century, after his discovery of the microscope,[2] did not significantly alter concepts about the nature of wound complications. All this changed, albeit slowly, when Koch and Pasteur convincingly introduced the "germ theory" at the end of the nineteenth century.[2] It is beyond the scope of this chapter to detail what has followed in the approach to treatment, much less prevention, of orthopedic wound infections. However, it is useful to think in terms of two "new" periods of medical treatment, with the realization that the common and most important modality of treatment remains surgical.[6-10] The first period, which lasted for some 50 to 60 years, might best be described as the years of specific chemical treatment, whereby various organic and inorganic powders, liquids, and pastes, and so on, were used as antiseptics or disinfectants.[2, 11] It culminated with the clinical introduction of sulfanilamide in the 1930s.[12] The second period started during World War II and continues as the era of antibiotics.

Thus, numerous chemical agents, including acidic solutions, organic dyes, and other substances, were introduced around the turn of the century to clear the specific wound "pathogen." Treatment was directed preponderantly toward *Staphylococcus aureus* following Ogston's discovery in 1881 of this bacterium as a cause of wound infection and the first report documenting experimental *S. aureus* infection in rabbits by Rodet in 1884.[13] With the exception of sulfonamides, these agents largely were used locally because no oral or parenteral forms were suitable. Also, many bacteria were

From the Department of Pathology and the Section of Infectious Diseases, Department of Medicine, Hennepin County Medical Center and the Musculoskeletal Sepsis Unit, Metropolitan Medical Center, Minneapolis, Minnesota.

considered nonpathogenic, e.g., *Staphylococcus epidermidis* and non-clostridial bacilli, so that disinfectants were directed toward pathogenic bacteria that caused infection in normal hosts. Even with the introduction in 1941 of penicillin, the first antibiotic, the emphasis was on "true pathogens." Changes in treatment at that time were followed by new antibiotics and correspondingly different routes of administration (e.g., oral, intramuscular, intravenous).[6, 14] When these efforts appeared to fail in spite of the appropriate antibiotic as determined by *in vitro* sensitivity studies, local application of antibiotics was introduced. Thus, an exposed wound was treated with various antibiotics alone or in combination by direct application or irrigation with or without suction.[14–16] Even regional perfusion with antibiotics for chronic bone infections was optimistically introduced.[17–19] Often local treatment was accompanied by an appropriate oral or parenteral course of antibiotics.

In spite of these efforts, bone and joint infections following traumatic fractures, even with prophylatic antibotics and in clean orthopedic surgery, remain a major clinical problem.[20–22] In addition, reparative and reconstructive orthopedic surgery led to the use of various metal appliances and synthetic polymers. Despite the remarkable progress in correcting the anatomical problems related to fractures and prosthetic joints, infections continued to be a complication, particularly in the presence of these foreign bodies.[22] Uncommon former "non-pathogens," such as coagulase-negative *Staphylococcus* (CNS) (prototype *S. epidermidis*), gram-negative bacillus (GNB), such as *Serratia marcesens,*[23] and even anaerobic bacteria, resulted in infections.[24–26] Some of these "non-pathogen" problems were reduced by the introduction of gentamicin into the bone cement.[27] What followed this success was inevitable. Gentamicin-impregnated bone cement was molded into "beads" in the operating room and placed in surgical wounds or joint spaces to obtain sustained high concentrations of this aminoglycoside.[28]

Thus, in 1973, Klemm introduced gentamicin-impregnated polymethyl methacrylate (PMMA) beads into sites of chronic bone infection.[28] Gentamicin delivered in this way was found to achieve high concentrations locally, with low levels in the serum and urine.[29, 30] Gentamicin levels in wound exudate from ten patients averaged 50 to 80 μg/ml over 4 days, while the maximum serum level did not exceed 0.5 μg/ml.[29] *In vitro* studies showed that a single bead eluted 400 μg, 120 μg, and 10 μg, respectively, on days 1, 10, and 80.[29] An animal study testing the efficacy of gentamicin beads in the treatment of *S. aureus* osteomyelitis demonstrated bacteriological, histological, and clinical cure in ten of 11 dogs treated with beads and in none of ten control animals that were not treated.[29] Although clinical experience utilizing antibiotic-impregnated beads is extensive in parts of Europe, the number of reports in the American literature is limited.[31–35] Vecsei and Barquet reported clinical success after a minimum of 3 years' follow-up in 22 of 25 patients with chronic osteomyelitis treated with gentamicin beads.[31] Two of the three patients for whom therapy had failed were later re-treated successfully. Seven patients received concomitant parenteral therapy for a maximum of 5 days. Hedstrom and co-authors compared therapy with gentamicin beads to suction-irrigation in a prospective randomized study of 48 patients.[32] After a mean of 24 months' follow-up and completion of therapy, there were two failures in 23 patients treated with gentamicin beads and four failures in 25 patients treated with suction-irrigation. However, in this study all patients received oral antibiotics for approximately 7 months postoperatively. Majid and associates reported on 50 consecutive patients with chronic osteomyelitis treated with gentamicin beads and intravenous antibiotics for 48 hours followed by oral therapy for 3 months.[33] There were four failures in the 43 patients who were followed for 1 to 24 months after discontinuation of all therapy. Grieben summarized the experience of 16 different investigators who treated 1045 patients with chronic osteomyelitis using gentamicin beads.[34] Primary postoperative control of infection was achieved in 85 percent of patients. Follow-up was available on 635 patients, and after 3 to 54 months 84 percent remained free of disease.

In the United States, commercial gentamicin beads have not been approved for general use. Also, gentamicin powder is available only in a reagent grade form that is not acceptable for use in patients. Therefore, surgeons have used powdered tobramycin, which is approved for use in the United States, as an alternative aminoglycoside to impregnate the PMMA beads. Although several reports have described the in vitro characteristics of tobramycin beads,[36, 37] there has been very little information published regarding its clinical use.[38]

The remainder of this chapter addresses two aspects of this innovative treatment undertaken at Hennepin County Medical Center. The first is the selected *in vitro* antibiotic elution studies done with PMMA antibiotic-impregnated beads, and the second is a review of the clinical experience with patients in whom such antibiotic beads have been used.

ANTIBIOTIC/PMMA BEAD IN VITRO ELUTION ASSAYS

Historically, aminoglycosides were the prototype antibiotics incorporated in bone cement. Because the only aminoglycoside available for patient use in the United States that comes in a powdered form is tobramycin sulfate, we elected to use it in clinical as well as in vitro evaluation. This powdered form of tobramycin enables uniform mixing with the powdered bone cement polymer before polymerization and hardening by added methyl methacrylate. In contrast, the only other approved aminoglycosides in the United States are in liquid form and do not mix or harden appropriately with the bone cement polymer. For in vitro comparison with tobramycin, both the powdered (reagent grade) and liquid (human use) forms of amikacin were tested. Two additional antibiotics, vancomycin hydrochloride and clindamycin hydrochloride, were studied in the PMMA bead model in vitro only. No patient in this study received PMMA beads impregnated with amikacin, vancomycin, or clindamycin.

Antibiotic-impregnated PMMA beads were made utilizing pharmaceutical tobramycin powder (Dista Products Co., Indianapolis, Ind.), liquid pharmaceutical amikacin, reagent grade amikacin sulfate powder (Bristol Labs, Syracuse, N.Y.), reagent grade vancomycin hydrochloride (Lilly, Indianapolis, Ind.), and reagent grade clindamycin hydrochloride (Upjohn, Kalamazoo, Mich.). With the exception of the liquid (1.0 gm) form of amikacin, which was mixed with the monomer, all antibiotic powder (1.2 gm tobramycin, 1 and 2 gm reagent grade amikacin, and 1 gm each vancomycin and clindamycin) and 20 gm polymer (Surgical Simplex P, Howmedica, Inc., Rutherford, N.J.) were pre-mixed for 3 to 6 minutes to ensure uniform distribution of the antibiotic (Table 8 – 1). Ten milliliters of liquid monomer was then added to the powder mixture and stirred until the mixture began to thicken. The paste was spread into custom-made plastic molds and allowed to cure for 10 to 15 minutes. One 20-gm batch of bone cement yielded three strands of 30 beads each, 6 mm in diameter.

The in vitro elution studies for the four antibiotics were done similarly and performed in triplicate. *A single bead* was placed in 2 ml of sterile phosphate-buffered saline (pH 7.4), that was removed, stored, and replaced daily over a 6-week period. The concentration of antibiotic in the aliquots was determined by fluorescence polarization immunoassay (TDX, Abbott Diagnostics, North Chicago, Ill.), or, in the case of clindamycin hydrochloride, by capillary gas chromatography (Analytical Biochemistry Laboratories, Inc., Columbia, Mo.).

The results (Fig. 8 – 1) show the average concentration in the aliquots *from a single bead* varied over time relative to the "therapeutic" serum level[39] for each antibiotic. The tobramycin beads eluted measurable and "clinically significant" levels for almost a month (Fig. 8 – 1A). Levels from beads made with 1 gm of amikacin, both clinical and reagent grade, fell below measurable levels by 1 week and below serum trough level by 3 days (Fig. 8 – 1B). However, beads made with 2 gm of reagent grade amikacin still eluted a measurable and clinically significant amount of antibiotic into the third week (Fig. 8 – 1B). Vancomycin elution concentrations were very high initially but fell rapidly over 2 days (Fig. 8 – 1C). Clindamycin was released at levels exceeding therapeutic serum levels for 5 days and continued to be released for the length of the experiment (Fig. 8 – 1D). The differences in the in vitro elution patterns for these antibiotics indicate that although PMMA beads are effective in delivering initial high levels of antibiotics, not all antibiotics have the same kinetics. Therefore, it would appear that each antibiotic should be evaluated in vitro before being incorporated into PMMA beads and used clinically.

CLINICAL EXPERIENCE WITH TOBRAMYCIN/PMMA BEAD THERAPY

The first 47 cases of patients with musculoskeletal infections who were treated and followed with tobramycin PMMA beads at the Hennepin County Medical Center and the Metropolitan Medical Center were reviewed (Table 8 – 2). During the review period (1980 – 1985), all patients admitted to the orthopedic service with osteomyelitis or infected joint prostheses received tobramycin beads as part of their therapy. There were 31 men and

TABLE 8–1. Amount of Antibiotics in Polymethyl Methacrylate (PMMA) Beads

Antibiotic	Grade/Form	Dose/20 gm PMMA	Available Antibiotic (6-mm Bead)
Tobramycin	Patient/powder	1.2 gm	11.6 mg
Amikacin			
Patient grade	Patient/liquid	2 gm/mg	7.8 mg
Reagent grade	Reagent/powder	1.0 gm/2.0 mm	7.4 mg/13.9 mg
Vancomycin	Reagent/powder	1.0 gm	8.6 mg
Clindamycin	Reagent/powder	1.0 gm	7.0 mg

15 women, ages 12 to 88. Not surprisingly, osteomyelitis following fracture was seen predominantly in a young male population, whereas the average age of patients with infected joint prostheses was 67.9 years. There were 20 cases of infected joint prosthesis, 20 cases of osteomyelitis following fractures, three cases of septic arthritis, two cases of soft tissue infection following hip replacement surgery, and one case each of hematogenous osteomyelitis and infection of a donor bone graft site.

Tobramycin beads were placed at the time of the initial surgical debridement. Beads were made in the *operating room* using 1.2 gm of tobramycin powder mixed with 20 gm of

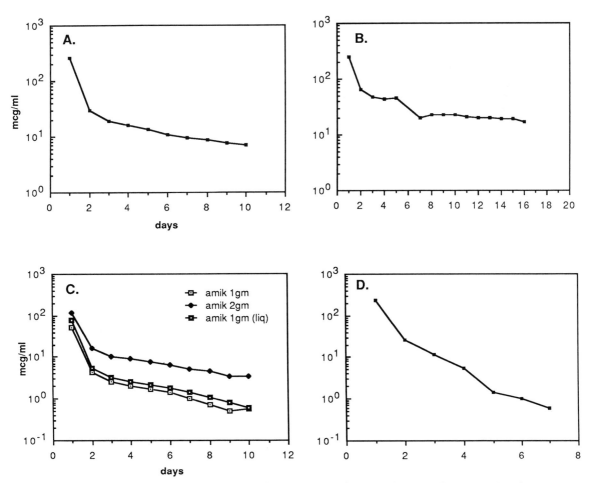

FIGURE 8–1. Single-bead elution kinetics of (*A*) tobramycin, (*B*) clindamycin, (*C*) amikacin, and (*D*) vancomycin.

TABLE 8–2. Results in Treatment of 46 Patients

	No. of Patients Treated	Infection Controlled	Treatment Failures
Infection after fracture	19	15	4
Prosthetic joint	20	15	5
Hip	12	9	3
Knee	8	6	2
Miscellaneous	7	7	0
Overall	46	37	9

* Observation period after therapy — 12.7 months (6–24 months).

PMMA, followed by the addition of the monomer. The beads were initially hand-made, but later a chain of 30 beads on a stainless steel wire was produced in a plastic mold. Typically, two to three chains of beads were placed in the infection site, depending on the extent and location of the infection. The wounds were closed to permit diffusion of the antibiotic from the bead to extend throughout the infected area, and an overflow drainage tube was placed to prevent buildup of excessive pressure within the wound.

The total duration of bead therapy ranged from 7 to 113 days (mean 37.7 days), with some patients receiving new beads sequentially when repeated surgical debridements were performed. Systemic antibiotic therapy was also given based on intraoperative culture results, with all cases of osteomyelitis and prosthetic joint infections receiving 6 weeks of high-dose parenteral antibiotics. However, systemic aminoglycoside therapy was administered in only one of the 47 patients in this review.

Intraoperative cultures were positive in 46 patients. The single exception was from a patient with a clinical infection of a total knee arthroplasty with drainage. There was a history of *Streptococcus* previously isolated, and the patient had been receiving chronic oral penicillin therapy until the time of surgery. A single pathogen was cultured in 27 patients, including 12 with *S. aureus,* five with CNS, and four with an anaerobic GNB. Of the five cases of CNS infections, four were patients with infected joint prostheses. There were 19 polymicrobial infections, which often included GNB (14 patients), *S. aureus* (ten patients), or CNS (11 patients) among the isolated organisms. Other bacteria that were frequently isolated include enterococcus (ten patients), *Streptococcus* (six patients), and anaerobes (five patients).

Tobramycin concentration was measured in the overflow drainage from the infection site in 12 patients (Table 8–3). Levels above the therapeutic serum range for tobramycin were maintained at 4 days after placement of beads, although there was considerable variation among patients. Almost all of the drainage tubes were discontinued at 3 to 4 days after bead placement. No fluid or tissue contiguous to the beads in the entire site of the infection was obtained for assay. However, it is reasonable to presume that the concentration of tobramycin at the tissue site was at least equal to the hemovac concentration.

In contrast to the perception that bone and joint infections involving GNB are difficult to treat,[40, 41] all four of our patients in whom GNB was isolated as a single pathogen and 11 of 14 patients in whom GNB was isolated in polymicrobial infections responded to therapy. On the other hand, our experience sug-

TABLE 8–3. Tobramycin Concentrations from Overflow Drainage in Patients with Implanted Beads

No. of Days After Implantation	Tobramycin (μg/ml)	Range (μg/ml)	No. of Patient Samples
1 Day	34.9	94.0–13.1	7
2 Days	19.3	40.0–3.1	7
3 Days	13.2	40.0–1.2	8
4 Days	13.0	16.4–3.1	5

TABLE 8–4. Treatment Failures in Patients with Tobramycin-Implanted Beads

Patient (Sex and Age)	Site	Bacterial Pathogen	Surgery	Systemic Antibiotics	Duration of Bead Therapy	Outcome	Comment
Man, 55 yr	Foot (calcaneus)	*Proteus mirabilis* CNS	Sequestrectomy Debridement	Cefoxitin	10 days	Chronic drainage	Osteomyelitis after fracture; asymptomatic for 26 yr prior to relapse
Man, 64 yr	Hip prosthesis	*Staphylococcus aureus*	Prosthesis removal	Cefazolin	66 days	Recurrent *S. aureus* infection	Osteoarthritis
Woman, 88 yr	Knee prosthesis	*S. aureus*	Prosthesis removal	Vancomycin	48 days	Recurrent *S. aureus* infection	Rheumatoid arthritis
Woman, 63 yr	Knee prosthesis	*S. aureus*	Prosthesis removal	Cefazolin	70 days	Recurrent *S. aureus* infection	Osteoarthritis
Man, 67 yr	Hip prosthesis Hip fusion	*S. aureus* *P. mirabilis*	Hip plate removal	Tobramycin Cefazolin	14 days	Chronic drainage	Prosthesis for traumatic fracture
Man, 75 yr	Hip prosthesis	CNS*	Prosthesis removal	Vancomycin	50 days	*Candida* hip infection	Prosthesis for fracture; CNS resistant to tobramycin
Man, 20 yr	Tibia	*S. aureus*	Debridement Fixation	Cefazolin	14 days	Chronic drainage; fracture healed	Traumatic fracture
Man, 34 yr	Tibia	*S. aureus*	Debridement Sequestrectomy	Penicillin G Oxacillin	19 days	Chronic drainage; anaerobes cultured; fracture healed	Traumatic fracture
Man, 28 yr	Tibia	*Serratia* *S. aureus*	Debridement Fixation	Cefotaxime	40 days	Infected nonunion	Traumatic fracture

Abbreviation: CNS = Coagulase-negative *Staphylococcus.*

* Abbreviation: CNS = Coagulase-negative *Staphylococcus.*

gests that tobramycin beads may be inadequate in some situations. A review of our nine treatment failures shows that *S. aureus* was the single pathogen isolated in four cases and was isolated as part of the polymicrobial flora in three other cases (Table 8–4). In contrast, therapy was successful in eight cases with pure *S. aureus* and in seven cases when it was isolated as part of a polymicrobial infection. In prosthetic joint infections, therapy was ineffective in three of four cases involving *S. aureus* as the single pathogen and ineffective in one of two cases when *S. aureus* was isolated as part of a mixed infection.

Because of the very high concentrations that can be achieved with local bead therapy, it is possible that an aminoglycoside may be effective against many bacteria that would be considered "resistant" by standard in vitro laboratory criteria, which are based upon achievable serum concentrations.[42] (See Chapter 5.) Others disagree and recommend that neither *Enterococcus*[43] nor "resistant" *Pseudomonas aeruginosa*[44] should be treated with gentamicin-impregnated PMMA beads. We found that CNS that are resistant to tobramycin (using standard in vitro criteria) are not inhibited (sensitive) by exceedingly high concentrations (100 gm/ml) in the laboratory. Therefore, it is unlikely that such infections will respond to tobramycin bead therapy. Unfortunately, the susceptibility of the CNS isolated in our patients to tobramycin is unknown. There were five cases of CNS isolated as a single pathogen, and four cases were treated successfully. Tobramycin has no activity against tested anaerobic bacteria and, in fact, has decreased activity against laboratory sensitive organisms when tested anaerobically. In our patients, anaerobes were cultured in five cases of polymicrobial infections (never as a single pathogen), of which three were successfully treated utilizing beads and an appropriate systemic anaerobic antibiotic.

Superinfection with highly resistant organisms is a potential complication of any form of antimicrobial therapy. This occurred in two of the 47 patients. In one patient, *Candida albicans* was isolated from the infected site after tobramycin treatment both parenterally and via PMMA beads was given. The second patient failure resulted in a *Bacteroides* species deep wound infection.

Since our success rate was no better than that with conventional therapy of osteomyelitis[45, 46] and concomitant systemic antibiotics are given to all our patients, no benefit can be attributed to local therapy with antibiotic-impregnated beads. However, we believe that there are significant advantages to this form of therapy which must be considered. Surgical dead space, which would otherwise be a potential site for an infected hematoma, is converted to an area of high antibiotic concentration. Early closure of the wound reduces the length of hospitalization and the extensive postoperative wound care required with alternative surgical options in the treatment of osteomyelitis (e.g., suction irrigation or open cancellous bone grafting.[1]) In addition and, most important, incorporating tobramycin into beads permits the delivery of high concentrations of a toxic antibiotic without the associated risk of auditory or renal side effects associated with conventional high-dose, prolonged parenteral aminoglycoside therapy. Less toxic antibiotics, such as beta-lactams, can then be given systemically to provide combination therapy which potentially is synergistic against several bacteria, including *S. aureus,* enterococcus, *Streptococcus viridans,* and GNB.

Tobramycin was the only antibiotic mixed into PMMA beads used in our 47 patients. It is leached from the beads over several days, resulting in prolonged high local concentrations. Antimicrobial activity is maintained in spite of the high temperature generated by the polymerization of the powdered mix of tobramycin and bone cement. Heat-labile antibiotics (e.g., the beta-lactam penicillins and cephalosporins, macrolides such as erythromycin, etc.) probably should not be used in PMMA beads because of potential loss of biologic activity. Furthermore, tobramycin is an antibiotic posing an extremely low risk of an allergic reaction. Thus, in contrast to the beta-lactams, it is safe to use in this repository manner. No allergic reactions have been reported by other physicians[47] or were seen in our patients. However, allergy, as a potential complication, must be considered. Although the activity and elution properties of several antibiotics in PMMA cement have been studied in vitro, the clinical efficacy of almost all antibiotics potentially useful in beads is largely unknown. The introduction of new antibiotics in beads, as emphasized above, should be approached in a systematic fashion to provide both in vitro data and clinical evidence of efficacy. Ineffective antibiotic-impregnated PMMA beads are potentially detrimental to the patient with infection. PMMA cement can serve as a foreign body nidus for persistent infection and has been shown to abolish the inhibitory effect of human serum on the growth of *S. epidermidis*[48] and to impair the bactericidal activity of phagocytic cells.[49]

SUMMARY

We were able to demonstrate a favorable outcome using tobramycin-impregnated PMMA bead therapy compared with other types of treatment of bone and joint infection. The in vitro antibiotic elution studies support this observation. The varied elution patterns of different antibiotics tested provide compelling reason to do in vitro testing of any antibiotic considered for use in PMMA beads. Additional benefit of this treatment included avoidance of intravenous tobramycin with the associated risk of toxicity as well as drug administration costs. Also, postoperative wound care was less.

Finally, the lesson we continue to learn about chronic bone and joint infections is the paramount inportance of surgery and that any form of antimicrobial therapy rarely will succeed without surgical intervention.

References

1. Majno G: The Healing Hand. Cambridge, Mass, Harvard University Press, 1975.
2. Cano RJ, Colome JS: Microbiology. St Paul, Minn, West Publishing Co, 1986.
3. Wells C: Bones, Bodies, and Diseases. London, Thames and Hudson, 1964.
4. Moodie RL: Paleopathology: An Introduction to the Study of Ancient Evidences of Disease. Urbana, Ill, University of Illinois Press, 1923.
5. Schopf JW, Barghoorn ES, Maser MD, Gordon RO: Electron microscopy of fossil bacteria two billion years old. Science 149:1365–1367, 1965.
6. Waldvogel FA, Medoff G, Swartz MN: Osteomyelitis: A review of clinical features, therapeutic considerations, and unusual aspects. N Engl J Med 282:198–206, 260–266, 316–322, 1970.
7. West WF, Kelly PJ, Martin WJ: Chronic osteomyelitis. I. Factors affecting the results of treatment in 186 patients. JAMA 213:1837–1842, 1970.
8. Shannon JG, Woolhouse FM, Eisinger PJ: The treatment of chronic osteomyelitis by saucerization and immediate skin grafting. Clin Orthop 96:98–107, 1973.
9. Cierny G, Mader JT: Adult chronic osteomyelitis. Orthopaedics 7:1557–1564, 1984.
10. Irons GB, Wood MB: Soft-tissue coverage for the treatment of osteomyelitis of the lower part of the leg. Mayo Clin Proc 61:382–387, 1986.
11. Wilensky AO: Osteomyelitis: Its Pathogenesis, Symptomatology and Treatment. New York, The Macmillan Co, 1934.
12. Spink WW: Sulfanilamide and Related Compounds in General Practice. Chicago, Ill, Year Book Medical Publishers, 1942.
13. Rodet A: Etude experimentale sur l'osteomyelite infectieuse. Compte Rend Acad de Science 99:569, 1884.
14. Norden CW: A critical review of antibiotic practice in orthopedic surgery. Rev Infect Dis 5:928–932, 1983.
15. Clawson DK, Davis FJ, Hansen ST Jr: Treatment of chronic osteomyelitis with emphasis on closed suction-irrigation technic. Clin Orthop 96:88–97, 1973.
16. Kelly PJ, Martin WJ, Coventry MB: Chronic osteomyelitis. II. Treatment with closed irrigation and suction. JAMA 213:1843–1848, 1970.
17. Jones RF, Barnett JA, Gregory CF: Regional perfusion with antibiotics for chronic bone infections. Arch Surg 106:142–144, 1973.
18. Hurley JD, Wilson SD, Worman LW, Carey LC: Chronic osteomyelitis. Arch Surg 92:548–553, 1966.
19. Ryan RF, Reemtsma K, Beddingfield GW, Creech O, Wickstrom J: Regional perfusion with antibiotics. Arch Surg 92:482–487, 1961.
20. Gustilo RB, Anderson JT: Prevention of infection in the treatment of one thousand and twenty-five open fractures of long bones. J Bone Joint Surg 58-A:453–458, 1976.
21. Gustilo RB, Mendoza RM, Williams DN: Problems in the management of type III (severe) open fractures: a new classification of type III open fractures. J Trauma 24:742–746, 1984.
22. Wilson PD Jr, Salvati EA, Agelietti P, Kutner LJ: The problem of infection in endoprosthetic surgery of the hip joint. Clin Orthop 96:213–221, 1973.
23. Kelly PJ, Wilkowske CJ, Washington JA II: Musculoskeletal infections due to *Serratia marcescens*. Clin Orthop 96:76–83, 1973.
24. Lewis RP, Sutter VL, Finegold SM: Bone infections involving anaerobic bacteria. Medicine (Baltimore) 57:297–305, 1978.
25. Raff MJ, Melo JC: Anaerobic osteomyelitis. Medicine (Baltimore) 57:83–103, 1978.
26. Brook I: Anaerobic osteomyelitis in children. Pediatr Infect Dis 5:550–556, 1986.
27. Buchholz HW, Engelbrecht E: Uber die depotwirkung einiger antibiotika bei vermischchung mit dem kunstharz palacos. Chirugie 41:511–515, 1970.
28. Klemm K: Septopal—a new way of local antibiotic therapy. In van Rens TJG, Kayser FH, eds: Local Antibiotic Treatment in Osteomyelitis and Soft-Tissue Infections. Amsterdam, Excerpta Medica, 1981, pp 24–37.
29. Wahlig H, Dingeldein E, Bergmann R, Reuss K: The release of gentamicin from polymethylmethacrylate beads. J Bone Joint Surg 60B:270–275, 1978.
30. Walenkamp G, Vree TB, Van Rens TJG: Gentamicin-PMMA beads: pharmacokinetic and nephrotoxicological study. Clin Orthop 205:171–183, 1986.
31. Vecsei V, Barquet A: Treatment of chronic osteomyelitis by necrectomy and gentamicin-PMMA beads. Clin Orthop 159:201–207, 1981.
32. Hedstrom SA, Lidgren L, Torholm C, Onnerfalt R: Antibiotic containing bone cement beads in the treatment of deep muscle and skeletal infections. Acta Orthop Scand 51:863–869, 1980.
33. Majid SA, Lindberg LT, Gunterberg B, Siddiki MS: Gentamicin–PMMA beads in the treatment of chronic osteomyelitis. Acta Orthop Scand 56:265–268, 1985.

34. Grieben A: Clinical results of Septopal in bone and soft tissue infections: a survey of clinical trials. In Van Rens TJG, Kayser FH, eds: Local Antibiotic Treatment in Osteomyelitis and Soft Tissue Infections. Amsterdam, Excerpta Medica, 1981, pp 144–154.

35. Boda A: Septopal change-exchange operation for the treatment of osteomyelitis cavities. Arch Orthop Trauma Surg 101:39–45, 1982.

36. Goodell JA, Flick AB, Hebert JC, Howe JG: Preparation and release characteristics of tobramycin-impregnated polymethylmethacrylate beads. Am J Hosp Pharm 43:1454–1460, 1986.

37. Kirkpatrick DK, Trachtenberg LS, Mangino PD, Von Graunhofer JA, Seligson D: In vitro characteristics of tobramycin-PMMA beads: compressive strength and leaching. Orthopaedics 8:1130–1133, 1985.

38. Cierny G, Couch LA, Mader JT: Clinical evaluation of antibiotic-impregnated polymethylmethacrylate beads in patients with osteomyelitis. In Proceedings of the 25th Interscience Conference on Antimicrobial Agents and Chemotherapy. Washington DC, American Society for Microbiology, 1985, p 253.

39. Hermans PE, Anhalt JP, Washington JA II: Pocket Guide to Antimicrobial Agents 1984. Philadelphia, Centrum, 1984.

40. Schurman DJ, Wheelen R: Gram-negative bone and joint infections. Clin Orthop 134:268–274, 1978.

41. Kelly PJ, Wilkowski CJ, Washington JA: Comparison of gram-negative bacillary and staphylococcal osteomyelitis of the femur and tibia. Clin Orthop 96:70–75, 1973.

42. Dingeldein E: Bacteriological studies in patients treated with gentamicin–PMMA beads. In Van Rens TJG, Kayser FH, eds: Local Antibiotic Treatment in Osteomyelitis and Soft Tissue Infections. Amsterdam, Excerpta Medica, 1981, pp 18–23.

43. Weise K, Weller S: Indication and use of Septopal in chronic osteitis. In Van Rens TJG, Kayser FH, eds: Local Antibiotic Treatment in Osteomyelitis and Soft Tissue Infections. Amsterdam, Excerpta Medica, 1981.

44. Callaghan JJ, Salvati EA, Brause BD, Rimnae CM, Wright TM: Reimplantation for salvage of the infected hip: rationale for the use of gentamicin-impregnated cement and beads. The Hip: Hip Society Awards Papers. St. Louis, CV Mosby, 1985.

45. Meyers BR, Berson BG, Gilbert M, Hirschman SZ: Clinical patterns of osteomyelitis due to gram-negative bacteria. Arch Intern Med 131:228–233, 1973.

46. Gentry LO: Role for newer beta-lactam antibiotics in treatment of osteomyelitis. Am J Med 78 (Suppl 6A):134–139, 1985.

47. Nelson CL, Bergman BR: Antibiotic-impregnated acrylic composites. In Eftekhar NS, ed: Infections in Joint Replacement Surgery: Prevention and Management. St. Louis, CV Mosby Company, 1984, pp 267–280.

48. Petty W: The effect of methylmethacrylate on the bacterial inhibiting properties of normal human serum. Clin Orthop 132:266–278, 1978.

49. Green AS: The effect of methylmethacrylate on phagocytosis. J Bone Joint Surg 57A:538, 1975.

J. Phillip Nelson, M.D.

Prevention of Postoperative Infection by Airborne Bacteria

INTRODUCTION

This chapter discusses the pathophysiology of postoperative wound sepsis, the part airborne bacteria may play in producing postoperative sepsis, the effectiveness of clean rooms and helmet-aspirator systems in reducing operating room airborne bacteria, and the data relevant to the influence of reduced airborne bacterial concentrations in the operating room on the incidence of deep postoperative infection in total hip arthroplasties. Because of their widespread use, preventive antibiotics are also considered. The information reported here is based upon our studies of the operating room environment and deep infection following total hip replacement[1-12] and upon several other pertinent reports.[13-15]

BACKGROUND

Subsequent to the development of total joint replacement 25 years ago, it has become apparent that the most important cause of irretrievable failure is deep infection. Charnley must be given credit not only for developing total hip arthroplasty but for focusing attention on the need for ever-improving bacteriologic control in the operating room. The principles of listerian antisepsis and precise surgical technique are even more important in implant surgery. The use of clean rooms and helmet-aspirator systems may be considered as an extension or refinement of surgical antisepsis because they reduce both airborne and contact intraoperative wound contamination.

The occurrence of postoperative wound in-

fection is the result of a complex interaction between host and bacteria. This interaction is influenced by the location and type of surgery, presence of foreign bodies, the functional state of host defenses, and the numbers and virulence of bacteria inoculated into the wound.

Wounds may be classified according to the estimated amount of preoperative or intraoperative bacterial contamination as (1) ultraclean, (2) clean-refined, (3) clean-contaminated, (4) contaminated, or (5) dirty. Even ultra-clean wounds are contaminated with bacteria to some degree at the conclusion of surgery. Surgical wounds may be contaminated with bacteria from patient (endogenous) or from environmental (exogenous) sources. Wound contamination from endogenous sources may originate from the skin, mucous membranes, an opened viscus, or local or distant sources of old or concurrent infection. Wound contamination from exogenous sources occurs from direct wound or sterile surface contact with contaminated gloves, instruments, or implants and from deposition of airborne bacteria into the wound. Traditional methods of surgical antisepsis and technique have been directed toward reduction of wound contamination from endogenous and exogenous contact routes with substantial success. Until recently, relatively little attention has been paid to the influence of airborne bacteria in the etiology of postoperative sepsis.

AIRBORNE BACTERIA

Airborne bacteria in the operating room seldom, if ever, exist independently. They reside on inorganic particles at least 2 microns (μ) in size. They are almost entirely gram-positive and originate almost exclusively from humans in the operating room. People shed bacteria

From Cherry Creek Orthopedic Surgery, Denver, Colorado.

into the air at rates up to 5000 per minute, and these come primarily from skin and hair. Individual rates of shed vary with each person and from time to time. Interestingly, humans shed more bacteria shortly after a shower than at any other time.

Some people carry more virulent organisms, and a few of these "carriers" intermittently or constantly disperse these more virulent strains into the air. Several epidemics of postoperative sepsis have been associated with "dispersers" of virulent, typeable bacteria. From their origin on humans, airborne particulates bearing bacteria rapidly disperse in an enclosed space as a result of air turbulence and convection currents. They settle or impinge on surfaces, and, provided that there has been no break in sterile technique, they are the only source of sterile surface contamination.

Active air samplers used in the standard operating room during surgery, with from four to eight people within, consistently show from 2 to 15 microorganisms per cubic foot. These operating rooms are associated with air turnover rates averaging 12 to 14 times per hour.

Traditional operating attire made of cotton muslin material is very porous, with hole sizes of 50 to over 200 μ, depending on how much the material has been washed. This porosity allows easy escape of shed skin scales and bacteria. Cotton is also a very "wettable" material and allows rapid transfer of bacteria from inner to outer surfaces, thereby contributing to contact contamination of other sterile surfaces.

Airborne bacterial concentrations in the operating room rise with increasing numbers and activity of operating room personnel. Concentrations are decreased by more effective garment barriers and by increasing the rate of air turnover in the room. Increasing air conditioning filter efficiency by itself does not reduce airborne bacterial concentrations unless there is a substantial increase in air turnover rate.

Because he observed that the initial total hip arthroplasty infection rate was high even though technique was unchanged from that for other major hip surgery, for which rates remained low, Charnley theorized that the implantation of large amounts of foreign material resulted in patients with total hip replacement being particularly prone to infection. Presumably, this could occur from smaller inocula of less virulent bacteria. The uncontrolled sources of this contamination in Charnley's

operating room were from airborne bacteria and bacterial penetration of gown materials. These observations led him to develop the operating room clean room and the helmet-aspirator system. In the United States, at about the same time in 1966, a slightly more efficient clean room was being tried at the Bataan Memorial Hospital under the guidance of W.J. Whitfield (the father of clean room technology in this country), Randolph Lovelace, and J.G. Whitcomb. At the present time, there are several hundred functional operating room clean rooms in the United States.

CLEAN AIR ROOM

In its present form, the operating room clean room is characterized by a bank of high-efficiency particulate air (HEPA) filters, which are usually 99.99 percent efficient for removal of particles 0.5 μ and larger. This degree of efficiency is not entirely necessary, since, as previously noted, bacteria reside on particles 2 μ in size or larger. Blowers force air into a plenum that pressurizes the filters. Air issuing from the filters is sterile and is kept flowing in one direction by walls. Air is usually recirculated at a rate of 300 or more times per hour. Air velocity is not perceptible. Depending on the positioning of the filter bank and walls, air flow may be horizontal or vertical. Installation costs range from about $20,000 for horizontal units to $40,000 for vertical units (Fig. 9–1).

The vertical units are slightly more efficient in reducing airborne bacterial concentrations than the horizontal units. Horizontal units are much easier to install and usually allow more flexible use of the operating room. Additional air conditioning capacity may be necessary to handle the 15,000 BTUs of heat generated from blower motors and from air movement. Noise from blower units and the movement of air is less than 64 decibels, which permits normal conversational speech. Including routine maintenance of blowers and filters and electrical charges, monthly upkeep is estimated to be $600. HEPA filter life should be at least 10 years. Except for wound drying, there are no known effects from clean rooms detrimental to patients or operating room personnel. A 10- × 10-foot enclosure is adequate for the performance of all orthopedic surgery, but a 12- × 12-foot enclosure is more spacious and satisfactory.

The helmet-aspirator system features gown materials made from papers, tightly woven

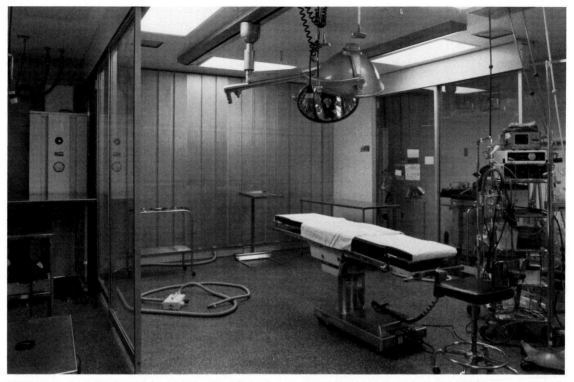

FIGURE 9–1. A 12- by 12-foot horizontal flow clean room with blower units at sides, plenum at back, and walls extended. The anesthesiologist sits at the head of the table downwind from surgery. Box on floor with hoses attached is a suction manifold.

cottons, or woven plastic polymers, all of which have much smaller pore sizes than muslin. In addition, the head is fully enclosed and a suction-aspirator produces negative pressure in the gown-body interspace. This allows for aspiration of shed bacteria and substantially reduces the possibility of gown penetration by shed bacteria. The suction also produces a cooling effect. The cost of a helmet-aspirator system to accommodate four people is approximately $1000. Those surgeons who use these systems have found that they are comfortable, vision is unimpaired, and there is no interference with the technical performance of surgery (Fig. 9–2).

DATA REVIEW

A substantial amount of information is now available regarding airborne bacterial concentrations, wound contamination rates, the comparative bacteriology of the operating room, and postoperative infection following total hip replacement. The data to be presented have been published in the 1977 Proceedings of The Hip Society[10] and the 1977 AAOS Instructional Course Lectures.

At Wound Airborne Bacterial Concentrations

In the regular operating room with regular garments, the average count was 5.4 (range 1.9 to 9.8) per cubic foot; in the clean room with regular garments, it was about 0.45 (range 0.2 to 1.4); and in the clean room with helmet-aspirator system, it was about 0.1 (range 0.004 to 0.4). In the clean room alone counts were reduced by 83 percent, and with the addition of the helmet-aspirator system for scrubbed personnel, counts were reduced by almost 99 percent. The vertical system was slightly more efficient than the horizontal system. Similar results were recorded when settle plates were used for sampling.

Wound Contamination Rates

In the regular operating room with regular garments, the average rate was 24.9 percent

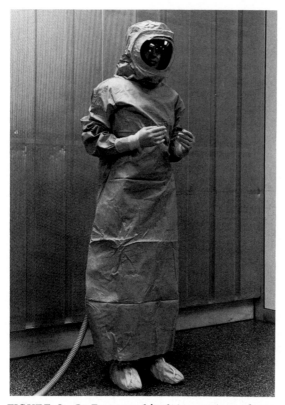

FIGURE 9–2. Personnel-isolator system showing full head enclosure with plastic shield, which snap-fits on a light-weight plastic welders head harness and the aspirator tubing exiting through the lower gown back.

3. *Staphylococcus aureus* (0.6, 0.5, and 1.9 percent) and gram-negative organisms (5.6, 0.7, and 2.8 percent) were found in small but persistent numbers in all three areas.

4. The proportions of bacterial types remained essentially constant in the regular operating room and clean room environments.

Total Hip Arthroplasty Infection Bacteriology

The bacteriology of 392 infections reported in eight separate series showed the following:

1. Sixty-three percent were caused by gram-positive organisms; 20 percent by gram-negative bacteria; and the remainder were classified as mixed (1 percent), sterile (9 percent), and cultures not valid (7 percent).

2. The predominant etiologic bacteria were *S. aureus* (28 percent), *S. epidermidis* (21 percent), *Escherichia coli* (8 percent), and *Proteus* (5 percent).

3. No conclusions could be reached concerning the effect of operating room environment on the bacteriology of infections.

The Incidence of Total Hip Infections

In the regular operating room with no preventative antibiotics used in 1880 cases reported by seven authors, 109 deep infections occurred for a rate of 5.8 percent (range 3.9 to 11.0). In the regular operating room with preventative antibiotics in 6791 cases reported by ten authors, the rate was 1.3 percent (range 0 to 3.1). In the clean room without preventative antibiotics in 2730 cases reported by three authors, the rate was 0.7 percent. In the clean room with preventative antibiotics in 2754 cases from six authors, the rate was 0.6 percent. The difference between the regular operating room–no antibiotic group and the remaining groups is very significant. The difference between the regular operating room–preventative antibiotic group is moderately significant. No statistically significant differences exist between the last two groups. The influence of helmet-aspirator systems could not be determined. These data indicate that at least 80 percent of postoperative total hip arthroplasty (THA) infections are caused by airborne bacteria.

The entire September 1973 issue of *Clinical Orthopaedics and Related Research* was devoted

(range 17.9 to 31.5); in the clean room with regular garments, the rate was 4.7 percent (range 3.9 to 5.1); and in the clean room with helmet-aspirator system for scrubbed personnel the rate was 3.9 percent (range 2.4 to 5.4). The clean room alone reduced rates of wound contamination by 81 percent, and the addition of the helmet-aspirator system resulted in a further, but statistically insignificant, drop to about 84 percent.

Comparative Environmental Bacteriology

Qualitative analysis of bacteria isolated from active air sampling, settle plates and the wound revealed the following facts:

1. Gram-positive organisms predominated in all three areas (88.2, 95.1, and 81.7 percent).

2. *Staphylococcus epidermidis* was isolated most frequently in all three cases (38.9, 37.4, and 39.9 percent).

to reports on total hip arthroplasty. An analysis of those series involving 16,807 cases revealed a reported infection rate of 2.4 percent for 11,377 cases done in a regular operating room as opposed to a rate of 0.5 percent for 5430 cases done in a clean room. The use of preventative antibiotics in a regular operating room was associated with an infection rate of 1.9 percent. Their use in the clean room had no effect on the incidence of infection in cases done in the clean room.

Other Pertinent Studies

The most important study confirming the efficacy of clean rooms and personnel-isolator systems was done under the auspices of the British Medical Research Council by Lidwell and associates[14] in 1982; 8055 total hip and total knee operations performed in 19 different hospitals were studied for the incidence of deep postoperative infection. The investigators concluded that the incidence of deep infection was 50 percent less in the clean room than in a standard operating room; this incidence was an additional 25 percent less when personnel-isolator systems were used. Preventative antibiotics further reduced the incidence of infection.

More recently, Howorth[13] published an excellent state-of-the-art review, which is highly recommended.

The only study known to the author that contradicts the data presented above is that done by Salvati and colleagues,[15] which showed an increased infection rate after total knee arthroplasty done in a horizontal flow clean room. The apparent explanation for this incongruity is that scrubbed personnel did not wear personnel-isolator systems and that bacteria shed by them were deposited by the laminar air flow in the wound and on sterile surfaces in concentrations sufficient enough to cause the increased rate of infection.

Infection Cost

In addition to concern for prevention of patient morbidity due to postoperative complications, physicians must also be cognizant of medical care costs. Analysis of the economic costs for hospital care of deep total hip arthroplasty infections in 14 of our patients revealed an average cost of approximately $12,000 in 1977. Eftekhar reports two patients for whom

these costs were $82,000 and $140,000, respectively. More current estimates for the cost of excisional arthroplasty, insertion of antibiotic impregnated beads, 6 weeks of intravenous antibiotics and then reinsertion of a total hip would be about $50,000. Physician charges, outpatient and nursing home costs, and economic loss due to lost wages and disability payments are not included in these calculations.

One of the major objections to the use of clean rooms has been their expense. If one assumes a figure of 100,000 total hip arthroplasties done yearly in the United States and a 2.4 percent deep infection rate for the regular operating room, 2400 deep infections per year could be expected. If the rate is 0.5 percent in the clean room, 500 infections per year could be expected. If 1900 infections can be prevented by the use of clean rooms, the yearly savings in medical care alone would be $95 million, assuming that the cost for additional care is $50,000 per case. Since the useful life of a clean room is at least 10 years, the savings in medical care costs alone over a 10-year period would allow purchase and maintenance of about 10,000 clean rooms.

SUMMARY

Wound infections result from wound contamination by bacteria and from the body's inability to kill these bacteria. Reduction of wound contamination and enhancement of normal antibacterial host defenses result in reduced rates of wound infection. Endogenous and exogenous contact wound contamination of clean wounds (e.g., the total hip replacement as a clean wound at high risk for infection) is readily controlled by traditional methods of sterile and surgical technique.

Airborne bacteria in the operating room are derived almost exclusively from people in the operating room. Airborne bacterial concentrations in the operating room may be reduced at least 80 percent using laminar-airflow clean rooms. Further reductions accompany the use of improved barrier technique such as personnel-isolator systems.

Wound contamination rates are reduced at least 80 percent when a clean room is used, indicating that most intraoperative wound contamination originates from airborne bacteria. Provided that traditional methods of sterile technique are scrupulously observed, wound contamination from contact sources or from environmental surfaces is rare.

The incidence and type of bacteria in the air, on environmental surfaces from fallout, and in the wound are very similar, with gram-positive organisms (*S. epidermidis*, diphtheroids, and *Bacillus subtilis*) isolated at least 80 percent of the time. *Staphylococcus aureus* and gram-negative bacteria were found infrequently.

Sixty-three percent of deep infections following total hip arthroplasty were caused by gram-positive organisms, with *S. epidermidis* and *S. aureus* predominating in approximately equal numbers. Approximately 20 percent of these infections result from gram-negative microorganisms. The increased virulence of *S. aureus* and gram-negative bacteria appears to account for their more frequent etiological role in postoperative sepsis as opposed to their relatively low occurrence in the operating room environment.

Analysis of postoperative infection rates shows that preventative antibiotics are very effective in reducing infection. The clean room with and without preventative antibiotics is at least as effective in preventing infection as the regular operating room with preventative antibiotics.

The sum of available data indicates that at least 80 percent of deep sepsis in total hip arthroplasty patients results from intraoperative wound contamination from airborne sources. Furthermore, these infections can be prevented using operating room clean rooms, personnel-isolator systems, and preventative antibiotics.

In conclusion, clean rooms and helmet-aspirator systems are very effective techniques for reduction of airborne bacteria in the operating room. There is substantial evidence that these innovations reduce rates of postoperative infection at least as effectively as preventative antibiotics. They have essentially no real or potential harmful effects on the patient, and they represent a technological improvement in traditional listerian antisepsis. Based on data presented from an extensive literature survey and costs of treatment of established total hip arthroplasty infection, they appear to be cost-effective.

References

1. Marsh RC, Nelson JP: Comparing surgical clean room filters. Contemp Surg 7:33–34, 1975.
2. Nelson JP: Deep infection following total hip arthroplasty. J Bone Joint Surg 59A:1042–1044, 1977.
3. Nelson JP, Glassburn AR Jr, Talbott RD, McElhinney JP: Clean room operating rooms. Clin Orthop 96:179–187, 1973.
4. Nelson JP: Five years experience with operating room clean rooms and personnel-isolator systems. J Med Instrum 10:277–281, 1976.
5. Nelson JP, Glassburn AR Jr, Talbott RD, McElhinney JP: Horizontal flow clean room, bacteriologic studies. Rocky Mt Med J 72:243–246, 1975.
6. Nelson JP: Horizontal flow operating room clean rooms. Workshop on Control of Operating Room Airborne Bacteria. Washington, DC, National Academy of Sciences, 1976, pp 243–251.
7. Nelson JP, Glassburn AR Jr, Talbott RD, McElhinney JP: Horizontal flow operating clean rooms. Cleve Clin Q 40:191–203, 1973.
8. Nelson JP: Operating room clean rooms and personnel-isolator systems. AAOS Instructional Course Lectures. St. Louis, CV Mosby Co, 1977, pp 52–57.
9. Nelson JP: The effect of operating room environment and preventive antibiotics on postoperative infection in a consecutive series of 711 total hip arthroplasties. Unpublished material, 1974.
10. Nelson JP: The operating room environment and its influence on deep wound infection. The Hip: Proceedings of the Fifth Open Scientific Meeting of the Hip Society, 1977. St. Louis, CV Mosby Co, 1977, pp 129–146.
11. Nelson JP: The prevention of orthopaedic surgical sepsis. Orthop Dig 4:14–24, 1976.
12. Wardle MD, Nelson JP, LaLime P, Davidson CS: A surgeon body-exhaust, clean air operating room system. Orthop Rev 3:43–51, 1974.
13. Howorth FH: Prevention of airborne infection during surgery. Lancet, February 16, 1985, pp 386–388.
14. Lidwell OM, Lowberry EJL, Whyte W, Blowers R, Stanley SJ, Lowe D: Effect of ultraclean air in operating rooms on deep sepsis in the joint after total hip or knee replacement: a randomised study. Br Med J 285:10–14, 1982.
15. Salvati EA, Robinson RP, Zeno SM, Koslin BL, Brause B, Wilson PD Jr: Infection rates after 3175 total hip and total knee replacements performed with and without a horizontal unidirectional filtered airflow system. J Bone Joint Surg 64A:525–535, 1982.

Phillip K. Peterson, M.D.
Dean T. Tsukayama, M.D.

CHAPTER

10

Bone and Joint Infections in Immunocompromised Patients

INTRODUCTION

In addition to its obvious structural function, the skeletal system plays a vital role in host defense, namely, protection of the bone marrow, the source of virtually all cells of the immune system (Fig. 10–1). Although the immune system is extremely complex, it is clinically useful to classify host defenses into three major components: (1) neutrophil defense, (2) humoral immunity, and (3) cell-mediated immunity. A deficiency in the production or function of any of the cells participating in these three aspects of host defense predisposes the host to infection by specific groups of opportunistic pathogens.[1]

During the past two decades the microbiology of bone and joint infections has changed considerably, and this phenomenon can be attributed in part to the increased number of immunocompromised patients being cared for in clinical practice.[2-4] Also, understanding of the basic mechanisms of immunity has increased dramatically in recent years, and techniques for studying the competency of cells of the immune system have become more readily available and applied in a variety of clinical circumstances. Thus, the list of patients found to have either primary or secondary defects in immune function has continued to grow (Table 10–1).

Because many of the diagnostic and therapeutic aspects of management of opportunistic infections of bones and joints in immunocompromised patients are covered in other sections of this book, the major focus of this chapter is on the pathogenesis of these infections.

NEUTROPHIL DISORDERS

Normally, over one hundred billion neutrophils are released from the bone marrow into the systemic circulation every day. These phagocytic cells remain in the bloodstream for about 6 hours but have the remarkable ability to respond quickly to microorganisms that have invaded the epithelial barrier of the host. The coordinated events involved in this process (adherence, chemotaxis, and opsonic recognition) have been the subject of intense investigation,[5, 6] and the mechanisms by which neutrophils kill engulfed microorganisms have been defined (Table 10–2).[7, 8]

Patients with one well-characterized neutrophil-killing disorder, chronic granulomatous disease (CGD), are especially prone to the development of osteomyelitis. Osteomyelitis is observed in almost one third of all CGD patients,[9] and for unexplained reasons infections usually develop in the small bones of the hands and feet.[10] *Staphylococcus aureus, Serratia marcescens, Aspergillus*, and *Nocardia* are the most frequently recovered pathogens.[9, 11, 12] As a result of a defect in the activation of cell membrane associated nicotinamide-adenine dinucleotide phosphate oxidase, neutrophils of CGD patients are unable to reduce molecular oxygen and thereby are incapable of generating microbicidal oxygen intermediates. Interestingly, the microorganisms that cause infections in these patients are uniquely protected from oxygen-independent killing mechanisms and produce catalase, which detoxifies hydrogen peroxide produced during their own oxygen metabolism.

From the Section of Infectious Diseases, Department of Medicine, Hennepin County Medical Center, and the Musculoskeletal Sepsis Unit, Hennepin County Medical Center and Metropolitan Medical Center, Minneapolis, Minnesota.

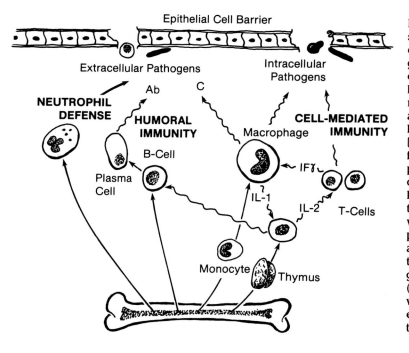

FIGURE 10-1. The immune system is a complex network of cells and cell products programmed to respond to microorganisms that have breached the epithelial barrier of the host. Neutrophils and humoral immunity (antibodies [Ab] and complement [C] proteins) are critical to defense against extracellular pathogens, whereas cell-mediated immunity (CMI) plays a key role in defense against intracellular pathogens. Activated macrophages are the principal effector cells of CMI, and T lymphocyte factors (interleukin-2 [IL-2], interferon-gamma [IFγ] and interleukin-1 [IL-1], a monokine, are involved in the sequence of events leading to cell activation.

Isolation of an unusual organism, such as *Serratia, Aspergillus,* or *Nocardia,* from a patient with osteomyelitis should raise the possibility of an underlying immune disorder, and CGD should be strongly considered. Although a primary neutrophil killing disorder is unlikely to be found in the vast majority of patients with staphylococcal osteomyelitis, one study[13] suggests that secondary killing defects may be common in patients with chronic *S. aureus* osteomyelitis and that this abnormality may play a role in the pathogenesis of this indolent infection.

Numerically, the most important group of patients with a deficiency in neutrophil defense are those with hematologic malignancy who are receiving cytotoxic chemotherapy. In the face of profound granulocytopenia (neutrophil counts of less than $500/ml^3$), infections caused by gram-negative bacilli, *S. aureus, Aspergillus,* and *Candida* become a major threat.[14] Surprisingly, bone and joint infections are relatively uncommon in this setting. Septic arthritis caused by *Candida* species has been identified as a problem in these patients,[15] and *Candida albicans* osteomyelitis has been reported in a patient with chronic lymphatic leukemia.[16] Neutropenia associated with aplastic anemia may also be a predisposing factor in the development of *Aspergillus* osteo-

TABLE 10-1. Deficiencies in Immunocompromised Patients (Partial List)

Neutrophil Disorders	Abnormalities of Humoral Immunity	Deficiencies of Cell-Mediated Immunity
Functional abnormalities	*Immunoglobulin deficiency*	*Primary defects*
Chronic granulomatous disease	Primary (Bruton's agammaglobu-	DiGeorge's syndrome, ataxia
Chédiak-Higashi syndrome	linemia, common variable	telangiectasia, chronic mucocu-
Job's syndrome	immunoglobulin deficiency)	taneous candidiasis
Diabetes mellitus	Secondary (multiple myeloma,	*Secondary defects*
Alcoholism	chronic lymphocytic leukemia,	Lymphoma, malnutrition, systemic
Quantitative deficiencies	asplenism)	lupus erythematosus, acquired
Cyclic neutropenia	*Complement deficiency*	immunodeficiency syndrome
Aplastic anemia	(C1, C2, C3, C4, C5, C6, C7, C8,	(AIDS), immunosuppression in
Cytotoxic chemotherapy	or factor B)	organ transplants, steroid
		therapy, and surgery; immuno-
		deficiency in the elderly

TABLE 10–2. Neutrophil Microbicidal Mechanisms

Oxygen-Independent Mechanisms	Oxygen-Dependent Mechanisms
Primary (azurophilic) granules	Free radicals
Cationic proteins	Hydroxyl radical ($\cdot$OH)
Hydrolytic enzymes	Superoxide (O_2^-)
Myeloperoxidase	Singlet oxygen ($^1O_2$)
Lysozyme	Hydrogen peroxide
Secondary (specific) granules	Myeloperoxidase–
Lactoferrin	hydrogen peroxide–
Lysozyme	halide
Defensins	

myelitis.[17] In more recent years, infections caused by the gram-negative bacillus *Aeromonas hydrophila* have been observed in patients receiving chemotherapy for cancer[18]; moreover, *A. hydrophila* septicemia and osteomyelitis have been reported in a leukemic child.[19]

ABNORMALITIES OF HUMORAL IMMUNITY

Two groups of plasma proteins play a crucial role in humoral immunity—immunoglobulins and complement factors. Patients with hypogammaglobulinemia or complement deficiency are at increased risk of infections caused by encapsulated bacteria (*Streptococcus pneumoniae, Haemophilus influenzae,* and *Neisseria*), and in the case of a deficiency of any of the early components of the complement cascade, *S. aureus* and gram-negative bacillary infections are also observed. Splenectomized patients share an increased risk of serious infections by encapsulated bacteria.[20] The basis for the increased susceptibility of these patients to infections caused by these specific microorganisms is related in part to the important role of immunoglobulins and complement factors in the opsonization and killing of these bacteria.[1]

Bone and joint infections appear to be relatively uncommon in patients with abnormalities of humoral immunity, although these pathogens should be considered in the evaluation of osteomyelitis or septic arthritis occurring in this clinical setting. *Mycoplasma pneumoniae*[21] and *Ureaplasma urealyticum*[22] have been recognized as the cause of septic arthritis in patients with hypogammaglobulinemia. Although the explanation for this finding is as yet unknown, special cultures of joint fluid for mycoplasmas should be performed in hypogammaglobulinemic patients with "culture-negative" septic arthritis.

DEFICIENCY OF CELL-MEDIATED IMMUNITY

Host defense against microorganisms that have the capacity to survive within cells of the mononuclear phagocyte system is dependent upon the cooperative interaction of T lymphocytes (primarily cells belonging to the helper/inducer or T4 lymphocyte subclass) and tissue macrophages. Macrophages that have been activated by the lymphokine interferon-gamma can kill a broad spectrum of intracellular pathogens, and patients with compromised cell-mediated immunity are at increased risk of infection caused by these same microorganisms (Table 10–3).

Patients with primary deficiencies of cell-mediated immune function are few in number, whereas patients with incompetent T lymphocytes due to immunosuppressive therapy (especially corticosteroids) or related to an underlying disease or infection are among the most frequently encountered immunocompromised hosts (see Table 10–1). Of the many intracellular pathogens that threaten these patients, mycobacteria, *Nocardia,* and certain fungi are the most common opportunistic infections involving bones or joints. *Salmonella* species[23] and a related gram-negative bacillus, *Arizona hinshawii,*[24] must also be considered in bone and joint infections occurring in patients with a secondary deficiency of cell-mediated immunity, such as lymphoma or organ transplantation. Although hematogenous dissemination may be the route by which many of these organisms gain access to the skeletal system, reactivation of a latent focus of infection appears to be common in most mycobacterial infections.

Patients with the newly recognized acquired immunodeficiency syndrome (AIDS) suffer from a thus far uniformly fatal defect of cell-mediated immunity, related in this disease to an uncontrolled infection of T4 lymphocytes. Osteomyelitis caused by *Nocardia asteroides* has been reported in one such patient,[25] and bone and joint infections caused by other intracellular opportunists can be anticipated in this rapidly growing group of patients.

TABLE 10-3. Opportunistic Intracellular Pathogens*

Bacteria	Fungi	Parasites	Viruses
Mycobacterium tuberculosis†	*Candida* species†	*Pneumocystis carinii*	Cytomegalovirus
Atypical mycobacteria†	*Aspergillus* species†	*Toxoplasma gondii*	Herpes simplex
Nocardia species†	*Mucor* species†	*Cryptosporidium*	Varicella zoster
Legionella species	*Histoplasma capsulatum*	*Strongyloides stercorales*	Epstein-Barr virus
Listeria monocytogenes	*Coccidioides immitis*		
Salmonella species†	*Cryptococcus neoformans*		

* Microorganisms that pose a special threat to patients with compromised cell-mediated immunity.
† Pathogens that must be considered in patients with osteomyelitis or septic arthritis.

SPECIAL PATIENT GROUPS

A contribution of an immunodeficiency state in the pathogenesis of osteomyelitis or septic arthritis has been suggested in a variety of clinical disorders (Table 10-4). Under certain circumstances, the recovery of unusual or opportunistic pathogens supports this concept, e.g., encapsulated bacteria from neonates and elderly patients with septic arthritis and the increased prevalence of *Pseudomonas aeruginosa* and *Salmonella* infections among heroin addicts and patients with sickle cell anemia, respectively. In patients with diabetes mellitus, multiple defects of immune function have been described and compromised host defenses may play a role in the bone and joint infections that occur in these patients. Obviously, other factors, such as alterations in the microflora colonizing various epithelial surfaces, increased exposure to opportunistic pathogens, and microvascular insufficiency, also are involved in the pathogenesis of many of these infections. Nonetheless, an abnormality of neutrophil defense, humoral immunity, or cell-mediated immunity can be implicated as a potentially important predisposing condition in a sizable proportion of cases of osteomyelitis and septic arthritis.

MANAGEMENT OF INFECTIONS IN IMMUNOCOMPROMISED PATIENTS

Principles similar to those employed in managing patients with normal host defenses are applied in the diagnosis and treatment of bone and joint infections in immunocompromised patients. Since therapy in both groups of patients will rely on the establishment of a specific etiologic agent, it is essential that proper culture techniques be performed. In addition to blood cultures, which are of greatest value in febrile patients, aspirates of bone or joint fluid should be processed promptly for appropriate stains and cultures. The types of staining tech-

TABLE 10-4. Special Patient Groups with Bone and Joint Infections

Patients	Host Defense Abnormality*	Common Pathogens
Extremes of age (neonates, young children)	Immunoglobulin deficiency,[26] neutrophil disorder	Group B *Streptococcus*,[27, 28] *Escherichia coli, Haemophilus influenzae*,[29] *Staphylococcus aureus*,[30] *Streptococcus pneumoniae*
Elderly	Neutrophil disorder	Group B *Streptococcus*,[31] *S. aureus*, gram-negative bacilli
Heroin addiction	Cell-mediated immunity deficiency, neutrophil disorder[32]	*Pseudomonas aeruginosa*,[33] *S. aureus, Candida albicans*[34]
Sickle cell disease (hemoglobin SS and SC)	Complement deficiency, hyposplenism	*Salmonella* species[23, 35]
Diabetes mellitus	Neutrophil disorders,[36-38] monocyte defect,[39] cell-mediated immunity deficiency[40]	Mixed aerobic and anaerobic bacterial infections,[41] Group B *Streptococcus*,[42] *S. aureus*

* Proposed immunologic defects that may play a role in increased susceptibility to infection.
Note: Superscripts indicate references appearing at the end of this chapter.

niques and culture conditions requested should be guided by assessment as to which pathogens are most likely. This decision is based upon knowledge of a specific immune defect and the related opportunistic pathogens as well as clinical conditions associated with specialized groups of microorganisms. Not infrequently, synovial or bone biopsy specimens are needed to establish an etiologic diagnosis.

In acute osteomyelitis or septic arthritis, antimicrobial therapy should be targeted at the most likely etiologic agent(s), pending the results of stains and cultures. In cases of chronic osteomyelitis or indolent septic arthritis, it may be desirable to await the results of initial diagnostic tests, since empiric therapy may interfere with subsequent culture results. Debridement of all devitalized bone and tissue is critical. Once an etiologic agent is established, antimicrobial therapy should be intensive and, in general, more prolonged than in the patient with normal host defenses. Under special circumstances, immunomodulators may be considered to be adjunctive therapy.

References

1. Peterson PK: Host defense abnormalities predisposing the patient to infection. Am J Med 76(5A):2–10, 1984.
2. Meyers BR, Berson BL, Gilbert M, Hirschman SZ: Clinical patterns of osteomyelitis due to gram-negative bacteria. Arch Intern Med 131:228–233, 1973.
3. Goldenberg DL, Brandt KD, Cathcart ES, Cohen AS: Acute arthritis caused by gram-negative bacilli: a clinical characterization. Medicine 53:197–208, 1974.
4. Waldvogel FA, Vasey H: Osteomyelitis: the past decade. N Engl J Med 303:360–370, 1980.
5. Gallin JI: Abnormal phagocyte chemotaxis: pathophysiology, clinical manifestations, and management of patients. Rev Infect Dis 3:1196–1220, 1981.
6. Winkelstein JA: Opsonins: their function, identity and clinical significance. J Pediatr 82:747–753, 1973.
7. Root RK, Cohen MS: The microbicidal mechanisms of human neutrophils and eosinophils. Rev Infect Dis 3:565–598, 1981.
8. Babior BM: Oxygen-dependent microbial killing by phagocytes. N Engl J Med 298:659–668, 1978.
9. Tauber AI, Borregaard N, Simons E, Wright J: Chronic granulomatous disease: a syndrome of phagocyte oxidase deficiencies. Medicine 62:286–309, 1983.
10. Wolfson JJ, Kane WJ, Laxdal SD, Good RA, Quie PG: Bone findings in chronic granulomatous disease of childhood. J Bone Joint Surg 51A:1573–1583, 1969.
11. Gallin JI (moderator): Clinical manifestations: recent advances in chronic granulomatous disease. Ann Intern Med 99:657–674, 1983.
12. Tack KJ, Rhame FS, Brown B, Thompson RC: Aspergillus osteomyelitis: report of four cases and review of the literature. Am J Med 73:295–300, 1982.
13. Perry CR, Felton CW, Palm JD, Burdge RE, Perry HM III: Decreased leukocyte cidal activity in patients with chronic osteomyelitis. Clin Res 33:846A, 1985.
14. Brown AE: Neutropenia, fever, and infection. Am J Med 76:421–428, 1984.
15. Fainstein V, Gilmore C, Hopfer RL, Maksymiuk A, Bodey GP: Septic arthritis due to Candida species in patients with cancer: report of five cases and review of the literature. Rev Infect Dis 4:78–85, 1982.
16. Estrov Z, Resnitzky P, Shenker Y, Berrebi A, Hurwitz N: Candidemia and sternal Candida albicans osteomyelitis in a patient with chronic lymphatic leukemia. Isr J Med Sci 20:711–714, 1984.
17. Simpson MB Jr, Merz WG, Kurlinski JP, Solomon MH: Opportunistic mycotic osteomyelitis: bone infections due to Aspergillus and Candida species. Medicine 56:475–482, 1977.
18. Harris RL, Fainstein V, Elting L, Hopfer RL, Bodey GP: Bacteremia caused by Aeromonas species in hospitalized cancer patients. Rev Infect Dis 7:314–320, 1985.
19. Lopez JF, Quesada J, Saied A: Bacteremia and osteomyelitis due to Aeromonas hydrophila: a complication during the treatment of acute leukemia. Am J Clin Pathol 50:587–591, 1968.
20. Francke EL, Neu HC: Postsplenectomy infection. Surg Clin North Am 61:135–155, 1981.
21. Johnston CLW, Webster ADB, Taylor-Robinson D, Rapaport G, Hughes GRV: Primary late-onset hypogammaglobulinemia associated with inflammatory polyarthritis and septic arthritis due to Mycoplasma pneumoniae. Ann Rheum Dis 42:108–110, 1983.
22. Webster ADB, Taylor-Robinson D, Furr PM, Asherson GL: Mycoplasma (ureaplasma) septic arthritis in hypogammaglobulinemia. Br Med J 1:478–479, 1978.
23. Ortiz-Neu C, Marr JS, Cherubin CE, Neu HC: Bone and joint infections due to Salmonella. J Infect Dis 138:820–828, 1978.
24. Quismorio FP Jr, Jakes JT, Zarnow AJ, Barber D, Kitridou RC: Septic arthritis due to Arizona hinshawii. J Rheumatol 10:147–150, 1983.
25. Masters DL, Lentino JR: Cervical osteomyelitis related to Nocardia asteroides. J Infect Dis 149:824–825, 1984.
26. Kuo KN, Lloyd-Roberts GC, Orme IM, Soothill JF: Immunodeficiency and infantile bone and joint infection. Arch Dis Child 50:51–56, 1975.
27. Fox L, Sprunt K: Neonatal osteomyelitis. Pediatrics 62:535–542, 1978.
28. Edwards MS, Baker CJ, Wagner ML, Taber LH, Barrett FF: An etiologic shift in infantile osteomyelitis: the emergence of the group B streptococcus. J Pediatr 93:578–583, 1978.
29. Granoff DM, Sargent E, Jolivette D: Haemophilus influenzae type b osteomyelitis. Am J Dis Child 132:488–490, 1978.
30. Weissberg ED, Smith AL, Smith DH: Clinical features of neonatal osteomyelitis. Pediatrics 53:505–510, 1974.
31. Laster AJ, Michels ML: Group B streptococcal arthritis in adults. Am J Med 76:910–915, 1984.
32. Tubaro E, Borelli G, Croce C, Cavallo G, Santiangeli C: Effect of morphine on resistance to infection. J Infect Dis 148:656–666, 1983.
33. Roca RP, Yoshikawa TT: Primary skeletal infections in heroin users: a clinical characterization, diagnosis and therapy. Clin Orthop Rel Res 144:238–248, 1979.

34. Dupont B, Drouhet E: Cutaneous, ocular, and osteoarticular candidiasis in heroin addicts: new clinical and therapeutic aspects in 38 patients. J Infect Dis 152:577–591, 1985.

35. Givner LB, Luddy RE, Schwartz AD: Etiology of osteomyelitis in patients with major sickle hemoglobinopathies. J Pediatr 99:411–413, 1981.

36. Mowat AG, Baum J: Chemotaxis of polymorphonuclear leukocytes from patients with diabetes mellitus. N Engl J Med 284:621–627, 1971.

37. Rayfield EJ, Ault MJ, Keusch GT, Brothers MJ, Nechemias C, Smith H: Infection and diabetes: the case for glucose control. Am J Med 72:439–450, 1982.

38. Repine JE, Clawson CC, Goetz FC: Bactericidal function of neutrophils from patients with acute bacterial infections and from diabetics. J Infect Dis 142:869–875, 1980.

39. Hill HR, Augustine NH, Rallison ML, Santos JI: Defective monocyte chemotactic responses in diabetes mellitus. J Clin Immunol 3:70–77, 1983.

40. Kolterman OG, Olefsky J, Kurahara C, Taylor K: A defect in cell-mediated immune function in insulin-resistant diabetic and obese subjects. J Lab Clin Med 96:535–543, 1980.

41. Fierer J, Daniel D, Davis C: The fetid foot: lower extremity infections in patients with diabetes mellitus. Rev Infect Dis 1:210–217, 1979.

42. Small CB, Slater LN, Lowy FD, Small RD, Salvati EA, Casey JI: Group B streptococcal arthritis in adults. Am J Med 76:367–375, 1984.

C H A P T E R

11

Management of Open Fractures

INTRODUCTION

An open fracture is one in which the bone ends have penetrated to the outside skin and there is injury to the underlying soft tissues of varying severity.

The initial treatment of the patient in general and of the open fracture in particular often determines the final outcome of the injury as to life, residual disability, and functional result of the involved extremity. Four essential features of open fractures must be recognized, and they serve as guidelines for treatment.

First, 30 percent of patients with open fractures are polytrauma victims. A polytrauma patient has two or more system injuries of the head, chest, abdomen, pelvis, or extremities. Cardiac arrest, respiratory failure, shock, head and spinal injury, arterial injuries, and fractures, including open ones, are listed in the order of severity and possible threat to the patient's life. Because of the complexities of the problem, a general surgeon with trauma training and experience must be in charge of the patient, with a team of specialists to assist with any specific problem. Obviously, the orthopedic surgeon must be consulted immediately to take care of the open fractures. Another very important participant in the management of the polytrauma patient is an anesthesiologist who has knowledge of trauma physiology and experience in maintaining the patient during the long hours required for emergency procedures without prior knowledge of the patient's medical history. After surgery, these patients often require respiratory assistance in the surgical intensive care unit. Repeated surgical procedures are frequently necessary, particularly in open fractures with severe extensive soft tissue injuries.

Cardiac arrest, respiratory failure, and shock demand immediate diagnosis and treatment, which is usually begun at the site of the accident, continued in the emergency stabilization room, and completed in either the operating room or the surgical intensive care unit. As these problems are resolved, determining the nature and severity of head injury is next in priority. In our institution, 75 percent of deaths of multiple trauma patients are due to head injury. In an unconscious patient whose condition has not been diagnosed, with focal neurological signs and increasing intracranial pressure, anesthesia for open fracture treatment is contraindicated. Computed tomography (CT) can usually be performed immediately and a definite diagnosis made a few hours from the time of admission.

Abdominal signs indicative of intra-abdominal injury, such as ruptured spleen, liver, or viscus, can easily be evaluated by means of a carefully done abdominal tap. In our institution, 20 percent of pelvic fractures secondary to vehicular accident are complicated by rupture of the bladder; hence, in such cases cystography is required to rule out a ruptured bladder.

Arterial injury is not uncommonly associated with open or closed fracture or dislocation, particularly in anatomical sites close to the knee, elbow, or hip joint. Any suspicion of circulatory insufficiency demands an emergency arteriogram or exploration of the injured vessels through the open wound during debridement.

When life-threatening problems are identified and surgically correctable, the patient is immediately brought to the operating room after consultation with members of the trauma team, including the anesthesiologist. Often, when the patient is under anesthesia to correct life-threatening problems, the open fractures can be treated at the same time by the orthopedic surgeon or by other trauma team members.

From the Department of Orthopaedic Surgery, Hennepin County Medical Center, Minneapolis, Minnesota.

Recognize life-threatening problems, and do not be in a hurry to bring a patient to surgery because of an open fracture. Open fractures will not kill the patient. We strongly advise that open fractures be taken care of within the first 8 hours, provided that all other emergent life-threatening problems are recognized and resolved.

The second essential feature of open fractures is that there are varying degrees of soft tissue damage and varying severity of bone involvement. It has been shown by Chapman* that the energy levels in open fractures from different mechanisms were as follows:

Mechanism	Energy Level
Fall from a sidewalk	100 ft-lb
Skiing injury	300–500 ft-lb
High-velocity gunshot wound	2000 ft-lb
Bumper injury at 20 mph	100,000 ft-lb

Classification of open fractures, based on the severity of soft tissue and skeletal injuries and the mechanism of injury, is therefore important because it determines the outcome of treatment and usually the course of events that follow. It allows one to prognosticate the eventual outcome with some degree of accuracy.

Third, an open fracture is a *contaminated wound*. Patzakis and co-workers[1] and our studies[3,4] revealed a 60 to 70 percent incidence of bacterial growth in open fracture wounds at the time of admission.

Fourth, open fracture wounds require emergency treatment. It is generally considered that an open fracture wound, if left untreated over an 8-hour period, will probably change from a contaminated wound to an infected wound.

CLASSIFICATION OF OPEN FRACTURES

Open fractures are classified into three major categories, depending on the mechanism of injury, soft tissue damage, and degree of skeletal involvement (Figs. 11–1 to 11–3).

Type I

A Type I open fracture is characterized by a puncture wound 1 cm or less in diameter and is relatively clean. Most likely, the spike of the bone pierces the skin from the inside without

---

*Unpublished data, 1980, San Francisco.

much muscle contusion or other soft tissue involvement and no crushing component. The fracture is usually a simple transverse, short oblique fracture with minimal comminution (Fig. 11–1A,B).

Type II

A Type II open fracture features a laceration more than 1 cm long, without extensive soft tissue damage, flaps, or avulsion, with a minimal to moderate crushing component. The fracture is usually a simple transverse, short oblique fracture with minimal comminution (Fig. 11–2A,B).

Type III

A Type III open fracture is one that involves extensive damage to the soft tissues, including muscle, skin, and neurovascular structures. It is often accompanied by a high-velocity injury or a severe crushing component (Fig. 11–3A–J). Special problems associated with Type III fractures include the following:

1. Open segmental fracture, irrespective of the size of the wound, indicating a high-velocity injury, usually caused by vehicular accident (Fig. 11–3C,D).
2. Gunshot wounds—high-velocity and short-range shotgun injuries (Fig. 11–3E,F).
3. Farm injuries with soil contamination, irrespective of the size of the wound (Fig. 11–3G,H).
4. Open fracture with neurovascular injury (Fig. 11–3I,J).
5. Traumatic amputations (Fig. 11–3K,L).
6. Open fractures over 8 hours old (Fig. 11–3M).
7. Mass casualties, e.g., war and tornado victims.

The Type III open fracture is a very broad classification and encompasses varying degrees of severity, with a wide discrepancy of prognoses and end results. It therefore has been subdivided into three subtypes:

Subtype IIIA. Adequate soft tissue coverage of a fractured bone despite extensive soft tissue laceration or flaps or high-energy trauma irrespective of the size of the wound. This includes segmental fractures or severely comminuted fractures (Fig. 11–3A,B).

Subtype IIIB. Extensive soft tissue loss with periosteal stripping and bony exposure. This is usually associated with massive contamination (Fig. 11–3G,H).

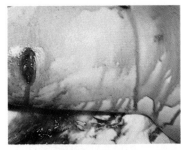
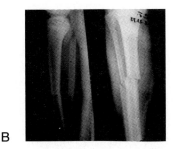

FIGURE 11–1. Type I open fracture. *A,* Small laceration, middle of leg. No crushing component or soil contamination. *B,* X-rays show simple transverse fracture, midshaft of tibia. (From Gustilo RB, ed: Principles of the management of open fractures. In Management of Open Fractures and Their Complications, Vol IV. Philadelphia, WB Saunders Co, 1982, p 21.)

Subtype IIIC. Open fracture associated with arterial injury requiring repair irrespective of degree of soft tissue injury (Fig. 11–3*I, J*).

As our study from 1975 to 1984 shows, (Tables 11–1 and 11–2) the treatment of each subtype varies greatly and the complication rates of wound sepsis, amputation, and nonunion differ significantly.

The type of open fracture considerably influences the plan of treatment and the subsequent course of events as well as the prognosis of the injury.

PRINCIPLES OF TREATMENT

The following principles are essential to the successful treatment of open fractures, in this order:

1. All open fractures treated as an emergency.

2. Thorough initial evaluation to diagnose other life-threatening injuries.

3. Appropriate and adequate antibiotic therapy.

4. Adequate debridement and irrigation.

5. Stabilization of the open fracture.

6. Appropriate wound coverage.

7. Early cancellous bone grafting.

8. Rehabilitation of the involved extremity.

THE OPEN FRACTURE AS A SURGICAL EMERGENCY

The three primary goals in the treatment of open fractures are (1) to prevent wound sepsis, (2) to obtain fracture healing, and (3) to restore normal or optimal function of the injured extremity.

Devitalized and avascular dead muscles provide an environment ideal for bacterial growth. Both conditions—dead muscles and

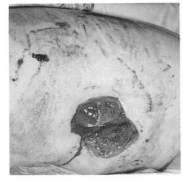
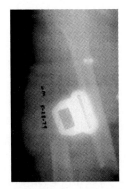

FIGURE 11–2. Type II open fracture. *A,* Open fracture, midshaft of left femur, with 2-inch laceration medially and spike of bone sticking out. *B,* X-ray shows simple transverse fracture, midshaft of left femur. (From Gustilo RB, ed: Principles of the management of open fractures. In Management of Open Fractures and Their Complications, Vol IV. Philadelphia, WB Saunders Co, 1982, p 21.)

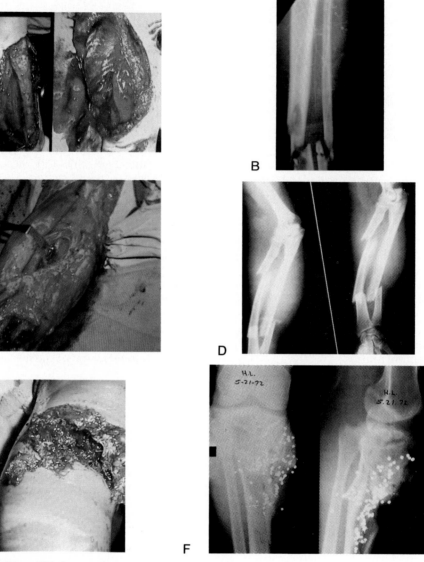

FIGURE 11-3. Type III injury.

A, Extensive soft tissue injury of leg.

B, X-ray shows fracture, lower third of tibia and fibula.

C, Extensive soft tissue injury of arm.

D, X-rays show segmental fracture, radius, and ulna.

E, Shotgun injury at close range with extensive soft tissue injury over proximal tibia.

F, X-rays show comminuted fracture, proximal tibia, with numerous pellets embedded in bone and soft tissues.

G, Farm injury. Extensive soft tissue injury of leg, with hay and dirt embedded in soft tissues and bone.

H, X-rays show comminuted fracture, midshaft of tibia, with free bone fragments.

I, Vascular injury secondary to knee dislocation, with large transverse laceration over upper end of tibia with connection into the joint, and marked instability of the knee joint in all directions.

J, Arteriogram shows complete disruption of the popliteal artery above the bifurcation.

K, Traumatic amputation, upper femur, following a car-motorcycle collision. Extensive soft tissue injury with extension into the rectum and bladder.

L, X-ray of injury in *K* shows severe disruption of symphysis pubis and sacroiliac (Malgaigne fracture).

M, Open fracture, lower third of the tibia, with 3 inches of bone sticking out. Injury is over 10 hours old; wound should be considered infected.

(From Gustilo RB, ed: Principles of the management of open fractures. In Management of Open Fractures and Their Complications, Vol IV. Philadelphia, WB Saunders Co, 1982, pp 21-23.)

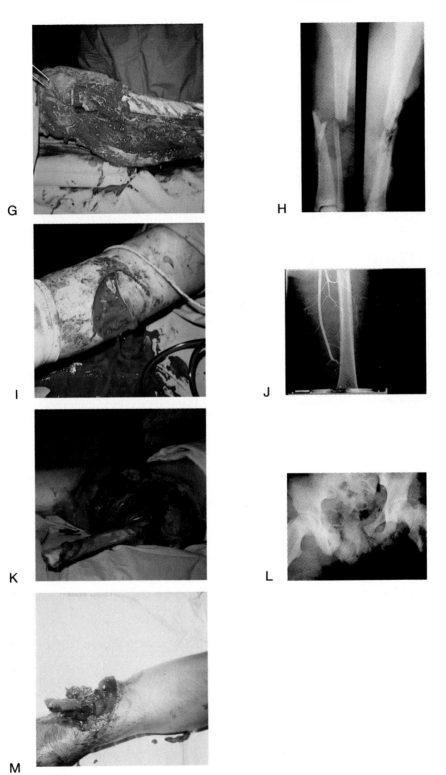

FIGURE 11–3 *Continued*

TABLE 11–1. Sepsis in 1846 Open Fractures: Cumulative Results at Hennepin County Medical Center (1955–1984)

Year	Reference*	Overall	Type I	Type II	Type III
1955–1960	11	11.8			
1961–1968	11	5.2			44
1969–1975	10	2.4	0	1.2	10.2
1976–1979	15	10.1	0	1.8	23.0
1980–1984		4.4	0	2.5	13.7

*References are listed at the end of this chapter.

bacteria—are always present in an open fracture at the onset of injury. It is logical, therefore, to begin treatment of open fractures immediately, if possible, in order to be successful in preventing wound sepsis.

In our hospital, the average time from injury to definitive treatment in the operating room is 3.2 hours. A trauma-designated hospital has to develop an efficient and effective ambulance and emergency room service to facilitate transfer and treatment of an open fracture patient. If one treats an open fracture that is 8 hours old or more, the wound should then be considered an infected one.

LIFE-THREATENING INJURIES IN OPEN FRACTURE PATIENTS

Ninety percent of open fractures are caused by accidents involving vehicles, including motorcycles. Related injuries and, therefore, other life-threatening problems are not uncommonly associated with them. Our evaluation of more than 1000 patients with open fracture at Hennepin County Medical Center, Minneapolis, revealed that *30 percent of open fracture patients had other system injuries.* Therefore, an accurate and thorough examination of the whole patient for other system injuries, especially of the head, neck, chest, abdomen, pelvis, and neurovascular structures, is imperative before treatment of the open fracture is undertaken. One must have clearance from the primary physician, usually the general surgeon in charge of the polytrauma patient in the emergency room, to begin definitive treatment of an open fracture. The surgeon must apprise the anesthesiologist of the patient's problem, including other probable injuries. The following procedures and laboratory examinations are done in the emergency room for open fracture patients on admission:

1. Establishment of two intravenous sites.
2. Chest and skeletal x-rays.
3. Complete blood count and urinalysis.
4. Blood typing and cross-matching.
5. Determination of blood gases and serum creatinine.
6. Determination of serum electrolytes.
7. Other appropriate x-rays and laboratory tests as indicated.

TABLE 11–2. Fracture Type Versus Sepsis, Amputation, and Nonunion (1980–1984)

Type	Total	Sepsis		Amputation		Nonunion	
		No.	PERCENT	No.	PERCENT	No.	PERCENT
I	120	0		0		3	2.5%
II	113	3	2.5%	0		10	8.8%
III	80	11	13.7%	15	18.7%	13/70‡	17.5%
IIIA	40	2	5.0%	1	2.5%	5	12.5%
IIIB	18	8	44.4%	1	5.6%	5	27.7%
IIIC	22	1	4.5%	12* - 3 (25%) 10† - Immediate		3	33.6%
TOTAL	313	14	4.4%	15	4.7%	26/300‡	8.6%

* Artery repaired.
† Immediate amputation at initial treatment.
‡ Less amputation.

The emergency room physician then examines the involved extremity; removes the splint that was applied at the site of the accident; uncovers the wound by removing the sterile dressing, using sterile technique; and, in writing and with sketches, describes the wound in detail — size, skin loss, degree of contamination (presence of foreign material), and exposed bone. A detailed examination of the neurovascular structure must be done at this time. The physician then covers the wound with sterile dressings. The wound must not be uncovered again until the patient is brought to the operating room and examined under sterile technique with gloves and adequate anesthesia prior to definitive treatment. Proper and accurate documentation of the history and physical findings on admission is very important, particularly in a patient with multiple system injuries.

APPROPRIATE AND EFFECTIVE ANTIBIOTIC THERAPY

Patzakis and associates,[1] in a randomized double-blind study of the effectiveness of antibiotic therapy in open fractures, compared placebo, penicillin/streptomycin, and cephalosporin (Keflin). The infection rate was 13 percent with placebo, 9 percent with penicillin/streptomycin, and 2.4 percent with cephalosporin. Rittman[2] noted the effectiveness of prophylaxis with cloxacillin in a double-blind study that showed a decrease of deep wound infection in Type III open fractures. Our previous studies[3, 4] showed an infection rate of 2.4 percent in over 1200 open fractures when appropriate and adequate doses of antibiotic were given for a short period of time. Our antibiotic coverage has changed, based on our analysis of open fractures from 1976 to 1984.

As shown in Table 11 – 3, the bacterial flora in the 1980 – 1984 series reverted back to predominantly gram-positive bacteria (55 percent) in contrast to 80 percent gram-negative in the 1976 – 1979 study. However, in the current series, there is only one infection with pure *Staphylococcus* coagulase-positive infection and 90 percent are either gram-negative or mixed infections.

Based on the bacterial flora in 1976 to 1979, we conducted a randomized prospective study using single cephalosporin versus combined cephalosporin and aminoglycoside in Type III open fractures during the 1980 – 1984 series. With single cephalosporin, the wound sepsis was 29 percent in contrast to 8.8 percent with combined antibiotic therapy; therefore, the study was stopped before the end of 1983.

TABLE 11 – 3. Bacterial Flora of Wound Infections in Type III Open Fractures: Prospective Study (1980 – 1984) Results

	Study Period		
	1980 – 1984	1976 – 1979	1969 – 1975
Staphylococcus coagulase-positive	6*	4	27
Enterococcus	3	3	0
Staphylococcus coagulase negative	3	0	3
Streptococcus viridans	3	0	0
Total gram-positive†	15 (55%)	7 (20%)	30 (64%)
Escherichia coli		5	4
Enterobacter cloacae	1	5	
Enterobacter aerogenes	1	3	
Klebsiella species	1	3	2
Pseudomonas species	7	2	3
Serratia marcescens	3	2	
Proteus morganii		2	
Proteus mirabilis		1	3
Proteus vulgaris		1	
Other (G-rod)		0	1
Total gram-negative†	13 (45%)	24 (80%)	13 (36%)
Negative culture	1	0	5

* There was only one wound infection with pure culture of *Staphylococcus* coagulase-positive. Ninety percent are either gram-negative or mixed infections (gram-positive and gram-negative) bacteria.

† Chi-square for gram-negative versus gram-positive cultures in two time periods is 13.71 with 1 degree of freedom ($P < 0.01$): 1976 – 1979 versus 1969 – 1975.

When we analyzed cases in this study period with combined antibiotic therapy only, our sepsis rate of Type III open fractures was 7.1 percent instead of 13.7 percent for the entire series, which included single-antibiotic therapy.

In the emergency room, we begin with an effective intravenous dose of the appropriate antibiotic. Our choice at the present time is cephalosporin, 2 gm intravenously, followed for 3 days by 1 to 2 gm every 4 to 6 hours, depending on the type of cephalosporin used. Cephalosporin is effective against all gram-positive bacteria and many gram-negative bacteria except *Pseudomonas*. Our bone level studies show that with 2 gm of cephalosporin as an initial dose an effective minimal inhibitory concentration (MIC) is obtained 100 percent of the time and two times more bone concentration in contrast with a 1-gram initial dose of cephalosporin.

In cases involving wounds contaminated by soil, we add 10 to 20 million units of penicillin daily. We also add aminoglycosides, 3 to 5 mg/kg of body weight in divided doses, in patients with Type II and Type III wounds. All antibiotics must be discontinued in 3 days unless the wound becomes infected. In such cases, the infecting bacteria are usually resistant to the antibiotic being given and routine culture and sensitivity studies must be done so that an appropriate alternative antibiotic can be given. If the infection has not been controlled in 3 days, continuing the same antibiotic therapy is not going to be successful. If an infection develops, it is better to know this when the patient is still in the hospital. When giving aminoglycoside therapy, one must be aware of the potential for renal shutdown, particularly in a polytraumatized patient. Careful monitoring of aminoglycoside blood levels and of renal and auditory function is mandatory to prevent nephrotoxic and ototoxic effects.

Antibiotic therapy is restarted for another 3 days under the following conditions:

1. During delayed primary or secondary wound closure.

2. When elective open reduction and internal fixation are performed.

3. When internal or external fixation is changed (for instance, when the external fixation device is discontinued and when an unstable fracture is plated) or when a plate is removed in favor of external fixation.

TETANUS PROPHYLAXIS[5]

Tetanus prophylaxis is indicated in all open fractures following the guidelines proposed in Table 11-4.

DEBRIDEMENT AND IRRIGATION (FIG. 11-4)

The patient is brought to the operating room, the wound still covered with the sterile

TABLE 11-4. Tetanus Prophylaxis in Open Fractures

Immunization Data	Action to Be Taken
Immunization completed previously; last booster within 1 year	None
Immunization completed within the previous 10-years; no subsequent booster dose	0.5 ml of tetanus and diphtheria toxoid, adult type (Td).
Immunization completed more than 10 years previously; last booster within the previous 10 years	0.5 ml of Td
Immunization completed more than 10 years previously; no booster within the previous 10 years; wound minor and relatively clean, treated promptly and adequately	0.5 ml of Td
Immunization completed more than 10 years previously; no booster within the previous five years; wound other than minor and clean and/or not minor and clean and/or not treated promptly	0.5 ml of Td and 250 to 500 units of human tetanus immune globulin (TIG[H]); 500 units if wound is clostridia prone, otherwise 250 units; give Td and TIG(H) by separate syringes and needles at separate sites
No history or record of immunization; wound minor and clean; wound surgery prompt and adequate	Begin immunization program with 0.5 ml of Td; schedule further immunization
No record of immunization; wound other than clean and/or treated promptly and adequately	250 units of human tetanus immune globulin (TIG[H]); begin immunization with 0.5 ml of Td
	Give 500 units of TIG(H) if wound is prone to *Clostridium*; otherwise give 250 units; give Td and TIG(H) by separate syringes and needles at separate sites

dressing applied in the emergency room. The anesthesiologist has examined the patient and given either regional or general anesthesia.

During elective open reduction and internal fixation of fractures, the principles of aseptic technique are strictly observed. A tourniquet is applied but not used unless there is severe arterial bleeding. The wounds are then uncovered under aseptic conditions, with the surgeon using mask and gloves. Samples for cultures are taken from the depth of the wound in Type II and Type III open fractures. The leg is elevated, washed and scrubbed with either pHisoHex and Betadine soap, and painted with Betadine solution around the edges of the wound but not in the wound. In a patient with farm injuries, one usually uses a brush to remove the dirt, hay, and other embedded materials from the soft tissues and bone of the involved extremity. The extremity is draped free in the usual manner.

Adequate debridement is the most important step in the treatment of open fracture. Debridement must be systematic, complete, and meticulous and it must be repeated. Intermittent pressure lavage must be used to deliver irrigating fluids in Type II and Type III open fractures (Fig. 11–5).

Debridement entails the removal of nonviable and devitalized tissues. To accomplish adequate debridement, the surgeon must not hesitate to extend the wound or give it an elliptical shape in order to remove dead skin, muscles, or foreign bodies. Exposure, however, must be lengthwise in order to facilitate internal fixation if that is needed to achieve fracture stability.

Structures to Be Debrided

The following structures are to be debrided:

- Skin
- Fascia and tendon
- Muscles
- Bones

SKIN

When debriding skin, be conservative but be certain to remove all nonviable and mutilated or macerated skin. Small wounds in Type I and Type II open fractures are elliptically enlarged, with dead or frayed skin edges excised. Skin circulation can be determined by skin color (pink versus pale or black); if in doubt, perform a tourniquet test. If the color remains pale during release of the tourniquet without a flush of initial pink or red, most likely that skin is dead. Obviously, when a margin of the skin is cut and does not bleed, it is dead or its circulation is impaired. A fluorescein test is occasionally used by the plastic surgeon to determine the viability of the skin. Fluorescein dye (1 to 2 gm in the adult) is injected intravenously. If there is no diffusion of dye to the skin as detected by a Wood's lamp, the skin is nonviable.

FASCIA AND TENDON

Fasciae are expendable. Excise contaminated and devitalized fascia completely without fear of causing a residual functional deficit. Paratenon contains the main blood supply of the tendon and must be preserved to maintain tendon viability. If excised or destroyed, exposed tendon will not survive for long. Early skin coverage, such as skin graft, primary closure, or muscle or skin flap, is necessary to preserve its viability.

MUSCLES

Scully and colleagues,[6] in an excellent clinical and histological study, determined four criteria of muscle viability:

1. *Consistency.* Live muscle is firm and resilient. A dead muscle picked up with forceps is seen to be friable and easily fragmented, lacking the firm and elastic consistency of a live muscle. If the muscle is severely crushed or infected, it is mushy and disintegrates easily.

2. *Contractility.* Live muscles will contract or retract or pull away when cut, pinched, or stimulated under low-power coagulation.

3. *Ability to bleed.* Live muscles will bleed when cut, but bleeding from muscles must be distinguished from bleeding from small arterioles or veins within the muscles or under muscle groups. Persistent oozing from the muscles indicates muscle viability.

4. *Color.* Proper lighting is needed for accurate recognition of color. With poor lighting, the color of even a viable muscle can look dark rather than pink or bright red. Therefore, be sure to have good lighting when debriding. Jet lavage can easily remove the blood clots overlying muscles that can give them a dark appearance instead of their normal red color.

Obviously, all foreign materials, particularly organic foreign bodies, must be removed if possible. Farm materials, such as hay, dirty clothing, and gunshot wadding, have to be removed meticulously. Gun pellets or bullets

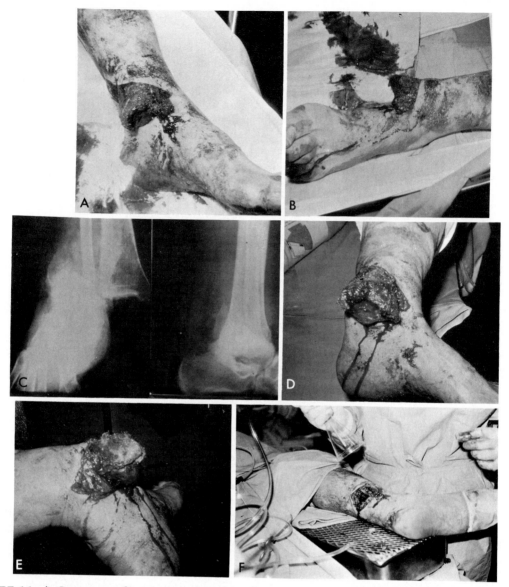

FIGURE 11–4. Sequence of treatment of an open fracture. Emergency treatment of the wound at the accident site includes covering the wound with sterile dressing, assessing neurovascular status, and splinting the fracture.

A, B, In the hospital emergency room the wound is uncovered, revealing a large laceration anteromedially over the lower leg, with the distal tibia at the ankle joint protruding out of the wound. The neurovascular status is determined, the extent of wound injury is illustrated on the chart, and antibiotics and tetanus prophylaxis are given.

C, X-rays show bimalleolar fracture dislocation of ankle joint.

D, E, In the operating room, with the patient under general anesthesia, the wound is uncovered again and examined with mask and gloves.

F, G, Adequate debridement of devitalized tissues, removal of foreign bodies, and copious irrigation are done with the aid of jet lavage, particularly in Type II and Type III open fractures.

H, After adequate debridement and irrigation, the wound and bone appear clean and vascular.

I, The protruding bone is inserted back inside the wound, and the intra-articular fractures are fixed with screws to secure fracture stability.

J, K, The wound is left open, then closed in three to five days in the absence of infection and without tension.

L, One year later, the wound and fractures have healed without sepsis or osteomyelitis. Notice again the internal fixation as shown in *I,* right.

(From Gustilo RB, ed: Principles of the management of open fractures. In Management of Open Fractures and Their Complications, Vol IV. Philadelphia, WB Saunders Co, 1982, pp 24–25.)

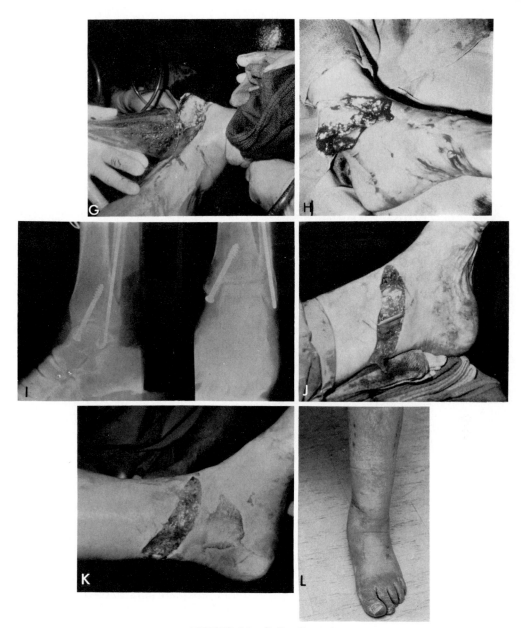

FIGURE 11–4 *Continued*

need not be removed unless they are causing pressure to vital structures or are intra-articular in location.

BONES

Small, free, devitalized cortical bone fragments should be removed. On the other hand, large bone fragments, even if completely devitalized, should be retained if they provide stability. Obviously, any bone fragment with a vascular soft tissue connection must be gently cleansed to preserve vascularity, debrided, and retained. Any free cancellous bone, if not dirty or contaminated, should be returned or preserved for possible use as a bone graft. Large bone fragments or whole segments of bone taken from the side wall must be discarded.

Fractured bone ends must be exposed so that any foreign materials, such as dirt, clothing, or other contaminated material, can be curetted out or removed. The use of jet lavage

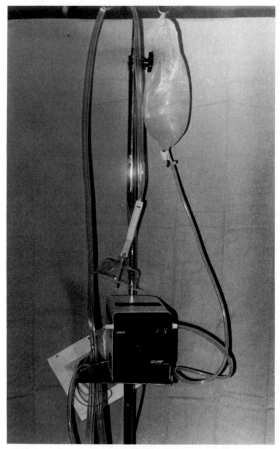

FIGURE 11–5. Intermittent pressure lavage—to be used routinely for all Type II and Type III open fractures during debridement and irrigation.

during the debridement process is helpful and effective in cleansing bone of embedded foreign material.

We recommend 1000 to 2000 ml of irrigating solution initially for Type I wounds and at least 5000 to 10,000 ml for Type II and Type III wounds, using normal saline solution or distilled water. For final irrigation, we usually use 2000 ml of a mixture of bacitracin and polymyxin in solution.

Amputation

EARLY AMPUTATION

When to amputate a severely mangled or crushed limb is a difficult decision. An early or even an immediate decision to amputate an injured limb at the time of initial debridement can save prolonged agony and expense of both the patient and the surgeon. Acceptance of the inevitable loss of the limb tends to be better initially than a few days or weeks later, when the patient has had a chance to form a mental reattachment to the limb (Fig. 11–6).

INDICATIONS FOR AMPUTATION

A limb should be amputated under these conditions:

1. There is complete loss of the neurovascular system, with severe crushing of both muscles and skin (e.g., farm injuries) (Fig. 11–7).

2. The neurovascular system is intact but with such severe muscular deficit and bone loss that reasonable function is unlikely (Fig. 11–8).

3. The vascular system is intact or damaged blood vessels may even be amenable to repair, but there is complete loss of movement and sensation in the injured limb without a possibility of primary or secondary nerve repair (Fig. 11–9).

Open Joint Injuries

An open fracture entering into the joint, or an open joint injury without a fracture, demands arthrotomy and cleansing of the joint. The wound incision must be large to facilitate exposure and thorough inspection of the joint for any foreign body. If one is dealing with a puncture wound and is not sure whether the joint has been penetrated or not, an arthrogram may be done and will show any connection of the wound with the joint by spillage of the dye into the entrance wound.

Debridement and irrigation must be repeated under adequate anesthesia during the next 24 to 48 hours and daily, if needed, for all Type III open fractures and a majority of Type II open fractures. It is our experience that in most instances one cannot do an adequate debridement at initial surgery, particularly for Type III open fractures, for two reasons:

1. Even for an experienced surgeon, it is difficult to recognize varying degrees of tissue viability.

2. Tissue that appears to be viable at first debridement and irrigation may become nonviable in 24 to 48 hours because of circulatory insufficiency from a crushing component, or circulatory deficit at either a microcirculatory or a macrocirculatory level. *When there is arterial injury, repair with interposition graft (not direct anastomosis) is accomplished within 4 to 6*

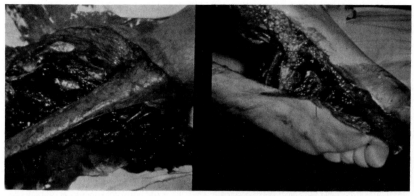

FIGURE 11–6. Decide on early amputation. (From Gustilo RB, ed: Principles of the management of open fractures. In Management of Open Fractures and Their Complications, Vol IV. Philadelphia, WB Saunders Co, 1982, p 30.)

hours. Adequate compartmental fasciotomies must be done at all times following an arterial repair in open fractures. It is mandatory to perform debridement again within 12 to 24 hours. Almost always, more necrotic muscles are found during the second debridement that were not recognized before. Two to 3 days later, it is too late for debridement to be effective; usually an infection has already developed.

STABILIZATION OF THE OPEN FRACTURE

Just as important as debridement and irrigation in the management of open fracture is achieving *fracture stability* (Fig. 11–10). Stable fracture fixation accomplishes the following:

1. Preserves the integrity of the remaining viable soft tissues, muscles, and neurovascular structures.

2. Facilitates the care of the wound as well as of the whole patient. At least one daily dressing is required for a Type III wound.

3. Preserves fracture alignment during manipulation or change of position of the extremity during dressing changes or repeated surgical procedures. Experimental studies by Rittman and Perren[7] and Friedrich and Klaue[8] have shown that stable fixation is a major contributor to prophylaxis against infection. Gristina and Rovere[9] reported in an *in vitro* study

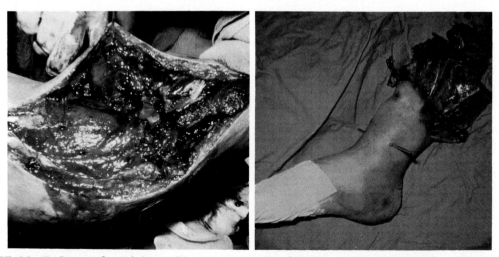

FIGURE 11–7. Severe farm injury with complete loss of the neurovascular system, requiring open amputation and delayed closure. (From Gustilo RB, ed: Principles of the management of open fractures. In Management of Open Fractures and Their Complications, Vol IV. Philadelphia, WB Saunders Co, 1982, p 30.)

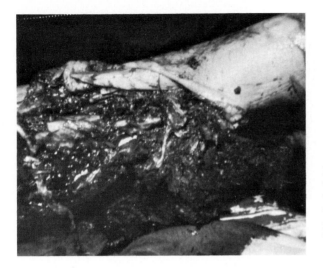

FIGURE 11–8. Intact neurovascular system, but with such severe muscular deficit and bone loss that reasonable function is unlikely. (From Gustilo RB, ed: Principles of the management of open fractures. In Management of Open Fractures and Their Complications, Vol IV. Philadelphia, WB Saunders Co, 1982, p 31.)

that metal itself does not promote bacterial growth and dissemination. Chapman and Mahoney[10] reported no increased incidence of infection following early internal fixation of Type III open fractures. Our preliminary studies during the past few years support this finding.

4. Provides greater ease and comfort to the patient during mobilization and transfer. Since 25 percent of these patients are multiple trauma victims, they require early and frequent mobilization to avoid respiratory problems. These patients also require frequent transfer into and out of the operating room or

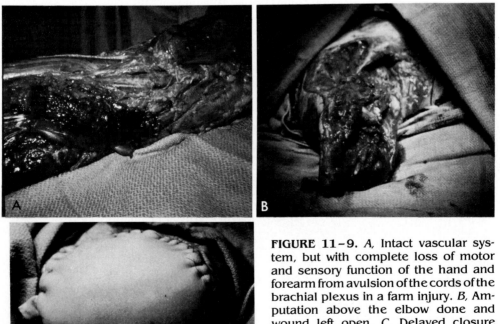

FIGURE 11–9. A, Intact vascular system, but with complete loss of motor and sensory function of the hand and forearm from avulsion of the cords of the brachial plexus in a farm injury. B, Amputation above the elbow done and wound left open. C, Delayed closure done without tension. (From Gustilo RB, ed: Principles of the management of open fractures. In Management of Open Fractures and Their Complications, Vol IV. Philadelphia, WB Saunders Co, 1982, p 31.)

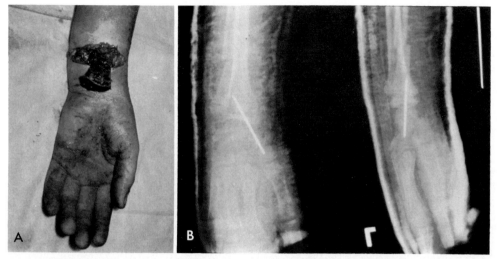

FIGURE 11 – 10. Stabilization of open fracture. *A,* Type II open fracture of the distal radius (Salter Type II) with distal radius protruding from the wound. *B,* After thorough debridement and irrigation, fracture stability is achieved by Kirschner wire fixation and application of anterior-posterior plaster splints. (From Gustilo RB, ed: Principles of the management of open fractures. In Management of Open Fractures and Their Complications, Vol IV. Philadelphia, WB Saunders Co, 1982, p 32.)

other diagnostic facilities. Fracture stability facilitates this total care.

5. Allows an isometric muscle exercise program and early joint motion, both active and passive, above and below the fracture site.

The general guiding principle is this: Choose the simplest method that provides fracture stability, allows access to and care of the wound, and preserves the integrity of the remaining viable soft tissue.

Plaster Immobilization

A plaster splint is indicated for stable Type I and Type II open fractures for the first 7 to 10 days (see Fig. 11 – 11). This splint allows inspection and care of the wound with ease and prevents circular compression in a traumatized limb. It is easy to apply, and, obviously, no additional trauma is needed. I repeat, however, that it is indicated only in stable Type I and Type II open fractures, usually when no additional procedure or care of the wound is required and post-injury swelling and treatment are no longer expected. Immediate application of a circular plaster cast after adequate debridement and irrigation is rarely indicated, and then only in a Type I open fracture with very minimal crushing components. The fracture must be stable and enough compression wadding can be applied to allow for

the swelling. If the fracture is unstable, external fixation or unreamed intramedullary nailing, provided fracture stability can be achieved, is the treatment method of choice.

Note: I believe there is no place for the immediate application of a walking plaster cast in open fractures. *Immediate application of a circular cast to an open fracture must be avoided if possible.*

Pins and Plaster Immobilization

During the initial debridement and irrigation, if the fracture is unstable and tends to angulate or shorten, pins and plaster immobilization may be used for Type I and Type II open fractures. A window can be made either at this time or a few days later to inspect the wound. The plaster window has to be placed back to prevent swelling; otherwise, the soft tissue around the wound herniates at the window margin, producing a constricting effect and further increasing the swelling. Serious problems may result. A transfixing Steinmann pin may be inserted obliquely across the fracture to maintain reduction during surgery and is removed after pins and a plaster cast have been applied. *Note: At the present time, if immobilization with pins and plaster is indicated, our choice would be an external fixation device.*

Skeletal Traction

Skeletal traction (Fig. 11–12) is indicated under the following conditions:

Isolated Type I and Type II. Femoral shaft fractures with no other system injuries: The wound is allowed to heal, followed by closed nailing or other definitive means of internal fixation in 10 days to 2 weeks. Closed nailing would be preferred to an open procedure. The other alternative (not my choice) is continued traction followed by cast bracing or spica cast treatment.

Isolated Type III. Open fractures of long bones (femur, tibia, and distal humerus) with a severely contaminated wound, such as a farm injury: Skeletal traction may be applied to provide temporary nonrigid immobilization for

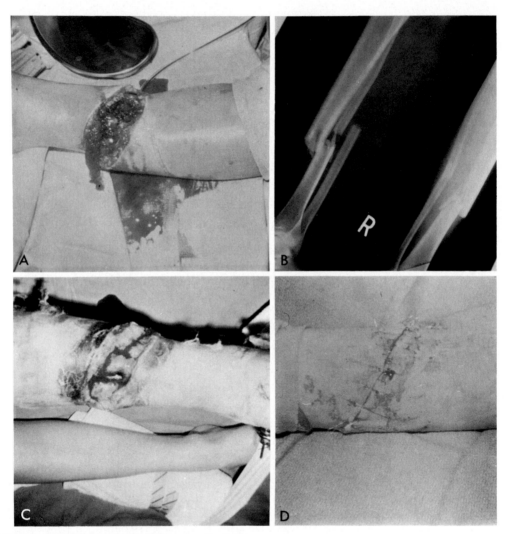

FIGURE 11–11. Cast treatment for open fracture.

A, Type II open fracture of lower leg with transverse laceration.

B, X-ray shows slightly comminuted transverse fracture, lower third of tibia.

C, Debridement and irrigation performed, wound left open, and wound dressed daily with 0.025 percent silver nitrate.

D, Delayed primary closure after 5 days.

E, Left and center, Cast applied after removal of sutures. *Right,* Six months later, fracture healed.

F, G, One year later, fracture has healed completely with no sepsis and the leg is restored to normal function.

(From Gustilo RB, ed: Principles of the management of open fractures. In Management of Open Fractures and Their Complications, Vol IV. Philadelphia, WB Saunders Co, 1982, pp 33–34.)

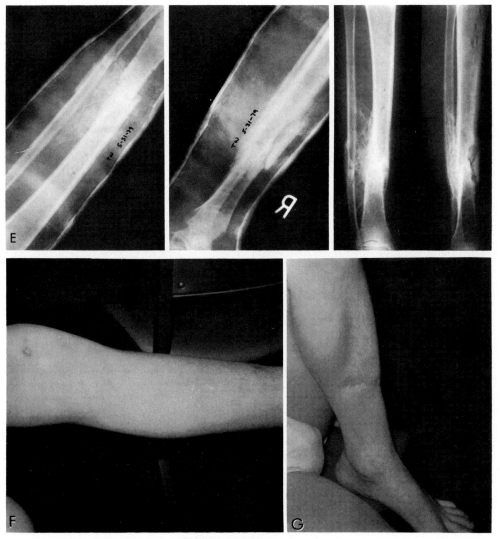

FIGURE 11–11 *Continued*

the first 3 to 5 days: The wound is debrided and left open, but the surgeon believes that debridement has not been adequate to allow application of a stabilizing internal fixation device. The extremity is therefore hung up in traction and debrided again; then, adequate stable internal fixation can be accomplished.

Note: Again, our choice for Type III open fractures of the tibia or humerus in which traction is indicated would be the use of an external fixation device.

Isolated Arterial Injury. Open fracture, particularly when there is a delay of over 6 hours prior to arterial repair: Skeletal traction may be used as a temporary stabilization treatment after repair of artery and vein in the following conditions:

1. An open supracondylar fracture with popliteal artery injury.
2. An upper femur fracture with femoral artery injury.
3. A humeral fracture with axillary or brachial artery injury.

Internal fixation is my preferred method of securing fracture stability in these cases.

Isolated Type II or Type III. Open fractures with severely comminuted intra-articular fractures, such as:

1. A T intercondylar fracture of the elbow.
2. A comminuted knee joint fracture.
3. A bursting fracture of the ankle.
4. An open pelvic or acetabular fracture.

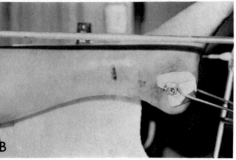

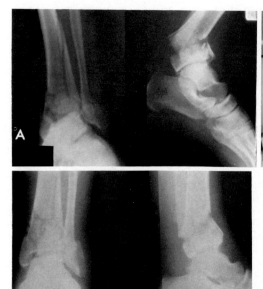

FIGURE 11-12. Skeletal traction. *A,* Open bursting fracture — Type III. Antero-posterior and lateral projections show comminution of the distal ankle. *B,* Calcaneal skeletal traction applied. *C,* Post-traction x-rays reveal satisfactory alignment of the fracture. (From Gustilo RB, ed: Principles of the management of open fractures. In Management of Open Fractures and Their Complications, Vol IV. Philadelphia, WB Saunders Co, 1982, p 35.)

A preliminary skeletal traction accomplishes the following:

1. Reduces the swelling in 3 to 5 days.
2. Possibly reduces the fracture.
3. Helps in identifying fracture fragments and determining their number and size; helps in decision-making and planning of delayed open reduction and internal fixation.

For these problem fractures above, open reduction and internal fixation can be accomplished under ideal conditions which include careful planning, expert surgical personnel, and satisfactory local wound conditions.

Use of Fracture Fixation Devices

INDICATIONS

Rigid fracture fixation with use of devices is indicated in the following injuries:

1. *Multiple trauma,* where primary internal fixation of open fractures allows for early immobilization, ease of transfer, and care of patients during frequent diagnostic and therapeutic procedures, better nursing care, and prevention of shock lung.
2. *Massive and mutilating soft tissue injury requiring repeated surgical procedures.* Stable internal fixation is an important factor for limb salvage in order to take adequate care of soft tissue injuries.
3. *Floating extremity* (ipsilateral fracture of

femur and tibia), including ligamentous knee instability, occasionally associated with displaced acetabular fractures.

4. *Arterial injury requiring repair.* In an isolated arterial injury, traction may be used instead of primary internal fixation for 4 to 6 weeks. A decision is then made as to whether to continue traction until the fracture is healed or to employ spica cast treatment, cast bracing, or delayed open reduction and internal fixation to achieve fracture stability.

5. *Intra-articular fractures.* Joint congruency must be restored by internal fixation followed by early mobilization. Open joint injury may be left open, then closed in 3 to 5 days.

CHOICE OF IMPLANTS

The choice of fracture devices is governed by these principles:

1. Choose the one that produces the least additional tissue trauma.
2. Incorporate the metallic implant without compromising the stability and viability of the fracture fragments and without compromising the circulation of the involved extremity.

The following devices are given in their order of preference.

Screws. Screws are the preferred method of internal fixation if enough stability can be provided (Fig. 11-13). Usually, however, because

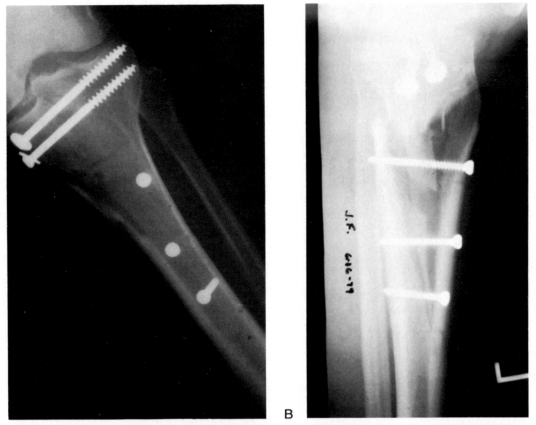

A   B

FIGURE 11–13. Use of screws to achieve fracture stability. *A, B,* Stability is achieved by multiple screw fixation, with minimal wound trauma and dissection. (From Gustilo RB, ed: Principles of the management of open fractures. In Management of Open Fractures and Their Complications, Vol IV. Philadelphia, WB Saunders Co, 1982, p 37.)

of the complexity of the fracture, particularly in Type III open fractures, screw fixation is not sufficient. Screw fixation is limited primarily to articular and metaphyseal fractures.

External Fixation Devices. These offer an advantage in cases of extensive soft tissue involvement in that the pins can be implanted away from the fracture site and render fracture stability. The use of half pins is oftentimes adequate for fracture stabilization. Rarely, one has to incorporate interfragmentary fixation, using screws or even plates, with external fixation (Fig. 11–14). The external fixation device may be removed as soon as the soft tissue problem has been resolved and enough fracture stability has developed for continued cast immobilization or continue with external fixation treatment until the fracture is healed.

Plate and Screws. Together these give better stability than any other type of fixation. However, infection is higher when compared

to external fixation or unreamed nailing. Plating is only indicated in intra-articular and metaphyseal open fractures. Ideally, it should be placed in an area where soft tissue coverage is available. Otherwise, local flaps or free vascularized muscle transfer is needed to cover the plate (Fig. 11–15).

Intramedullary Fixation. Reamed intramedullary fixation is contraindicated in Type II and Type III injuries because it destroys the intramedullary circulation in an environment where there is already compromised periosteal and muscular circulation, particularly in the tibia. In a floating knee, when there is a concomitant open fracture of both the femur and the tibia, unreamed intramedullary nailing of the femur may be done for Type I and Type II fractures (Fig. 11–16). Intramedullary nailing with reaming can be accomplished as an elective procedure when the soft tissue wound has healed, in 3 to 6 weeks.

WOUND COVERAGE

Wound coverage in open fractures has always been the subject of controversy between those who advocate primary closure and those who favor delayed primary or secondary closure.[3, 6-8, 11-13] Our study[3] relating the incidence of infection to types of open fracture, primary closure, and delayed secondary closure leads us to conclude that primary closure may be accomplished in Type I fractures without increased incidence of infection. *However, our study of gas gangrene cases sent to our institution, following Type I open fractures, revealed 80 percent primary closure of the open wound. The safe approach would be to leave the wound open.*

Primary Closure in Open Fractures

The indications for primary closure (Fig. 11–17) are rare and only for these conditions:

1. Type I open fracture wounds only, after *adequate debridement* and irrigation have been done.

2. Wound closure can be accomplished without tension.

3. No evidence of soil contamination or crushing component.

4. The open fracture wound has not been left open for more than 8 hours.

In my opinion, *a surgeon who only occasionally manages an open fracture wound should leave all wounds open and perform a delayed primary closure. If it is not certain that adequate debridement and irrigation have been done, the wound should be left open.* The incidence of infection following primary closure in Type I open fractures without the use of early metallic fixation has been less than 1 percent in our experience. In all types of open fractures, when open reduction and primary internal fixation are performed to stabilize the fracture, particularly in a polytrauma patient, then the *wound must be left open* and delayed primary closure must be done.

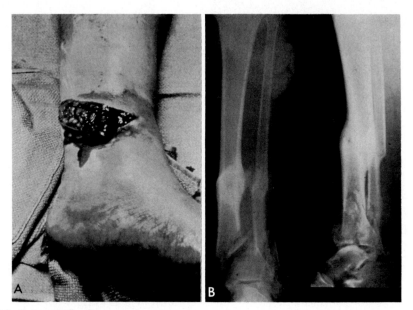

FIGURE 11–14. External fixation.

A, Type III open fracture of the lower tibia. Patient was found in a sewer more than 12 hours following injury.

B, X-ray showed comminuted fracture of the lower third of the tibia with intra-articular involvement.

C, External fixator applied after adequate debridement and irrigation; wound left open; fracture fixed with screws and Kirschner wires.

D, Delayed primary closure without tension.

E, X-ray shows fracture in good alignment held in place by screws and external fixation. External fixation device removed in 8 weeks.

F, G, One year later, fracture healed; good foot and ankle motion.

(From Gustilo RB, ed: Principles of the management of open fractures. In Management of Open Fractures and Their Complications, Vol IV. Philadelphia, WB Saunders Co, 1982, p 39.)

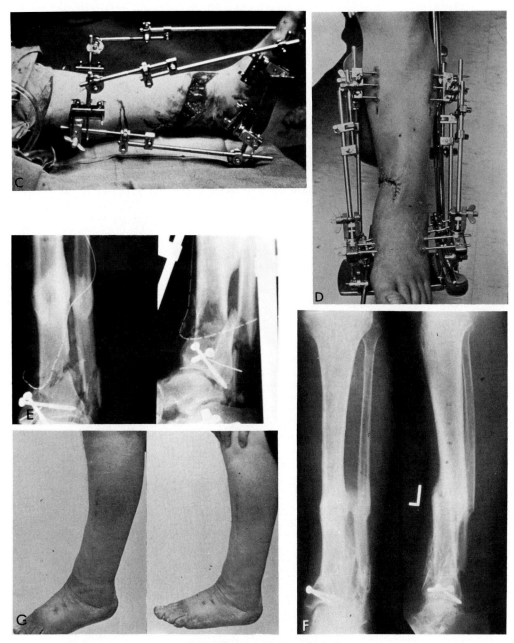

FIGURE 11–14 *Continued*

Delayed Primary Closure

Delayed primary closure is defined as closure of an open fracture wound in 3 to 10 days, either with or without early appearance of granulation tissue. First, a clinical decision has to be made that indeed there is no infection. The wound looks healthy, with or without early granulation either by direct skin suture or by delayed primary skin graft. There is no indication for primary skin grafting in any open fracture wounds, except probably hand injuries. Delayed primary closure has to be accomplished without tension; if there is tension, either a relaxing type incision or a primary split-thickness skin graft must be done (Fig.

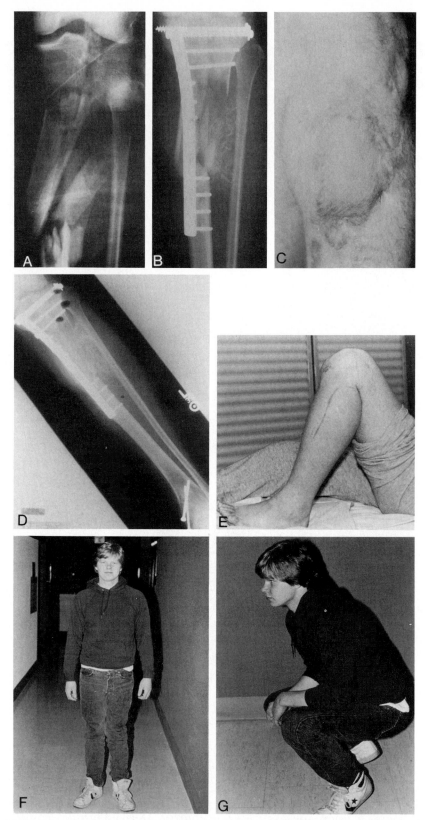

FIGURE 11 – 15. Plating intra-articular and metaphyseal fracture of proximal tibia to achieve fracture stability.

   A, Anteroposterior (AP) x-rays showed severely comminuted intra-articular and metaphyseal fracture of proximal tibia (Type IIIB). There was severe soft tissue, and bone was exposed.

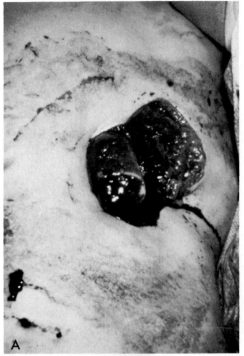

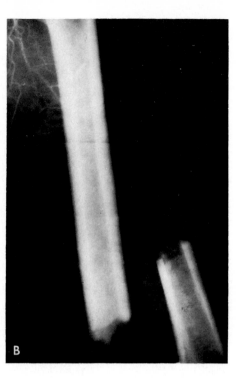

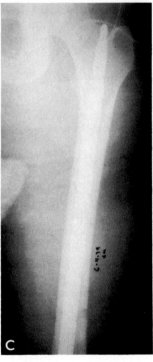

FIGURE 11–16. *A,* Type II wound: open fracture of the femur. *B,* Anteroposterior x-ray shows displaced transverse fracture of the midshaft of the femur. *C,* Primary nailing done and wound left open. Patient also had a severe Type III open fracture of the proximal tibia on the same side. (From Gustilo RB, ed: Principles of the management of open fractures. In Management of Open Fractures and Their Complications, Vol IV. Philadelphia, WB Saunders Co, 1982, p 45.)

FIGURE 11–15 *Continued*

B, After adequate debridement and irrigation, the plate was applied to achieve fracture stability (AP x-rays). The wound was left open.

C, Localized gastrocnemius flap to cover plate was done 5 days later. Six weeks after injury, the wound has nicely healed.

D, Autogenous cancellous bone grafting was done 6 weeks after wound coverage, through a separate posterolateral incision (AP x-rays).

E, F, Five months later, the fracture has completely healed.

G, The patient has regained normal motion and function of the knee.

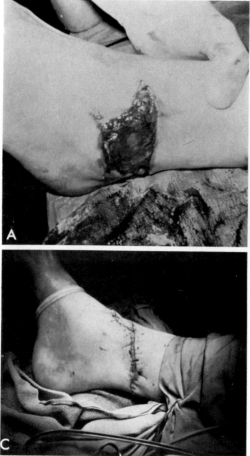

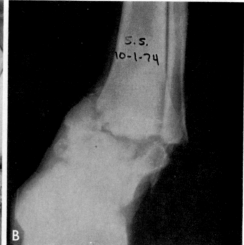

FIGURE 11–17. Primary closure for Type I and occasional Type II open fractures. *A,* Type II open fracture of the lower tibia with a 1½-inch laceration. *B,* X-rays show slightly comminuted displaced fracture of the lower end of the tibia. *C,* Following *adequate debridement and irrigation* of open fracture, the wound closed with interrupted sutures 5 days later *(never continuous)* and *without* tension. (From Gustilo RB, ed: Principles of the management of open fractures. In Management of Open Fractures and Their Complications, Vol IV. Philadelphia, WB Saunders Co, 1982, p 46.)

11–18). Occasionally, with a large area of exposed bone or bone loss, a cross-leg flap (Fig. 11–19) or free vascular bone–muscle composite transfer can be done. Our study indicates that wound closure must be accomplished in 5 to 10 days by whatever method to reduce wound sepsis.

To repeat:

1. Delayed primary closure, secondary closure by skin graft, or healing by secondary intention or by localized muscle flap or free vascular muscle transfer is indicated in all Type II and Type III open fractures. Meshed skin graft is extensively used in open fractures with extensive soft tissue loss (Fig. 11–20).

2. In any type of open fracture, if primary or early open reduction and internal fixation with metal is performed, *the wound must be left open* and secondarily closed.

CANCELLOUS BONE GRAFTING IN OPEN FRACTURE

From 1974 to 1977, Anderson and Gustilo[14] conducted a study of 109 open fractures of the tibia with extensive soft tissue injury at Hennepin County Medical Center with the following objectives:

1. To assess soft tissue management.
2. To assess fracture management.
3. To evaluate the temporary relationship between soft tissue and fracture management and eventual healing in the hope of coordinating the total care of the patient and minimizing the time required for complete healing of both soft tissue and bone.

The conclusions drawn from this review are as follows:

1. In Type III open fractures of the tibia

associated with extensive soft tissue loss, a large area of exposed bone, severe fracture comminution, and bone loss, there was a non-union rate of 60 percent.

2. These injuries are severe, with a high rate of infection regardless of the method of treatment employed, although eventually all our patients achieved soft tissue coverage and bone union. The time involved was frequently significant. The average time for complete soft tissue healing was 3 months and for complete fracture healing, 12 months.

3. In patients who received bone graft, the average time of bone grafting was 7 months

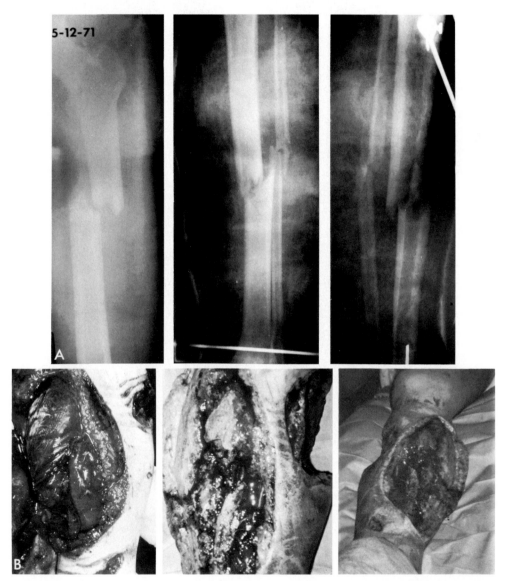

FIGURE 11–18. Wound closure by split-thickness skin graft. *A,* Open fracture of the left tibia and severe soft tissue injury (Type III) in a 22-year-old man involved in a vehicle accident. The patient also had a closed fracture of the left femur. *B,* Left, extensive soft tissue injury on admission. Middle and right, 5 and 10 days later, following debridement and irrigation. *C,* Left, split-thickness skin graft. Middle and right, wound healed a year later. *D,* X-rays of both femur and tibia 4 months later show healed fractures. There is normal function of the left lower extremity. (From Gustilo RB, ed: Principles of the management of open fractures. In Management of Open Fractures and Their Complications, Vol IV. Philadelphia, WB Saunders Co, 1982, pp 47–48.)

Illustration continued on following page

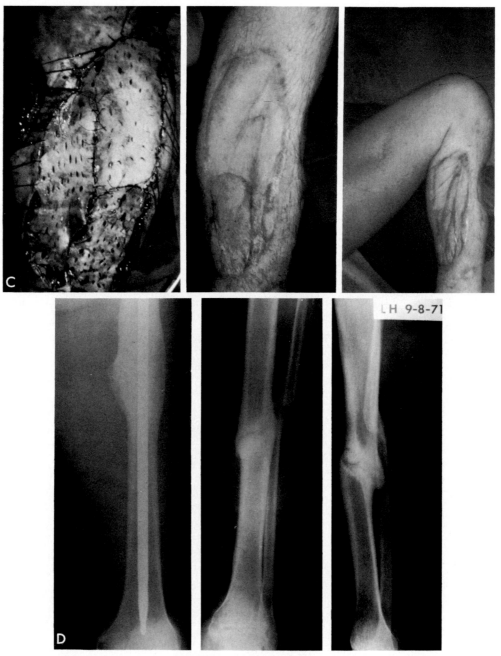

FIGURE 11-18 *Continued*

after injury, the earliest being at 5 months. This finding made it clear that a delay existed between soft tissue coverage and aggressive treatment directed towards fracture healing in fractures that did not consolidate within 6 to 9 months following injury.

We looked for early, reliable, predictive factors in the stages of fracture healing. Since soft tissue healed at an average of 6 weeks, we analyzed the x-ray appearance of the fracture at that time in all patients. The absence of callus, visible on x-ray films 3 months after injury, uniformly indicated delayed or nonunion. Therefore, early cancellous bone grafting is recommended for patients with extensive soft tissue injury, great exposure of bone, bone

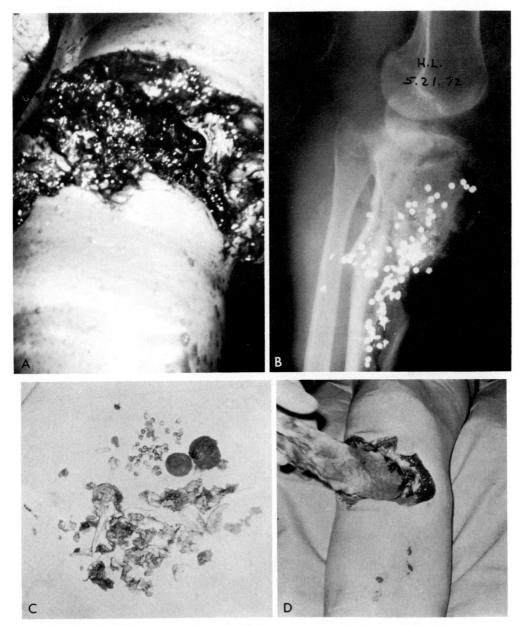

FIGURE 11–19. Wound coverage by cross-leg flap.

A, Gunshot injury (short range) over proximal tibia, causing extensive tissue injury and bone loss.

B, X-ray shows comminuted open fracture involving about 3 inches of proximal tibia, and numerous pellets.

C, Adequate debridement and irrigation done; wadding and pellets meticulously removed.

D, Large cavity packed with wet dressing.

E, Ten days later, cavity filled with cancellous bone.

F, G, Anteroposterior (AP) and lateral projections show bone defect filled with cancellous bone graft.

H, One week later, cross leg flap graft performed.

I, Three years later, AP and lateral projection show fracture completely healed.

J, K, Follow-up examination 3 years later shows that patient has full extension and 115 degrees flexion.

(From Gustilo RB, ed: Principles of the management of open fractures. In Management of Open Fractures and Their Complications, Vol IV. Philadelphia, WB Saunders Co, 1982, pp 47–51.)

Illustration continued on following page

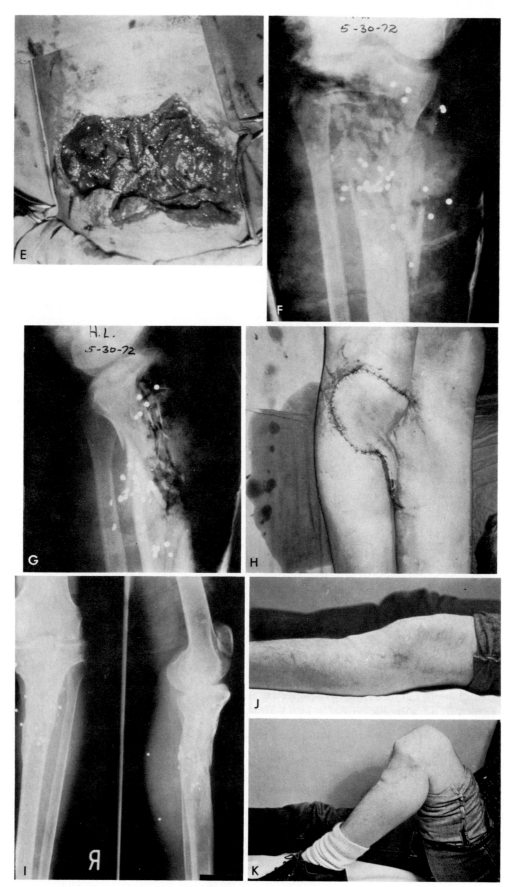

FIGURE 11–19 *Continued*

loss, and no x-ray evidence of callus formation at the end of 3 months, provided the following conditions are present:

- No active or florid infection
- Early or good granulation tissue
- Achievement of fracture stability

Following cancellous grafting, the wound may be left open and granulation tissue may be allowed to develop over it, followed by split-thickness skin grafting or healing by secondary intention.

What are the indications of bone grafting in open fractures?

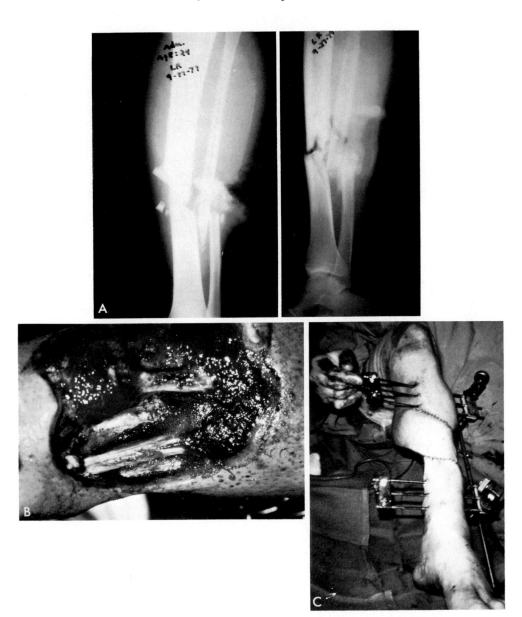

FIGURE 11–20. Use of myocutaneous flap to cover defect.

  A, Anteroposterior (AP) and lateral X-rays show severe open comminuted fracture of the midshaft of the tibia, with extensive soft tissue injury.

  B, Granulated wound with exposed tendon, bone, and muscles.

  C, Myocutaneous flap to cover large defect.

  D, Meshed graft to cover wound posteriorly.

  E, Fracture stabilized with external fixation device, and the butterfly fragment with circlage wire.

  (From Gustilo RB, ed: Principles of the management of open fractures. In Management of Open Fractures and Their Complications, Vol IV. Philadelphia, WB Saunders Co, 1982, pp 52–53.)

Illustration continued on following page

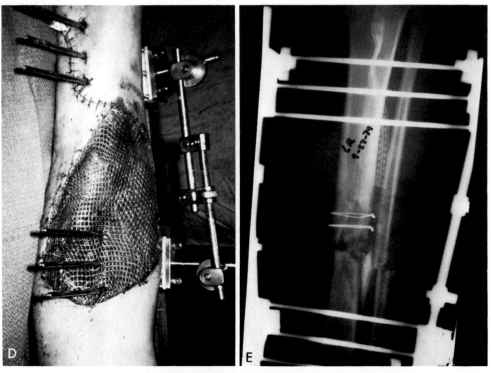

FIUGRE 11–20 *Continued*

1. All Type II and III open fractures.
2. Bone loss.
3. Comminuted open fractures.

When is cancellous grafting done?

1. At time of delayed primary closure in 5 to 10 days for Type I and II open fractures.

2. In 4 to 6 weeks after the wound has completely healed and there is no clinical evidence of wound infection and in Type III open fractures when the fracture site has attained its optimal vascular environment.

3. Definitely, when there is no evidence of callus at the fracture site with motion in all types of open fractures at 3 months.

REHABILITATION

The Involved Extremity

At the very outset of the treatment of open fracture, the rehabilitation of the extremity must be planned and started. Early fracture stabilization allows early joint motion above and below the fracture site and also allows muscle exercise as soon as possible with minimal discomfort. An exercise program of the involved extremity can be followed by the patient, either actively or with the assistance of the physical therapist. Other extremities are also strengthened at the very outset in order to facilitate the ambulation program later. Rehabilitation accomplishes three objectives:

1. Prevention of muscle atrophy and disuse.
2. Prevention of joint stiffness.
3. Improvement of circulation in the extremity and around the fracture site.

The Patient

In our institution, the average hospital stay of patients with Type III tibial fractures and extensive soft tissue injuries is 67 days. With Type I open fracture it is 5 to 7 days, and with Type II open fracture it is 12 to 14 days. Thirty percent of patients with open fractures are multiple trauma victims. The patients and family members have to be informed at the very beginning of treatment of the economic and social implications of the serious injury. For instance, possible job implications, such as continuance at work, modification, or a complete change, must be discussed early. Prolonged rehabilitation and functional limitation of the involved extremity must also be discussed.

Comprehensive discharge planning should be started when the patient is admitted to the hospital. A well-organized discharge planning and rehabilitation program at the very early treatment of the injury will go a very long way in returning the injured patient to a functional status and gainful employment.

References

1. Patzakis JJ, Harvey JP, Ivler D: The role of antibiotics in the management of open fractures. J Bone Joint Surg 56A:532, 1974.
2. Rittmann WW: Use of cloxacillin in open fractures. Personal communication, 1985, Switzerland.
3. Gustilo RB: Use of antimicrobials in the management of open fractures. Arch Surg 114:804, 1979.
4. Gustilo RB, Anderson JT: Prevention of infection in the treatment of one thousand and twenty-five open fractures of long bones. J Bone Joint Surg 58A:453, 1976.
5. Sandusky WR: Prophylaxis of infection in trauma. In Mandell GI, Douglas RG, Bennett JE, eds: Principles and Practice of Infectious Disease. New York, John Wiley & Sons, 1979.
6. Scully RE, Artz C, Sako Y: An evaluation of the surgeon's criteria for determining viability of muscle during debridement. AMA Arch Surg 73:1031, 1956.
7. Rittmann WW, Perren SM: Cortical Knochenhelung nach Osteosynthese und Infektion, Biomechunik und Biologie. New York, Springer, 1974.
8. Friedrich B, Klaue B: Mechanical stability and post-traumatic osteitis: an experimental evaluation of the relationship between infection in bone and internal fixation. Injury 9:23, 1977.
9. Gristina AG, Rovere GD: An in vitro study of the effects of metal used in internal fixation on bacterial growth and dissemination. J Bone Joint Surg 58A:435, 1976.
10. Chapman MW, Mahoney M: The role of early internal fixation in the management of open fractures. Clin Orthop 138:120, 1979.
11. Davis AG: Primary closure of compound fracture wounds. J Bone Joint Surg 30A:405, 1948.
12. Rittmann WW, Schibli M, Matter P, Allgower M: Open fractures: long-term results in 200 consecutive cases. Clin Orthop 138:132, 1979.
13. Veliskaskis KP: Primary internal fixation in open fractures of the tibial shaft. J Bone Joint Surg 41B:342, 1959.
14. Anderson JT, Gustilo RB: Immediate internal fixation in open fracture. Orthop Clin North Am 11:569, 1980.
15. Gregory CF: Open fractures. In Rockwood CA, Green DP, eds: Fractures, Vol I. Philadelphia, JB Lippincott Co, 1975.

Thomas F. Varecka, M.D.

CHAPTER

12

Soft Tissue Coverage in Open Fractures

INTRODUCTION

Loss of soft tissue integrity in conjunction with a fracture can result in a number of real and potential problems for the treating surgeon. The most obvious is the need to include in the overall treatment plan an appropriate and achievable means of wound closure.[1-3] Other common and sometimes less obvious, but no less challenging, problems include dealing with possible wound contamination and/or preventing late infection,[2] identifying the degree and extent of soft tissue and osseous destruction and devitalization, and recognizing the compromised local vascularity and its influence on bone healing[4] as well as securing stabilization of the fracture in such a way as to allow for adequate access to and treatment of the soft tissues. All of these problems are obviously intertwined, and just as the occurrence of one frequently stems from another and can lead to a third, the prompt recognition of their common origin, namely the loss of the protective and supportive function of the skin and soft tissues, and early attention to this situation, can lessen considerably or eliminate entirely the many complications associated with open fractures.[2] This chapter addresses the issue of securing adequate soft tissue coverage.

THE PROBLEM

Any fracture has the potential for being an open fracture. Fortunately, for us and our patients, most of our skeletal structures are covered with thick layers of muscle and other soft tissues (the femur, for example), or they break sufficiently easily that soft damage is not in-curred (the ankle, for example). The one bone that, unfortunately, does not fit these descriptions is the tibia, and it is probably the single most vexing bone to treat when it sustains an open fracture. Accordingly, most of the following discussion deals with open fractures of the tibia, although the treatment principles outlined can just as easily be applied to other open fractures.

Triangular in shape, the tibia is very much disadvantaged with respect to a soft tissue envelope, with virtually the entire medial surface being subcutaneous. Moreover, large portions of its lateral surface also have scant soft tissue padding, if not being entirely subcutaneous. Consider also that the pretibial skin has a very precarious blood supply, with few or no perforating nutrient arteries from an underlying muscle; rather, it derives its vascular supply from longitudinally oriented vessels running tangentially to the deep dermal surfaces.[3] Skin so supplied is at high risk when injured because such blood supply is readily interrupted by shearing or lacerating mechanisms, thus producing potentially large areas of avascularity. Crushing mechanisms can be especially damaging because of the hard "anvil" provided by the underlying tibial surface for the forceful, crushing "hammer" of the injuring object. Vessels of the pretibial skin fall easy prey to such injury. In addition, as swelling and edema accumulate, pretibial vessels are readily compressed, adding further to the ischemic problem, as volume of blood flow is reduced. The venous structures tend to be equally exposed to traumatic risks. It can be readily seen, therefore, that the soft tissues surrounding the tibia provide tenuous protection at best and cannot be reliably expected to dissipate much force if the tibia is injured.

To compound this situation, the tibia itself is quite vulnerable to injury in today's modern,

From the Department of Orthopaedic Surgery, Hennepin County Medical Center, Minneapolis, Minnesota.

mechanized society. We as orthopedic surgeons are only too familiar with the forces to which the otherwise unprotected tibia is exposed, as when a motorcyclist comes to an abrupt halt against a highway guardrail or a car fender. Farm machinery, all-terrain vehicles, minibikes, and so on, are other somewhat less traumatic but no less ominous instruments of injury to the tibia. Moreover, the substantial bony deformity and displacement accompanying a tibial fracture can add secondarily to soft tissue destruction. As vessels are avulsed, lacerated, or crushed in response to the fracture deformity, further soft tissue damage, above what may have been primarily inflicted by the injury mechanism, is sustained.

As noted earlier, the problems become intertwined as the violation of skin and soft tissues opens the way for external bacterial contamination of the fracture; compromises local vascularity; leads to the accumulation of devitalized tissue and other debris, which favor sepsis; and challenges the surgeon to provide satisfactory soft tissue closure. This, in essence, is the problem.

THE PLAN

Addressing the task of treating an open tibial fracture, as with any job, is more easily done when a logical and orderly plan or approach is implemented. Such methodology is adequately discussed elsewhere in this volume, yet certain points are to be restated.

It is imperative that a patient with an open fracture be brought to the operating room as quickly as possible. In our institution, open fractures are considered bona fide emergencies and the patient is taken to the operating room within the first few hours. This initial surgical procedure is used not only for a thorough irrigation and debridement but also as an opportunity to adequately assess the extent of soft tissue injury. With reference to the soft tissues, the basic decision that must be made is simply whether the wound is one that can be closed directly or one that will necessitate a later soft tissue reconstruction.

In the classification of open fractures proposed by Gustilo and colleagues[5] Type I and Type II fractures are typically associated with wounds amenable to direct closure. By definition, both of these fracture types are characterized by wounds that are small and not accompanied by large flaps and extensive underlying, or widespread devitalization. Copious irrigation and sharp debridement in a Type I wound not grossly contaminated usually allow for direct closure; frequently, these procedures can be accomplished at the time of the initial surgery. Type II wounds are handled similarly, although closure is usually delayed for 48 to 72 hours to ensure that any devitalized tissue, not recognized at the initial debridement, can be removed and will not be retained in the wound.

Type III wounds pose the most challenging problems. Gustilo's initial classification recognizes this, as does the modified classification of Byrd and associates.[1] Few, if any, fractures within this category are amenable to direct closure. Therefore, alternative means of closure must be considered. Of necessity, such alternative measures usually involve rearrangement of skin or soft tissue, either locally obtained or harvested from a distant source.

ALTERNATIVE MEANS OF CLOSURE

Wound Granulation

The simplest and most readily available method of secondary closure of severe open fractures is through the process of wound granulation. Trueta[6] and Orr[7] were quite successful with this method, but it must be borne in mind that the majority of their patients were victims of gunshot wounds, in which overall soft tissue injury is modest in extent and limited devascularization occurs. Patients with such injuries still seem to do well with plaster immobilization and wound granulation. However, the typical motorcycle victim has a much more extensive wound, with the high-energy impact being diffusely applied to the leg, tearing and crushing soft tissue extensively, fracturing the tibia, and frequently leaving viable but severely impaired skin surrounding the wound margins. Treatment by granulation, therefore, becomes a very lengthy and time-consuming process requiring the body to heal sometimes massive defects under suboptimal conditions as well as permitting the potential for secondary infection. It is the method that, for the most part, must be considered obsolete and reserved as a salvage procedure when all other techniques have failed or are not applicable.

Split-Thickness Graft

Split-thickness skin grafting can be considered a corollary procedure to granulation. It has many of the inherent limitations of granulation, in that it provides rudimentary coverage through which subsequent bone reconstruction can be carried out only with great difficulty, if at all. Furthermore, wound granulation, with its great expense in terms of time, very often has to precede the use of split grafts. Like granulation, split grafting also can be considered a metabolic drain, because much of the body's resources are directed to the support of the graft and thus are diverted away from the task of bone healing.[4] Split grafting, nonetheless, can be an excellent delaying procedure for temporarily closing the wound and thus preventing infection while one is awaiting the performance of a more satisfactory reconstruction. Open fractures in which periosteum is preserved in the face of other soft tissue loss can readily be closed with split grafts. Such closure usually provides very unstable soft tissue, which is susceptible to repeated breakdowns over the long run, and is unsatisfactory for secondary bone procedures, such as grafting, internal fixation, and so on. In most instances of Type III fractures, split grafting must be considered a temporizing procedure.

Skin Flaps and Myoplasty

From the foregoing discussion, it can be concluded that Type III open fractures, in which there is a lack of sufficient, viable local skin to permit direct closure, are best closed by a means that allows for good quality soft tissue, either from a local or a distant site, to be brought into place over the fracture. Soft tissue so obtained should be durable, should allow for secondary procedures, and, preferably, should have its own blood supply. There are two soft tissue techniques that fall into this broad set of indications. One is the use of skin flaps, either by local rotation or distal mobilization. The other is the so-called myoplasty, again either by local rotation or distal mobilization.

SKIN FLAPS

For reasons discussed earlier, the simple use of skin flaps alone can prove to be unsatisfactory.[1] The blood supply to the intact skin adjacent to the fractured tibia may have been injured as a result of the mechanism producing the fracture. Thus, while the skin survives in situ, any attempts to mobilize it by undermining, relaxing incisions, or flap elevation can provide the final blow that leads to skin necrosis. Moreover, the vagaries of the blood supply to otherwise healthy pretibial skin make it a poor candidate for such mobilization techniques in the first place. Distant skin flaps, such as cross-leg flaps or tube and pedicle flaps, can provide satisfactory coverage of the fracture and allow for later reconstruction. Like granulation methods, however, they require a considerable investment in time. The elevation of the cross-leg flap requires multiple, staged, delaying procedures; lengthy immobilization of both legs while the flap is in place; plus several staged procedures as it is divided and inset. Tube flaps and pedicles from the thigh and abdomen are even more time-consuming. In today's climate of cost containment, the expense of cross-leg or tubed pedicle flaps can be considered so prohibitive that these procedures are not considered primary treatment methods, but, like granulation methods, should be relegated to the realm of salvage procedures.

MYOPLASTY

Myoplasty is a reconstructive technique in which muscle is used as a means of establishing soft tissue closure. This muscle can be either locally obtained or distantly harvested. The procedure was first described in the orthopedic literature by Stark as a method of dealing with chronic bone infection.[8] He recommended the use of gastrocnemius rotational flaps in such instances. The use of myoplastic flaps has gained wide clinical acceptance after its reintroduction by Ger.[2] The myocutaneous flap, as first introduced, involved rotating a single head of the gastrocnemius along with an overlying paddle of skin. This method eventually proved to be somewhat cumbersome, as the resultant donor defect required additional grafting and the rotated skin paddle was very often much thicker than the surrounding skin of the recipient bed. Both sites tended to be cosmetically unappealing. The currently favored myofascial flap, therefore, consists of a single head of the gastrocnemius with surrounding fascia only. The overlying skin of the posterior surface of the tibia is left undisturbed and usually provides no problems. Each head of the gastrocnemius has an independent, proximal, axially oriented blood supply, coming from either the medial or lateral sural arteries, respectively, which then courses longitudinally in the muscle belly. Thus, each half of the muscle is independently supplied and thereby allows for transfer of either half, without jeopardizing its viability or that of its non-mobilized partner. Moreover, the single-vessel, axial pattern of blood supply allows the muscle belly to bring a fresh, abundant blood flow into the injured area when transferred, and consequently aids in the re-establishment of a more physiologic, healthier milieu.[4] At the same time, none of the soft tissue surrounding the injury is deprived of nutrition.

The coverage thus supplied is very durable and forms an excellent bed for later bone reconstructive procedures. The disadvantage of the gastrocmyoplasty is its limited area of application. It is most useful in a range from the supracondylar region of the femur through the knee and as far distal as the mid-tibia. Soft tissue reconstruction beyond this region can be accomplished with a soleus myoplasty but frequently is better handled through myoplasty by means of a free tissue transfer.[9, 10] Many donor muscles are available, fulfilling the criteria of expendability and axial blood supply, including the rectus abdominus, latissimus dorsi, gracilis, and a tensor fasciae latae. The latissimus frequently proves to be the most useful. The advantages of using free tissue transfer are the same as those of the gastrocmyoplasty. Although technically more demanding than the gastrocnemius, when performed by teams of trained microsurgeons, the procedure can be accomplished in reasonable time and with a high degree of reliability.

Myoplasty procedures, furthermore, have one more additional advantage that separates them from all other methods of soft tissue closure. Namely, when the treating surgeon knows that adequate soft tissue reconstruction of even large proportions can be reliably and readily accomplished, he or she is much less hesitant to adequately and aggressively debride the initial wound. No procrastination is necessary in deciding whether to debride or defer on the removal of questionably devitalized tissue. All muscle that has poor color, consistency, contractility, or circulation can be appropriately removed instead of "waiting to see" if it survives (in the frequently foolish hope that it will), and thus large wounds can be considered to be significantly less menacing. All grossly contaminated tissue can be removed, thereby avoiding sepsis. All crushed and avulsed skin can be debrided, thereby facilitating good wound toilet. All the principles of appropriate wound care can be confidently followed because the treating surgeon, knowing that a future myoplasty procedure will pro-vide adequate soft tissue reconstruction, need not be intimidated by a large defect. It is easy to understand why these procedures are currently considered the treatment of choice for soft tissue reconstruction.

TISSUE EXPANSION

A relatively new technique of providing soft tissue coverage is that of tissue expansion. Utilizing the viscoelastic properties of skin and subcutaneous tissues, it employs deflated silicone bladders, which are inserted under the skin and are then slowly inflated, thereby slowly stretching the skin. When enough skin relaxation and redundancy are then achieved to allow for atraumatic mobilization of skin flaps, the bladders are removed, the unsatisfactory skin excised, and a "delayed primary" closure accomplished. The theoretical appeal of this technique is enormous; its practical application is yet to be fully tested. It would obviously be difficult to utilize such a technique in acute injury, where the emphasis is frequently on the avoidance of introducing foreign material. Delay in wound closure inherent in the technique makes it subject to many of the same limitations associated with the use of distant skin flaps requiring delaying procedures. Its ultimate application may be as a means of supplanting unsatisfactory tissue used for an earlier closure, for example, a split-thickness skin graft, and when sepsis has been successfully avoided.

PREFERRED TREATMENT METHODS

Having become familiar with methods of wound closure, the treating surgeon must choose the method that will most satisfactorily allow achieving the goals of early closure, avoidance of sepsis, establishing durable soft tissue coverage, facilitating future reconstructive surgery, and containing costs. With these goals in mind, the following are protocols followed at the Hennepin County Medical Center for severe, open Type III wounds:

1. The injured patient is brought to the operating room as quickly as possible, after hemodynamic stabilization is achieved.

2. The wound is aggressively and widely debrided, as noted; wound size is not a reason to be intimidated and thus to avoid adequate debridement. All nonviable and suspicious tissue is removed.

3. Antibiotic prophylaxis is instituted.

4. The patient is returned to the operating room for a second debridement within 36 to 48 hours to ensure that no devitalized tissue has been left behind. Plans for wound closure/soft tissue reconstruction are made at this time.

5. Soft tissue procedures are completed, optimally by the fifth to seventh post-injury day and not later than the tenth day. If delay is necessary for some reason, the patient is returned to the operating room every 48 hours for additional irrigation and debridement.

In over 125 fractured tibias treated this way, of which 89 patients have received free tissue transfers, wound care has been greatly simplified. Wounds are able to be closed without soft tissue sepsis, without secondary bone infection, and without protracted clinical courses. Soft tissue homeostasis can usually be achieved by 3 to 4 weeks, so that bone grafting and other osseous procedures are able to be done. Ultimate bony union has been greatly facilitated, with most of the patients healing within 8 months. In cases of free flap failure, other salvage techniques have been employed. No gastrocnemius failures have been encountered.

SUMMARY

The importance of good, durable, versatile soft tissue coverage has been discussed, and methods of achieving this have been reviewed. Good soft tissue coverage is a prerequisite to further management of the severe, open tibial fracture.

References

1. Byrd HS, Cierny G, Tebbetts JB: The management of open tibial fractures with associated soft tissue loss: external pin fixation with early flap coverage. Plast Reconst Surg 68:73–82, 1981.
2. Ger R: Muscle transposition for treatment and prevention of chronic post-traumatic osteomyelitis of the tibia. J Bone Joint Surg 59A:784–791, 1977.
3. Henderson NJ, Dixon PL, Godfrey AM, Duthie RB: Rigid fixation and myoplastic techniques for the salvage of major tibial injuries. Int Orthop 6:71–77, 1982.
4. Mathes SJ, Alpert BS, Chang N: Use of the muscle flap in chronic osteomyelitis: experimental and clinical correlation. Plast Reconstr Surg 69:815–829, 1982.
5. Gustilo RB, Anderson JT: Prevention of infection in the treatment of one thousand and twenty-five open fractures of long bones. J Bone Joint Surg 58A:453–458, 1976.
6. Trueta T: The treatment of war fractures by the closed method. Proc R Soc Med 33:65–74, 1939.
7. Orr HW: Compound fractures: with special reference to the lower extremity. Am J Surg 46:733–737, 1939.
8. Stark WJ: The use of pedicled muscle flaps in the surgical treatment of chronic osteomyelitis resulting from compound fractures. J Bone Joint Surg 28:343–349, 1946.
9. Serafin D, Sabatier R, Morris R, Georgiade N: Reconstruction of the lower extremity with vascularized composite tissue: improved tissue survival and specific indications. Plast Reconstr Surg 66:230–241, 1980.
10. Swartz WM, Mears DC: The role of free tissue transfer in lower extremity reconstruction. Plast Reconstr Surg 76:364–373, 1985.

Ramon B. Gustilo, M.D.

13

Management of Acutely Infected Fractures

The germ is nothing. It is the terrain or environment in which it grows which is everything.
LOUIS PASTEUR

INTRODUCTION

It behooves every surgeon to understand fully the implications of Pasteur's statement, for indeed it applies to the treatment of infected fractures. The increase in incidence and severity of open injury to bone and surrounding soft tissues from vehicular accidents, and the aggressive surgical approach of open reduction and internal fixation of closed fractures, contribute to a definite rise in acute wound infection in fracture management. There are two main objectives in the management of infected fractures: (1) to diagnose infection early and (2) to treat it effectively and thereby prevent the infection from spreading into bone.

The incidence of wound infection in open fractures reported from five major institutions ranged from 0 to 23 percent (Table 13–1), depending on the types of open fractures. The infection rate in our institution—5 percent from 1961 to 1968, 12 percent from 1955 to 1961, 23 percent from 1976 to 1979, and 4.5 percent from 1980 to 1984—clearly shows the relevance of classifying the severity of open fractures into Types I, II, and III. The incidence of infection in Types I and II open fractures adequately treated by debridement, irrigation, and appropriate antibiotics was less than 2.5 percent. However, the incidence of wound infection in Type III open fractures

remained high at 13.7 percent (1980–1984). Others report wound sepsis rates in Type III open fractures varying from 10 to 50 percent.[1-11e] Prevention of infection in open reduction and internal fixation or early internal fixation of open fractures presents a compelling challenge to every surgeon. The primary aim in fracture treatment is to obtain a healed fracture and a normally functioning limb without infection. An infected wound following treatment of an open fracture or open reduction and internal fixation of a closed fracture signifies increased morbidity and may result in a lifetime bone infection, limited function, and loss of a limb and possibly life.

Early diagnosis is based on easily recognizable signs and symptoms of inflammation. Our main "hangup" is that we consider infection our failure and unconsciously forget that it is the most common potential complication in the management of open fractures or in any elective open reduction and internal fixation of a fracture. A good history is needed—when, where, and how the trauma occurred; the type of fracture; the initial treatment; whether adequate debridement and irrigation were done; who performed the surgery; what antibiotics were given; what type of internal fixation device was used; and when the wound was closed. When did the patient develop an elevated temperature? Any elevation of temperature during the first 2 or 3 days would suggest respiratory problems, such as atelectasis or fat emboli syndrome. Gas gangrene, however, can develop as early as in the first 24 to 48 hours. Any temperature elevation occurring from the third day after surgery or thereafter should arouse strong suspicion of a wound infection.

After a complete history has been taken, one looks for abnormalities in the cardinal signs and for symptoms of an infected wound:

From the Department of Orthopaedic Surgery, Hennepin County Medical Center, Minneapolis, Minnesota.

TABLE 13–1. Incidence of Wound Infection in Open Fractures

Authors	Total Cases	Type I	Type II	Type III	Type IIIA	Type IIIB
Gustilo et al (1980–1984): Hennepin County, Minneapolis[3]	311	0 %	2.5%	13.7%	5.0%	44.4%
Chapman and Mahoney (1979): U of California–Davis, Sacramento[12]	495	1.1%	3.0%	14.8%	8.1%	15.6%
Patzakis: U of California, Los Angeles[8]	1390	1.4%	3.6%	22.7%		
Edwards: U of Maryland, Baltimore[2]	203 (tibias only)		13.3% (all types)			
Behrens: St. Paul–Ramsey, St. Paul[38]	88 (tibias only)		18.0% (superficial) 7.0% (deep) (all types)			

1. Increased temperature.
2. Increased pain.
3. Redness.
4. Increased discharge, from serous to purulent.
5. A foul smell.
6. Toxic signs of septicemia or bacteremia.
7. Abnormal laboratory tests such as elevated white blood count and erythrocyte sedimentation rate (ESR).
8. X-ray finding of periostitis, bone lysis, sequestrum formation.
9. Abnormal bone scan.
10. Results of smear and culture of wound drainage.

In taking a culture, one must be sure that the deeper part of the wound is sampled for both aerobic and anaerobic cultures. Otherwise, superficial wound cultures give false information about the actual infecting organisms. Once the diagnosis has been made, two main goals should be accomplished:

1. Eradicate the infection and prevent the onset of acute or chronic osteomyelitis.
2. Obtain bony union.

As a corollary to the Louis Pasteur principle of the relationship between bacteria and environment or host is this fact: *Fracture healing can occur completely even when there is infection of soft tissue and bone, provided that there is decreased bacterial activity and that a viable vascular environment has been provided.*

The following principles are advocated in the treatment of acute infection in open fractures or following open reduction and internal fixation of a closed fracture (Fig. 13–1):

- Radical debridement of necrotic soft tissue and dead bone
- Appropriate antibiotic therapy
- Local antibiotic beads
- Maintenance of fracture stability
- Wound left open
- Delayed primary or secondary closure
- Cancellous bone graft

SURGERY: RADICAL DEBRIDEMENT AND COPIOUS IRRIGATION
(Fig. 13–2)

Under general or regional anesthesia, with the use of sterile technique, the wound should be opened widely through a generous longitudinal incision, following Henry's extensile exposure. An adequate and appropriate surgical exposure should be carefully planned. Remaining nonabsorbable suture material should be removed. Pus must be evacuated completely. Necrotic, infected soft tissues and devitalized and sequestrated bone should be completely excised. The wound is irrigated copiously with 5000 to 10,000 ml of normal saline solution, using intermittent pressure lavage followed by another 2000 to 3000 ml of 0.1 percent bacitracin-polymixin solution. The wound must be left open. Antibiotic beads, impregnated with tobramycin (60 to 90 6-mm) are left in place and covered with sterile dressing. Primary closure of infected open fractures, even after adequate debridement and irrigation and use of a closed suction irrigation system at the initial operation, is fraught with a high incidence of wound breakdown

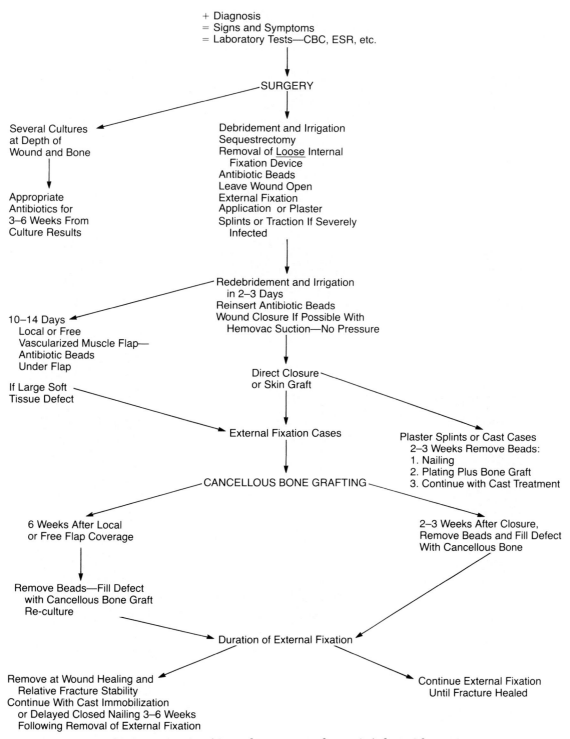

FIGURE 13–1. Algorithm of treatment of acutely infected fractures.

and eventual bony involvement (osteomyelitis). There is nothing to gain by primary closure except saved time and reduced expense. Debridement is repeated in 2 to 3 days. At this time wound closure without tension is done with antibiotic beads, again inserted in the wound. Hemovac suction is inserted without pressure. In Type IIIB wounds, local or free flaps for coverage are done in 5 to 14 days when early granulating wound has developed.

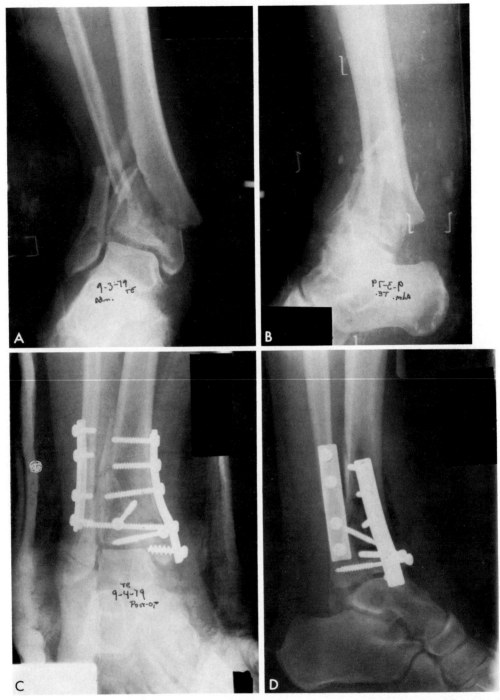

FIGURE 13–2. Acute wound infection following open reduction and internal fixation of a closed ankle fracture in a 33-year-old man who had fallen from a ladder. The plate and screws became loose. Culture revealed coagulase-positive *Staphylococcus.*

A, B, Anteroposterior (AP) and lateral x-rays show a closed bursting fracture of the left ankle.

C, D, Immediate open reduction and internal fixation with lateral and medial plate and screw fixation. AP and lateral x-rays show anatomical reduction of the fracture.

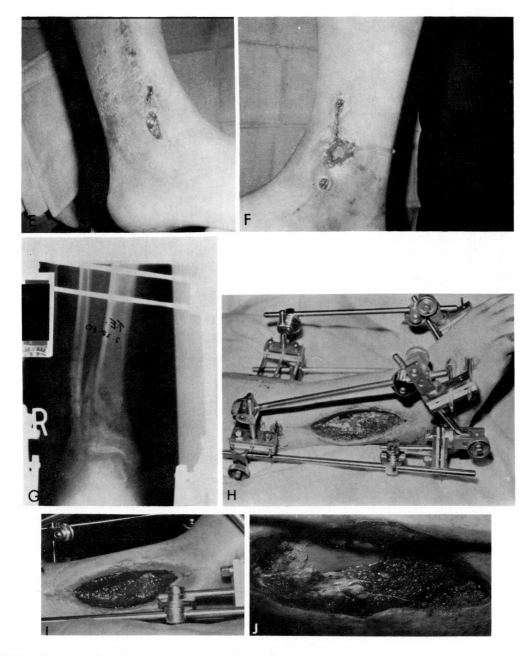

FIGURE 13–2 *Continued*

E, F, Two and a half weeks later, both the lateral and the medial wounds revealed signs of infection, drainage, and wound breakdown.

G, Incision and drainage was done immediately. The wound was left open. The plate and screws were loose and were removed. External fixation was applied to maintain stability. Wound culture revealed coagulase-positive *Staphylococcus* sensitive to penicillin. Intravenous penicillin, 12 million units daily, was given for 3 weeks.

H, I, J, Three weeks after incision and drainage, both wounds showed good granulation tissue except on the medial side, where dead cortical bone was exposed. Dead bone was removed, and cancellous graft was placed 2 weeks later on granulation tissue (Papineau procedure).

Illustration continued on following page

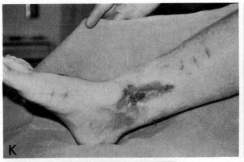

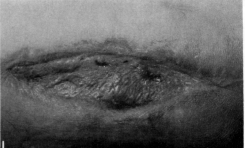

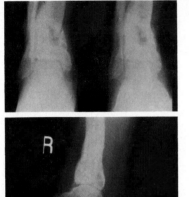

FIGURE 13–2 *Continued*

K, L, Three months later, the whole cavity was covered with granulation tissue, and there was subsequent epithelialization.

M, AP and lateral x-rays 11 months later show healed fracture and moderate narrowing of the ankle joint. There is full weight bearing with slight difficulty.

(From Gustilo RB, ed: Management of infected fractures. In Management of Open Fractures and Their Complications, Vol IV. Philadelphia, WB Saunders Co, 1982, pp 149–151.)

Antibiotic beads are placed for 4 to 6 weeks when bone grafting is done after complete wound healing.

MAINTAINING AND ACHIEVING STABILITY (Fig. 13–3)

Achieving fracture stability reduces wound sepsis, and an unstable fracture promotes wound sepsis; this has been experimentally and clinically reported.[12-14] When primary internal fixation, such as plating or intramedullary nailing, has been achieved at initial treatment, it should be left alone if it continues to provide fracture stability and the device is not loose. If the internal fixation device is loose, it should be removed and an external fixation device can be used to achieve fracture stability. Skeletal traction may be used temporarily in severely infected fractures, but not as a definitive method for achieving fracture stability. Occasionally, a pin or plaster technique can be substituted for an external fixation device, if not available, to achieve stability. Primary *internal fixation,* such as *plating* or *nailing,* should be avoided at the time of initial incision and drainage in cases of florid infection or when there are severe systemic symptoms of bacteremia or septicemia. Internal fixation may be done in 4 to 5 days when acute signs and symptoms of severe infection and local wound reaction have subsided greatly.

Choice of Implant

An *external fixation device* can be used in almost all cases of infected fractures to achieve rigid stability and to allow the surgeon to care for the soft tissue problem with ease. This is particularly indicated in tibial fractures. The femoral shaft fracture presents a slightly more difficult problem in achieving stability because of the abundant soft tissues and vital structures medially.

The advantages of external fixation devices are these:

1. They are easy to apply without additional major surgical trauma to soft tissues.

2. They allow daily wound inspection and care.

3. They allow secondary procedures, such

as skin grafting and other plastic procedures for wound coverage.

4. They enable the surgeon to achieve stability and compression.

5. They enable the surgeon to reduce angulation and displacement without much surgical trauma.

The disadvantages are as follows:

1. Infection around the pin sites remains very high (5 to 50 percent).

2. Secondary intramedullary rodding or plating results in increased wound sepsis following removal of external fixation that has infected pins in spite of antibiotic therapy for pin tract infection. Intramedullary nailing must be avoided in infected external fixator pins.

Maintenance of fracture stability can be accomplished by other means, such as cast immobilization with weight bearing or by elective closed nailing when the wound is completely healed in 3 to 6 weeks or more, provided the pins were not previously infected. Plating will be the internal fixation method in this instance. My choice would be to return to an external fixation device for fracture stabilization (Fig. 13–4).

Plating

Studies by Rittmann and Perren,[14] Rittmann and co-workers,[15] Mueller and Thomas[16] and Rosen[17] show the superior results of plating infected nonunions of both femur and tibia. Plating provides absolute stability and anatomical reduction, if possible, as well as compression. Plating can also maintain the length and still provide stability of the fracture. Early cancellous bone grafting may be done in 5 to 7 days to fill the bone gap if there is adequate soft coverage. Immediate soft tissue coverage of the plate is desirable, although not absolutely essential. Direct closure of the skin without tension or muscle transfer to cover the implant may be done in 5 to 14 days, when the infection is well under control. If muscle transfer is done for soft tissue coverage of exposed bone and/or plate, bone grafting should be delayed for 4 to 6 weeks, when the wound is completely healed. The other alternative is to leave the plate open for several weeks until either early granulation tissue develops over it or sufficient fracture healing has occurred to provide stability so that the plate can be removed and another type of immobilization substituted, such as an external fixation device

or cast. The efficacy of plating infected fractures has been well demonstrated by Meyer and co-workers,[18] Mueller and Thomas,[16] and Rosen.[17] They achieved 93, 87, and 83 percent good results, respectively.

Intramedullary Nailing

When an intramedullary nailing becomes infected and is loose, it should be removed. When infection is minimal with slight drainage, reaming and then re-insertion of a larger nail may be performed. Macausland and Eaton[19] and Kostuik and Harrington[20] reported a high percentage of union in spite of the fact that drainage or infection persisted in a great number of cases. However, one risks the potential hazard of pandiaphyseal osteomyelitis with this technique. This is quite rare, however, and I have not seen one. Intramedullary nailing, however, remains a viable alternative for achieving and maintaining rigid stability, particularly in the midshaft of the femur or tibia. In bones that are osteoporotic because of disuse or prolonged immobilization, nailing again provides good stable fixation.

Intramedullary nailing in the treatment of infected fractures of the tibia is fraught with more complications because of the sparsity of soft tissue surrounding the tibia. Moreover, the tibia has only a short segment of the shaft where good stability by intramedullary nailing is effective. Lottes[21] reported a 70 percent rate of union in nailing infected tibias; however, 12.5 percent of that author's cases ended in amputation. Our current treatment approach is to ream the entire intramedullary canal of an infected tibia, irrigate copiously, and follow with insertion of tobramycin beads. Stability is secured by an external fixator. At the end of 2 to 3 weeks, we remove the tobramycin beads and do cancellous bone grafting, and until the fracture is healed or if there is enough fracture stability, the external fixator can be removed and be substituted with a cast brace or a patellar tendon weight-bearing cast. The other choice is to continue with external fixation until the fracture is healed.

The other alternative is to remove the tobramycin beads, perform additional reaming, and insert a larger nail to secure fracture stability in either femur or tibia, if possible. If stability is not achieved by nailing, additional fixation, such as locking screws or cast immobilization, is recommended.

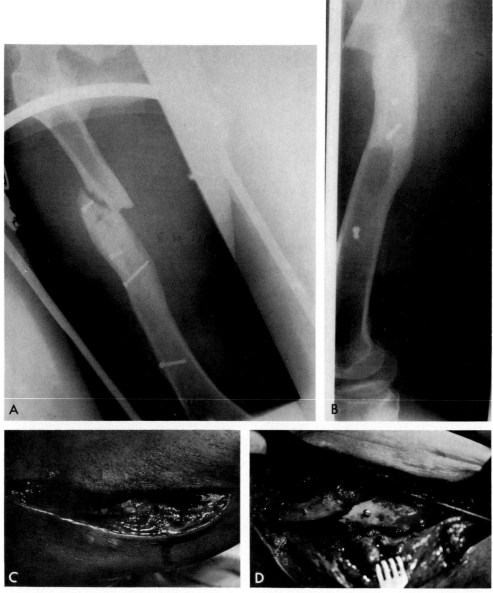

FIGURE 13 – 3. Acute exacerbation of an old osteomyelitis following a closed fracture of the right femur of a 56-year-old man. The patient was a pedestrian and had been hit by a car. Wound culture revealed coagulase-positive *Staphylococcus* resistant to penicillin.

A, B, X-rays showed a displaced fracture of the upper third of the right femur in traction, and also revealed an old fracture with four remaining screws. Twenty-two years previously, the patient had sustained a closed fracture of the right femur, which was treated by open reduction and internal fixation (plating). The injury subsequently became infected and took over 2 years to heal. There was no drainage for the next 20 years.

C,D, A septic course developed 5 days later. The patient had a temperature of 103° F, a leukocyte count of 19,000, and a very tender, swollen right thigh. Incision and drainage revealed a copious amount of pus. The fracture site was debrided and irrigated. The screws were removed and the wound was packed open. Culture revealed coagulase-positive *Staphylococcus* resistant to penicillin. The patient was given intravenous oxacillin, 8 gm daily for 4 weeks, followed by oral dicloxacillin, 4 gm daily for 3 months.

E, Six days later, stability was achieved by plating. Cancellous bone grafting was also done.

F, Anteroposterior (AP) and lateral x-rays showed fracture reduction with plate.

G, On discharge, the patient was walking with crutches and the wound was almost completely healed by secondary intention. The wound was not primarily closed.

H, I, AP and lateral x-rays 20 months later showed complete healing of the fracture.

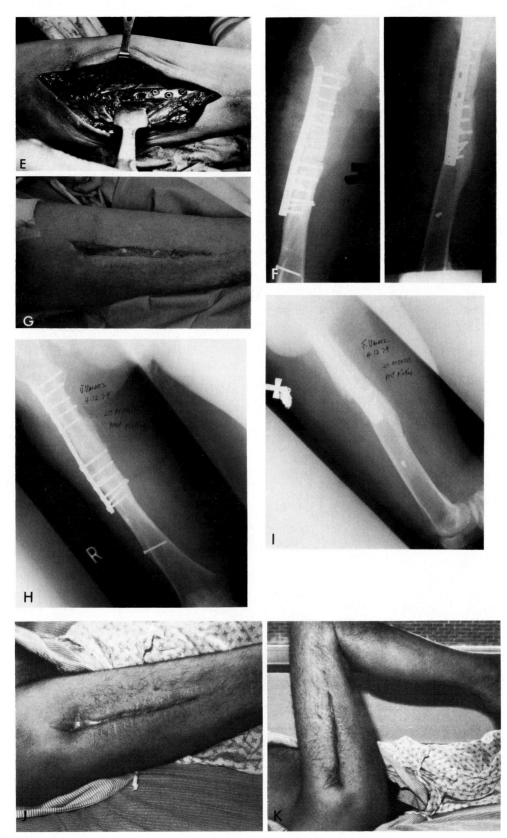

FIGURE 13–3 *Continued*

J,K, Wound completely healed, hip and knee function satisfactory.

(From Gustilo RB, ed: Management of infected fractures. In Management of Open Fractures and Their Complications, Vol. IV. Philadelphia, WB Saunders Co, 1982, pp 154–156.)

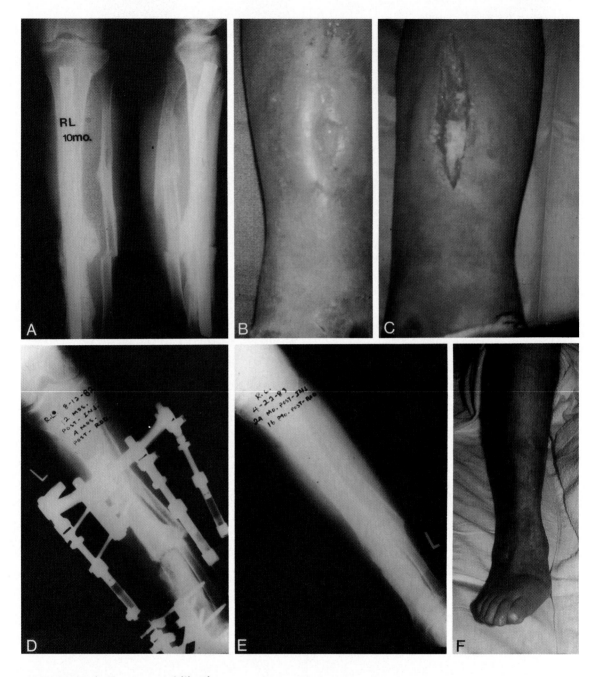

FIGURE 13–4. Fracture stabilization.

  A, The patient sustained an open fracture of the left tibia 10 months previously and had healed with malunion. Osteotomy was done to correct the malunion, and an intramedullary nail was inserted for stabilization. Anteroposterior and lateral x-rays of the tibia following nailing.

  B, Three weeks later, wound sepsis developed. The wound is red, swollen, and draining.

  C, Debridement and irrigation were done. Wound culture revealed coagulase-positive staphylococci.

  D, External fixation was applied to secure fracture stability. The wound was left open.

  E,F, Delayed closure, delayed cancellous bone. Grafting was performed, and 4 weeks of parenteral antibiotics done. Sixteen months following treatment, the fracture healed without recurrence of sepsis.

Skeletal Traction

Skeletal traction is recommended only as a temporary measure for 5 to 10 days until the wound looks clean or until early granulation tissue has developed. It is indicated if (1) there is a florid type of infection locally or (2) if there are severe systemic symptoms and signs of septicemia or bacteremia. When these two conditions have been corrected or significantly controlled, external or internal fixation should replace skeletal traction to provide more fracture stability.

The disadvantages of traction in treating an infected open fracture of the femur or tibia are these:

1. It is difficult to manage the wound effectively, particularly when frequent trips to the operating room or daily dressing changes in the patient's room are required.

2. It is difficult both to maintain alignment of the fracture for angular deformity with frequent dressing changes and surgery and to maintain satisfactory length without distraction at the fracture site.

3. Principally, it does not provide stability of the fracture—a deterrent to fracture and wound healing.

WOUND COVERAGE IN INFECTED OPEN FRACTURES

The prerequisites to wound closure are twofold:

1. The infection must be well under control, and all active signs of inflammation must have disappeared. There is no purulent drainage, redness, or swelling surrounding the wound. Beginning granulation tissue may or may not be present. Cultures may still be positive.

2. The patient has no systemic signs or symptoms of infection, such as fever, chills, restlessness, or increased pain. The white blood cell count must be within normal limits.

There are four types of problems of wound coverage in infected open fractures. These are now described.

Adequate Bone and Soft Tissue Coverage. Skin closure can be achieved, usually in 5 to 7 days, by direct skin suture without tension. Skin closure is accomplished by using interrupted wire or a nonabsorbable synthetic material, without tension. Continuous sutures should definitely not be used. The sutures are left in place for at least 2 weeks. Hemovac suction drainage is inserted without pressure if tobramycin beads are used for 2 to 3 days to allow egress of excessive dermatoma. Otherwise, suction can be removed in 48 hours, when the drainage is less than 25 ml in a 24-hour period.

Exposed Bone with Inadequate Soft Tissue Coverage but No Bone Loss. When bone is exposed with intact periosteum, the underlying cortical bone usually survives and granulation tissue develops over it from the periphery. When cortical bone is exposed without periosteum, usually the exposed cortical bone does not survive. The superficial cortical dead bone should then be removed down to the bleeding area or cancellous bone unless it provides stability. Cancellous bone stimulates formation of granulation tissue. Depending on the size of the exposed bone area, a 1-inch square usually takes 4 to 6 weeks to be covered completely by granulation tissue. Split-thickness skin grafting can be performed over granulation tissue. The alternative is to allow the wound to heal completely by secondary intention and epithelialization of the skin. Occasionally, one may resort to either a direct rotational skin flap or a local muscle transfer, a cross-leg flap, or a free vascular flap. An experienced plastic or microvascular surgeon should be consulted when such intricate reconstructive wound coverage procedures are required.

Exposed Bone with Inadequate Soft Tissue Coverage and Loss of Bone Continuity (Gaps) or Partial Defect. If there is bone loss with discontinuity of bone ends or if there is severe comminution causing marked instability, early or delayed primary cancellous bone grafting should be accomplished in order to fill the defect over good granulation tissue, using the Papineau technique. The granulation tissue is allowed to develop over the entire cancellous graft area. At a later date, if needed, skin grafting can be done. The other alternative that I favor is to achieve fracture stability by external fixation, free vascularized muscle transfer for wound coverage, antibiotic beads under the flap, and, in 6 weeks, removal of antibiotic beads and a massive cancellous bone grafting. External fixation is continued until the fracture is healed or until there is enough fracture stability so that a walking cast or weight-bearing cast brace can be applied.

Exposed Metal. In plating, adequate soft tissue coverage is desirable, although not absolutely essential. When metal is exposed, the surgeon either can wait long enough for the granulation tissue to cover it or can resort to reconstructive plastic surgery procedures for soft tissue coverage, such as muscle transfer with skin grafting or cross-leg flap. It would be preferable to accomplish soft tissue coverage followed by cancellous bone grafting in 4 to 6 weeks. Some patients can be sent home at the end of 4 to 6 weeks with exposed metal or bone, provided daily wound care can be accomplished by the patient or a visiting nurse. The other alternative for a very large open area with metal exposed is to wait until fracture healing is adequate to provide bone stability or until the infection is well under control. The plate can then be removed, and other methods of immobilization, such as external fixation or pins and plaster, or spica cast or long leg cast can be substituted. Our choice now would be to remove the plate if exposed and change to external fixator for securing fracture stability. The wound and fracture care can be provided as previously outlined. In selected cases, tibiofibular synostosis is recommended if there is recurrent infection of external fixation pins and other forms of internal fixation devices are contraindicated.

CANCELLOUS BONE GRAFTING

Our analysis of Type III open fractures (1980–1984) with severe soft tissue injuries showed a delayed union or nonunion rate of 60 percent. (Cancellous bone grafting is recommended when the wound is completely healed 4 to 6 weeks after a soft tissue coverage procedure.) In infected open fractures with large soft tissue defects and bone loss, cancellous bone grafting is recommended in 2 to 4 weeks with early healthy granulation tissue, as advocated by Papineau.[22, 23] Granulation is allowed to take place over cancellous bone, followed by split-thickness skin grafting over the granulation tissue, or to wait for complete healing by secondary infection.

Posterolateral bone grafting is indicated in the lower two thirds of infected tibia in the following conditions: (1) skin is tenuous anterolaterally either from direct skin closure or split-thickness skin graft, and (2) residual minimal draining sinus anteriorly. Posteromedial bone grafting in the upper one third of the tibia is recommended for similar indications.

In summary, soft tissue coverage of infected fractures has often presented a difficult problem. However, with appropriate treatment,[15, 18] in over 90 percent of infected open fractures one can accomplish either direct skin suture or split-thickness skin graft over granulation tissue. Our choice of treatment for large soft tissue loss and large bone exposed is to achieve wound coverage either by local flap or free vascular transfer, i.e., latissimus dorsi, in 2 to 3 weeks after initial debridement, intravenous antibiotics, and tobramycin beads. Then we go back and do cancellous bone grafting in 4 to 6 weeks, either through a posterior approach or by lifting one edge of the flap for insertion of the cancellous bone.

CLOSED SUCTION IRRIGATION

According to early reports by Goldman and colleagues[24] in 1960 and McElvenny[25] in 1961, continuous or intermittent closed suction irrigation treatment in conjunction with debridement produced a high rate of cure in 17 cases of osteomyelitis. However, later reports by various investigators revealed an incidence of recurrent drainage ranging from 17 to 52 percent.[26-31] The majority of the studies were of osteomyelitis with healed fractures. Kelly[30] reported a failure rate of 34.8 percent in 23 cases of nonunion with debridement, antibiotics, and closed suction irrigation, compared with 19 percent in 21 cases of infected nonunion treated in the same manner but with no closed suction irrigation system.

Is there an indication for closed suction irrigation treatment in acutely infected fractures? The answer is yes, in a very limited duration: first, if there is a large potential space or cavity with skin closure; and second, if a large amount of drainage or bleeding is expected when the wound is closed.

Irrigation systems must be used for a short time, 3 to 5 days, not 3 to 4 weeks as oftentimes used in the past, to prevent the hazard of super-infection with gram-negative organisms.[30, 32, 33] Jergesen[34] describes a method of intermittent pressure suction irrigation system with a single tube rather than the continuous flow systems advocated by many others.[26-31] However, there are no controlled comparative studies to show which system is more effective as an adjunct therapy for infected wounds or osteomyelitis. *We do not use suction-irrigation systems to deliver antibiotics locally. Our choice is local antibiotic beads.*

ANTIBIOTIC THERAPY

Antibiotic therapy is not started until appropriate wound cultures are taken from the deeper part of the wound. Wound cultures taken superficially or inside the sinus tract can be misleading as to the real infecting organism inside the deep part of the wound. There is no place, in the treatment of infected open fractures or infected wounds following open reduction and internal fixation of closed fractures, for antibiotic therapy as the only treatment of the problem. Wound cultures and smears taken of infected open fractures in our institution revealed 60 percent gram-positive and 40 percent gram-negative or mixed gram-positive and gram-negative bacteria. The predominant organisms were coagulase-positive *Staphylococcus* organisms, *Klebsiella, Enterobacter, Escherichia coli, Proteus,* and coagulase-negative *Staphylococcus. Pseudomonas* infection is increasing, particularly in wounds that are exposed for a long time.

Sensitivity studies showed cephalosporin to be the antibiotic of choice in most cases. When appropriate cultures have been taken, we give cephalosporin, 2 gm initially and 1 to 2 gm every 4 to 6 hours, depending upon the severity of the infection. Once the bacteria have been identified and sensitivity studies done, appropriate intravenous antibiotic therapy is given for 3 to 4 weeks. If we are dealing with an acute wound infection, the prognosis is relatively good, as opposed to chronic wound infection with bony involvement. When we are dealing with an infection that has not been recognized in the first 3 to 6 weeks, we must assume, after this length of time, that we are dealing with bone involvement. Intravenous antibiotics should be given for at least 4 weeks. Whether prolonged, massive antibiotic therapy will prevent osteomyelitis or recurrent osteomyelitis in the future has not been supported or contradicted by any reliable controlled studies. Kelly and associates,[35] however, reported a failure rate of 28 percent in the treatment of 50 cases of osteomyelitis with gram-negative rod infection, or mixed infection with gram-negative rods and coagulase-positive staphylococcal infection, in contrast to a 100 percent success rate with coagulase-positive *Staphylococcus* in 32 cases. Both groups were treated in the same manner — debridement, suction irrigation in the majority of cases, and appropriate antibiotic therapy — the only difference being that prolonged antibiotic therapy of infection with gram-negative rods was not possible because of the nephrotoxic and ototoxic properties of aminoglycosides, which are effective against those bacteria. Gentamicin or tobramycin beads applied locally obviate these potential problems.

LOCAL ANTIBIOTIC BEAD THERAPY (Fig. 13–5)

The release of gentamicin from polymethylmethacrylate beads in high concentration and its penetration to surrounding tissues, including cortical and cancellous bone as shown by Wahlig[36] and Hoff[37] and their associates, leads to a superior delivery of local antibiotic therapy, particularly aminoglycosides. Tobramycin beads, 6 mm in diameter (60 to 90 in number), are placed inside the intramedullary canal and wound area. The dose is 1.2 gm of tobramycin powder in 20 gm of bone cement. The antibiotic beads are left in place for 2 to 3 weeks and are removed when cancellous bone grafting or intramedullary nailing is done. Our own experience showed an 87 percent success rate with a minimum of 1 year follow-up.

SUMMARY

The principles in the treatment of acute infection of open reduction and internal fixation of fractures have been detailed:

1. Early diagnosis.
2. Prompt surgical incision and drainage with adequate debridement and copious irrigation.
3. Bacteriological diagnosis by means of Gram stain, smear and culture, and sensitivity tests.
4. Appropriate and adequate antibiotic treatment, based on culture and sensitivity studies, for a minimum of 3 weeks and as long as 6 weeks.
5. Insertion of antibiotic beads.
6. Secure stability of the fracture.
7. Leaving the wound open initially.
8. Delayed or secondary closure, either by direct suture or by split-thickness skin graft, or when those measures are not possible, either a cross-leg flap or a muscle rotational flap or free vascularized muscle transfer in 2 to 3 weeks.
9. Cancellous bone grafting to fill up large defects or severe comminution in 4 to 6 weeks.

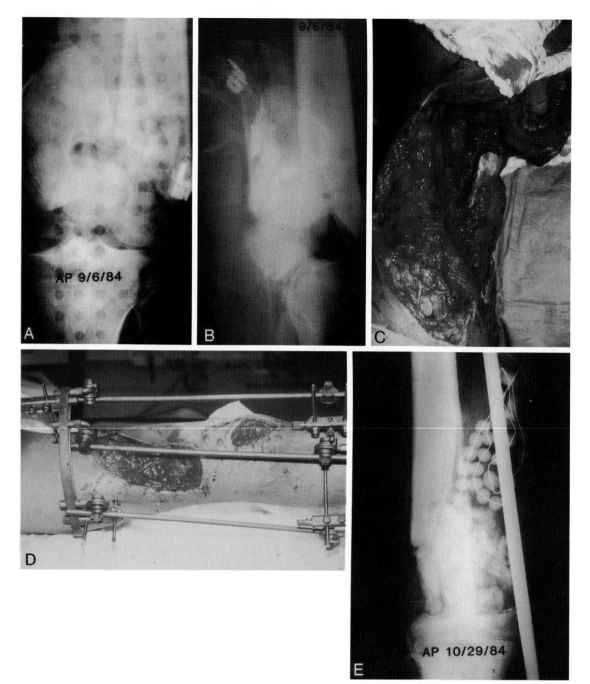

FIGURE 13–5. Antibiotic bead therapy.

A, B, Anteroposterior (AP)view. The patient sustained a Type IIIB open fracture of the distal femur. AP and lateral x-rays showed a comminuted, markedly displaced open fracture of the distal femur.

C, Seven days following injury, the wound became infected with both gram-positive and gram-negative bacteria.

D, Radical debridement and irrigation were performed. External fixation was applied to severe fracture stability. Tobramycin beads were inserted in the wounds.

E, F, Delayed primary knee arthrodesis with extensive bone was performed. Tobramycin beads were inserted under flaps for 4 weeks. AP and lateral x-rays of distal femur and knee joint showed arthrodesis with bone grafting and antibiotic beads.

G, Delayed closure by skin grafting was done following an early arthrodesis.

H, AP and lateral x-rays 2 years after injury showed solid knee fusion.

I, J, The patient has been employed as a cook, and the wound is nicely healed without recurrent sepsis 2 years after injury.

136

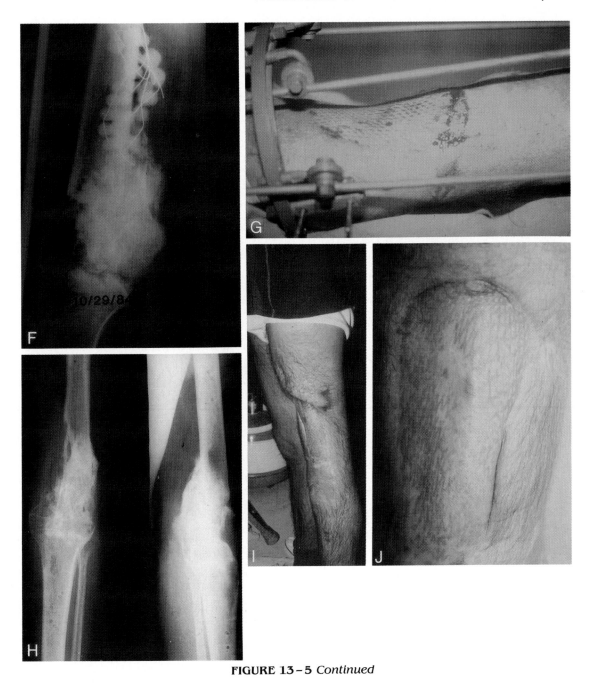

FIGURE 13–5 *Continued*

References

1. Chapman MW: Personal communication. University of California–Davis Hospitals, Sacramento, California.
2. Edwards C: Personal communication. University of Maryland Hospitals, Baltimore, 1985.
3. Gustilo RB, Gruninger R, Davis T: Classification of type III (severe) open fractures relative to treatment and results. Orthopedics 10:1781–1788, 1987.
4. Hasenhuttl K: The treatment of unstable fractures of the tibia and fibula with flexible medullary wires. J Bone Joint Surg 63A:921–931, 1981.
5. Karlstrom G, Olerud S: External fixation of severe open tibial fractures with the Hoffman frame. Clin Orthop 180:68–77, 1983.
6. Karlstrom G, Olerud S: Stable external fixation of open tibial fractures. Orthop Rev 6:25, 1977.
7. Olerud S, Karlstrom G: Tibial fractures treated by

A-O compression osteosynthesis. Acta Orthop Scand (Suppl) 140:3, 1972.

8. Patzakis MJ: Personal communication. University of California, Los Angeles, 1985.

9. Velazco A, Whitesides TE, Fleming LL: Open fractures of the tibia treated with the Lottes nail. J Bone Joint Surg 65A:879–885, 1983.

10. Velazco A, Fleming LL: Open fractures of the tibia treated by the Hoffman external fixator. Clin Orthop 180:125–132, 1983.

11. Velazco A, Fleming LL, Nahai F: Soft-tissue reconstruction of the leg associated with the use of the Hoffman external fixator. J Trauma 12:1052–1057, 1983.

11a. Anderson JT, Gustilo RB: Immediate internal fixation in open fractures. Orthop Clin North Am 11:569, 1980.

11b. Anderson LD, Hutchins WC, Wright PE, et al: Fractures of the tibia and fibula treated by casts and transfixing pins. Clin Orthop 99:179, 1974.

11c. Clansey BJ, Hansen ST, Jr: Open fractures of the tibia: a review of 102 cases. J Bone Joint Surg 60A:118, 1978.

11d. Gustilo RB, Anderson JT: Prevention of infection in the treatment of one thousand and twenty-five open fractures of long bones. J Bone Joint Surg 58A:453, 1976.

11e. Merianos P, Cambouridis P, Smyrnis P: The treatment of 143 tibial shaft fractures by Enders nailing and early weight bearing. J Bone Joint Surg, 67B:576–580, 1985.

11f. Patzakis MJ, Wilkins J, Moore TM: Consideration in reducing the infection rate in open tibial fractures. Clin Orthop 178:36–41, 1983.

12. Chapman MW, Mahoney M: The role of early internal fixation in the management of open fractures. Clin Orthop 138:132, 1979.

13. Friedrich B, Klaue P: Mechanical stability and post-traumatic osteitis: an experimental evaluation of the relation between infection of bone and internal fixation. Injury 9:23, 1977.

14. Rittmann WW, Perren SM: Corticale Knochenheilung nach Osteosynthese und Infektion. Biomechanik und Biologic. Berlin, New York, Springer-Verlag, 1974.

15. Rittmann WW, Schibli M, Matter P, et al: Open fractures: Long term results in 200 consecutive cases. Clin Orthop 138:132, 1979.

16. Mueller ME, Thomas RJ: Treatment of nonunion in fractures of long bones. Clin Orthop 138:141, 1979.

17. Rosen H: Compression treatment of long bone pseudoarthroses. Clin Orthop 138:154, 1979.

18. Meyer S, Weiland AJ, Willenegger H: The treatment of infected nonunion of fractures of long bones. J Bone Surg 57A:836, 1975.

19. Macausland WR, Jr, Eaton RG: Sepsis following fixation of fractures of the femur. J Bone Joint Surg 45A:1647, 1963.

20. Kostuik JP, Harrington IJ: Treatment of infected un-united femoral shaft fractures. Clin Orthop 108:90, 1975.

21. Lottes JO: Medullary nailing of infected fractures of the tibia. J Bone Joint Surg 45A:1543, 1963.

22. Papineau LJ: L'excision-greffe avec fermeture retardée délibérée dans l' ostéomyélite chronique. Nouv Presse Med 2:2753, 1973.

23. Papineau LJ, Alfageme A, Dalcourt JP, et al: Ostéomyélite chronique: excision et greffe de spongieux a l'air libre aprés mises a plat extensives. Int Orthop 3:165, 1979.

24. Goldman MD, Johnson RK, Grossberg NM: A new approach to chronic osteomyelitis. Am J Orthop 2:63, 1960.

25. McElvenny RT: Circulation and suction, Part II. Am J Orthop 3:154, 1961.

26. Clawson KK, Davis FJ, Hansen ST, Jr: Treatment of chronic osteomyelitis with emphasis on closed suction-irrigation technique. Clin Orthop 96:88, 1973.

27. Compere EL, Metzger WI, Mitra RN: The treatment of pyogenic bone and joint infections by closed irrigation (circulation) with a nontoxic detergent and one or more antibiotics. J Bone Joint Surg 49A:614, 1967.

28. Dombrowski ET, Dunn AW: Treatment of osteomyelitis by debridement and closed wound irrigation-suction. Clin Orthop 43:215, 1965.

29. Horwitz T: Surgical treatment of chronic osteomyelitis complicating fractures. Clin Orthop 96:118, 1973.

30. Kelly PJ, Martin WJ, Coventry MB: Chronic osteomyelitis. II. Treatment with closed irrigation and suction. JAMA 213:1843, 1970.

31. Lawyer RO, Jr, Eyring EJ: Intermittent closed suction-irrigation treatment of osteomyelitis. Clin Orthop 8:80, 1972.

32. Wade PA, Campbell RD: Open versus closed methods in treating fractures of the leg. Am J Surg 95:599, 1958.

33. Waldvogel FA, Medoff G, Swartz MN: Osteomyelitis: a review of clinical features, therapeutic considerations, and unusual aspects (second of three parts). N Engl J Med 282:260, 1970.

34. Jergesen F, Jawetz E: Pyogenic infections in orthopedic surgery: combined antibiotic and closed wound treatment. Am J Surg 106:152, 1963.

35. Kelly PJ, Wilkowski CJ, Washington JA II: Comparison of gram-negative bacillary and staphylococcal osteomyelitis of the femur and tibia. Clin Orthop 96:70, 1973.

36. Wahlig H, Dingeldein E, Bergmann R, Reuss K: The release of gentamicin from polymethylmethacrylate beads: an experimental and pharmacokinetic study. J Bone Joint Surg 60B:270–275, 1978.

37. Hoff SF, Fitzgerald RH, Kelly PJ: The depot administration of penicillin G and gentamicin in acrylic bone cement. J Bone Joint Surg 63A:798–804, 1981.

38. Behrens F: Personal communications. St. Paul Ramsey Medical Center, St. Paul, Minnesota 1985.

CHAPTER

14

Management of Infected Nonunion

The fact is, infection is not a cause of nonunion. If nonunion is allowed to occur, it is due not to infection, but to inadequate immobilization permitted by reason of infection.

SIR REGINALD WATSON-JONES

INTRODUCTION

Infected nonunion is defined as that state existing after considerable time (4 to 6 months) has elapsed when there is no evidence that the fracture will heal and infection still exists. Therefore, other methods of treatment must be undertaken in order to achieve fracture healing. Infection may predispose to nonunion because of the frequent interruptions of immobilization (casting) that are necessary in the care of the infected wound. Treatment of infected nonunion of long bones becomes difficult because there are two problems to be solved simultaneously: (1) nonunion and (2) infection.

The problems become even more difficult when one is dealing with long-standing, established, infected nonunion, for these reasons:

1. Usually, the patient has been operated on at least two to three times, with resultant scarring and cicatrization of the surrounding soft tissue, rendering the environment around the fracture site avascular.

2. A sinus tract has usually formed by the end of 6 months, leading into the fracture site. It indicates, either dead bone or sequestrum inside.

3. Osteomyelitis has usually developed, in-

volving a considerable length of bone and resulting in a thrombosis of the blood vessels of the haversian canals with resultant bone sclerosis and dead bone. Delineation between dead and living bone becomes very difficult. X-rays usually show sclerosis of bone ends of varying length. There is usually an interval of scar tissue, which is avascular, between the sclerosed bone ends. The application of differential bone scanning or magnetic resonance imaging (MRI) may help in delineating the extent of the infectious process.

4. Limited joint motion or stiffness is not unusual, because of prolonged immobilization or repeated surgical procedures with resulting scarring of the muscles involved, particularly close to the joint. The extremity may well be dystrophic following a long period of infected nonunion.

5. Mixed and drug-resistant infecting organisms, of both gram-positive and gram-negative bacteria, develop after the patient has been on antibiotics for a long time.

Kelly and associates[1] showed a treatment failure rate of 28 percent in osteomyelitis with gram-negative rods or mixed gram-negative rods and coagulase-positive *Staphylococcus* in contrast to a success rate of 100 percent in patients with pure coagulase-positive staphylococcal infections. The bacterial pathogens of infected open fractures at the Hennepin County Medical Center changed dramatically during the years 1975 to 1984.[2, 3] Eighty-seven percent of infected Type III open fractures were due to gram-negative bacteria or mixed infection compared with 24 percent reported 10 years earlier.[2, 3] Our most current series (1980–1984) revealed 55 percent gram-positive bacteria and the rest either gram-negative or mixed.

From the Department of Orthopaedic Surgery, Hennepin County Medical Center, Minneapolis, Minnesota.

PRINCIPLES OF TREATMENT

Remember the words of Louis Pasteur: "The germ is nothing; it is the terrain in which it grows which is everything."

Fracture healing can occur when there is decreased bacterial activity, provided there is stability of the fracture with a surrounding vascular environment. Therefore, three conditions must be met in order for the treatment of infected nonunion to be successful: (1) achievement of a vascular or viable environment around and at the fracture site, (2) fracture stability, and (3) early and massive bone grafting, to be repeated if necessary.

Figure 14–1 illustrates the overall treatment for infected nonunion of the tibia.

SURGERY: RADICAL DEBRIDEMENT
(Fig. 14–2)

Excision of the sinus tract and of avascular scarred and infected soft tissue is performed to produce active bleeding in the area of the margins surrounding the fracture site. Excision sometimes involves skin, subcutaneous tissue, fascia and muscles, and intervening scar tissue between the fracture ends and bone. The longitudinal incision must be generous to accomplish complete debridement. Viable skin should be left in place. Apprehension over not being able to close the skin should not and must not be a determining factor during the excision of infected and scarred tissues.

Removal of necrotic bone and sequestrum is often difficult to achieve in infected nonunion because of the surgeon's inability to differentiate between normal and dead bone. Also, one becomes apprehensive about removing too much bone and creating marked instability or loss of bone continuity. However, there is no other choice in the treatment of infected nonunion if one expects to cure the infection and achieve healing. An avascular environment or sequestrum or both allows bacteria to grow and multiply and causes persistent drainage. Dead bone must be removed with sharp rongeurs or osteotomes. The intramedullary canal or the ends of the sclerosed bones must be curetted to remove necrotic debris inside the canal. Cultures must be taken at the fracture site, proximal and distal intramedullary canal, and surrounding soft tissues. At intervals, copious irrigation by jet lavage, with bacitracin-polymixin solution or normal saline solution, is essential. Bleeding bone surfaces and bleeding soft tissue around and at the fracture site must be obtained. Repeat debridement under general anesthesia is mandatory, in 2 to 3 days, to ensure that complete removal of dead bone and infected tissue has been accomplished.

Intramedullary Reaming (Fig. 14–3)

In chronic diaphyseal osteomyelitis with nonunion, there is marked sclerosis and long segmental avascular bone. It is very difficult to determine the extent of endosteal or intramedullary extension of infection. Magnetic resonance imaging may be of help in determining endosteal involvement. Lidgren and Torholm,[4] in justifying intramedullary reaming in chronic osteomyelitis, believe it diminishes interosseous pressure and revascularizes the bone, thereby improving the endosteal circulation. They obtained satisfactory results in 16 of 18 cases in which intramedullary reaming was done in conjunction with other treatment modalities. We have been reaming 2 mm over size when the reamer touches or bites into the endosteal wall of the intramedullary canal. In infected nonunion, intramedullary reaming is accomplished at the bone ends proximally and distally. Our preliminary results were encouraging, with an 82 percent success rate and 18 to 24 months follow-up.

FRACTURE STABILITY (Fig. 14–4)

After removal of infected and nonviable tissue, stability of the fracture is the second most important factor in achieving union of an infected, nonunited fracture.

In experimental animals, Rittmann and Perren[5] and Friedrich and Klaue[6] demonstrated that the benefits of fracture stability achieved by metallic fixation outweighed the disadvantages of the foreign body effect by markedly reducing wound sepsis. Also, Gristina and Rovere[7] have shown that metal per se does not promote bacterial growth in vitro.

Frequent interruption of the immobilization of the fracture for wound care is the primary reason for nonunion. After complete debridement and irrigation of infected soft tissue and removal of dead bone, stability of the fracture must be achieved by either an external or an internal fixation device.

If the patient has signs and symptoms of bacteremia or septicemia, or if during surgery

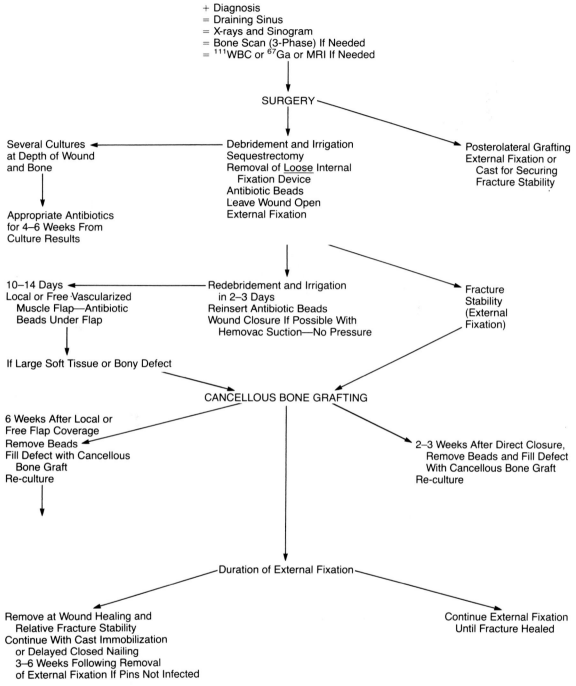

+ Diagnosis
= Draining Sinus
= X-rays and Sinogram
= Bone Scan (3-Phase) If Needed
= ^{111}WBC or ^{67}Ga or MRI If Needed

SURGERY

Several Cultures
at Depth of Wound
and Bone

Debridement and Irrigation
Sequestrectomy
Removal of <u>Loose</u> Internal
    Fixation Device
Antibiotic Beads
Leave Wound Open
External Fixation

Posterolateral Grafting
External Fixation or
Cast for Securing
Fracture Stability

Appropriate Antibiotics
for 4–6 Weeks From
Culture Results

10–14 Days
Local or Free Vascularized
    Muscle Flap—Antibiotic
    Beads Under Flap

Redebridement and Irrigation
    in 2–3 Days
Reinsert Antibiotic Beads
Wound Closure If Possible With
    Hemovac Suction—No Pressure

Fracture
Stability
(External
Fixation)

If Large Soft Tissue or Bony Defect

CANCELLOUS BONE GRAFTING

6 Weeks After Local or
Free Flap Coverage
Remove Beads
Fill Defect with Cancellous
    Bone Graft
Re-culture

2–3 Weeks After Direct Closure,
    Remove Beads and Fill Defect
    With Cancellous Bone Graft
Re-culture

Duration of External Fixation

Remove at Wound Healing and
    Relative Fracture Stability
Continue With Cast Immobilization
    or Delayed Closed Nailing
    3–6 Weeks Following Removal
    of External Fixation If Pins Not Infected

Continue External Fixation
Until Fracture Healed

FIGURE 14 – 1. Algorithm for infected nonunion of the tibia.

there is evidence of severe infection with copious purulent drainage, the wound should be
packed open without internal fixation. External fixation may be applied, provided pins can
be inserted away from the infected area. Our
preference would be to place the extremity in

traction or in a splint for 4 to 5 days until the
local or systemic infection has subsided. The
patient is then given massive doses of the appropriate antibiotics intravenously. The
wound is inspected and irrigated daily. Usually, in 48 hours the patient is returned to the

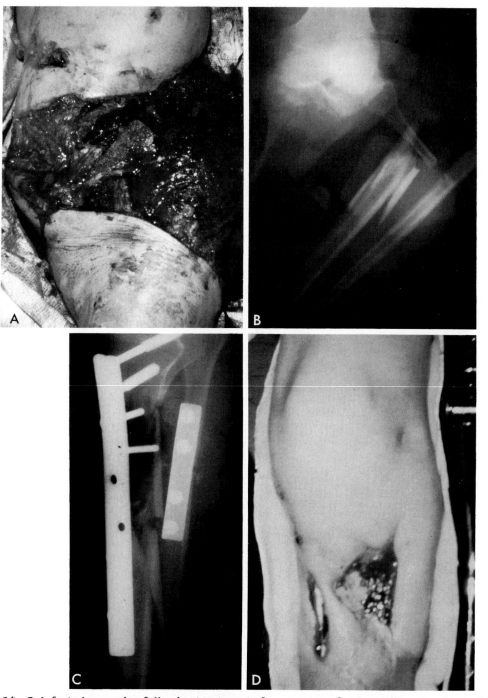

FIGURE 14 – 2. Infected nonunion following treatment of severe open fracture with extensive soft tissue injuries in a young woman. Culture revealed coagulase-positive *Staphylococcus.*

A, Severe soft tissue injuries and comminuted segmental fracture of the upper tibia.

B, Anteroposterior (AP) x-ray on admission shows severely comminuted displaced fracture of the upper tibia and fibula.

C, Early plating done to achieve wound stability; wound left open.

D, Four months later, wound is infected and not healed; plate is exposed and draining.

E, Debridement, sequestrectomy, and irrigation performed. Loose fibula plate removed. X-rays show large gap at fracture site.

F, G, Plate became loose and was removed: external fixation device applied to achieve fracture stability.

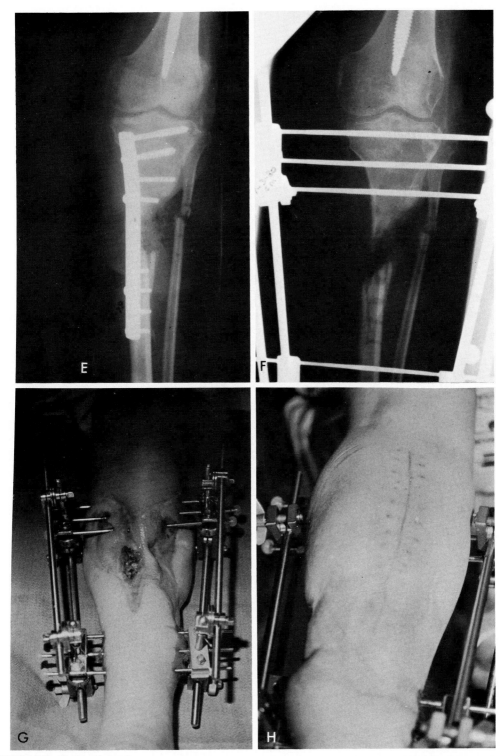

FIGURE 14–2 *Continued*

H, Three weeks later following application of external fixator, cancellous bone graft done posteriorly.

I, AP and lateral x-rays 15 months after injury and 9 months after bone graft show progressive healing of the fracture site.

J–L, The wound is completely healed 15 months after injury. The patient is ambulatory, with good knee and ankle motion.

(From Gustilo RB, ed: Management of infected nonunion. In Management of Open Fractures and Their Complications, Vol IV. Philadelphia, WB Saunders Co, 1982, pp 177–179.)

Illustration continued on following page

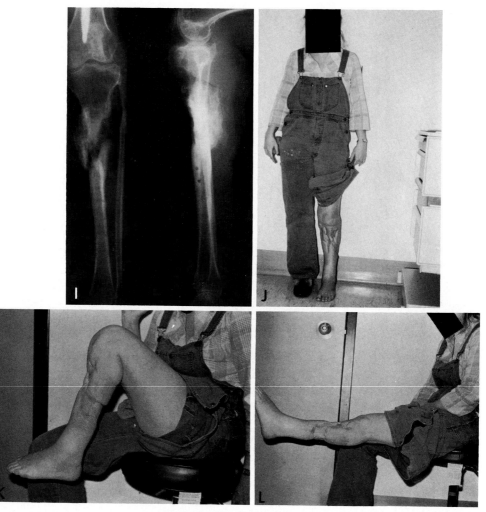

FIGURE 14-2 *Continued*

operating room for repeat debridement and irrigation. If the wound looks clean and infection is under control, a definitive stabilizing procedure is performed. Otherwise, wait another 5 to 7 days.

External Fixation

The alternative to traction is the immediate application of an external fixation device, with half pins 5 to 6 mm in diameter placed away from the infected area. This is the preferred method of immobilizing a fracture with extensive osteomyelitis and soft tissue injury, particularly of the tibia. The external fixation device is better than the pins and plaster technique for four reasons:

1. It provides better stability.
2. The larger area of the extremity is exposed, facilitating care of the infected wound by daily dressings and irrigation.
3. It allows surgical procedures, such as skin graft, rotation flaps, or cross-leg flaps, to be done more easily than pins and plaster cast immobilization.
4. It provides ease of application without additional trauma to soft tissues.

However, there are disadvantages:
1. Infection through pin tracts may occur.
2. The femur is not ideal for achieving rigid stability because of increased pin infection. There is inherent danger of application (bicortical pins) because of vital structures located medially.
3. There is a high incidence of infection fol-

lowing nailing, when an external fixator has been previously applied.

If the wound is completely healed, cast immobilization and early weight bearing may be substituted for external fixation. Late angulation may result if there is not enough fracture stability. Green and Dlabal[8] reported success in 13 of 15 patients with an external fixator providing stability until complete fracture healing is obtained with an average of 7.5 months. Lifeso and Al-Saati[9] reported success in 95 percent (35 out of 37 cases) in active, infected nonunion treated with sequestrectomy, external fixator, and bone grafting. The external fixator was removed following bone grafting, and a patellar tendon weight-bearing cast was applied.

Plating infected fractures would have been heresy 20 years ago, particularly among surgeons trained in the United States and England, where the influence of Watson-Jones in fracture treatment was overwhelming. "Moreover, special care should be taken to avoid fixation by metal screws and plates which serve as foreign bodies causing persistent infection and sinus formation."[10] The apprehension, however, over using plates to achieve stability of a fracture with or without compression, in infected nonunion, has been proven wrong by various reports.[5, 11, 12] Meyer and co-workers[11] and Mueller and Thomas[12] used primarily plates in a large series of cases of infected nonunion and achieved success rates of 93 percent and 87 percent, respectively, with union and control of infection. In 24 cases of infected nonunion, Rosen,[13] using primarily plates with cancellous bone grafting, achieved 83 percent excellent results with union and no drainage. In the past, whenever metal was used in the treatment of either open fractures or infected nonunion, the wound was primarily closed with or without a suction irrigation setup. The rate of wound breakdown has been alarmingly high. Primary wound closure with plating of infected nonunions accounts for the high failure rate in the past.

Compression plating is accomplished only after resection of the sclerosed portion of the fracture and the intervening scarred and infected soft tissue. With plating, one must try to maintain length and avoid undue shortening of more than 1 inch. Where length must be maintained, the plate is used as a holding device and the gap between bone ends is filled with cancellous bone, over granulation tissue, in 10 to 21 days.

Plating may be done either at the time of original debridement and irrigation or 5 to 7 days after the second or third debridement. The wound is left open; in 5 to 7 days, secondary closure by direct suture may be done to cover the plate and a suction irrigation system may be instilled for 3 to 5 days if a large cavity is present or potential excessive drainage is expected. If there is inadequate soft tissue coverage, the wound is left open and granulation tissue is allowed to develop for several weeks until the plate is completely covered. Closure may be completed with split-thickness skin grafting, or the wound may be allowed to heal completely by secondary intention or local or free muscle flap coverage. Cancellous bone grafting may also be done at the time of plating or 5 to 7 days later at wound closure.

Intramedullary Nailing (Fig. 14 – 5)

If an internal fixation device, such as a plate or a nail, has been applied at the original time of surgery, it must be left in place if it maintains stability. If it is loose, the internal fixation device is removed and stability is achieved by either an external fixation device or plating or renailing with a larger nail. Occasionally, if the infection is relatively benign with slight drainage, immediate reinsertion of a larger nail following reaming may be done immediately. Reports by Macausland and Eaton[14] showed excellent results with 100 percent union in treating 14 femurs with intramedullary nailing, where rigid stability was secured. Kostuik and Harrington[15] in 1979 obtained union of 80 percent of 16 fractures treated by intramedullary nailing and a few cases in which additional external immobilization was used when rigid stability was not accomplished. However, 11 out of 20 patients had persistent drainage.

Lottes[16, 17] reported a 70 percent success rate in the nailing of 24 infected tibias, but with a 12.5 percent (three patients) rate of amputation.

With intramedullary nailing, one also risks the potential hazard of massive osteomyelitis involving the entire shaft of the long bone, which I personally have not observed. Intramedullary nailing, however, remains a viable alternative for maintaining stability of infected long bones, particularly in the femur, because of the amount of surrounding soft tissue in a fracture located in the middle third of the femur. Intramedullary nailing provides excellent stability at this particular site and early, full weight bearing. In long bones that are os-

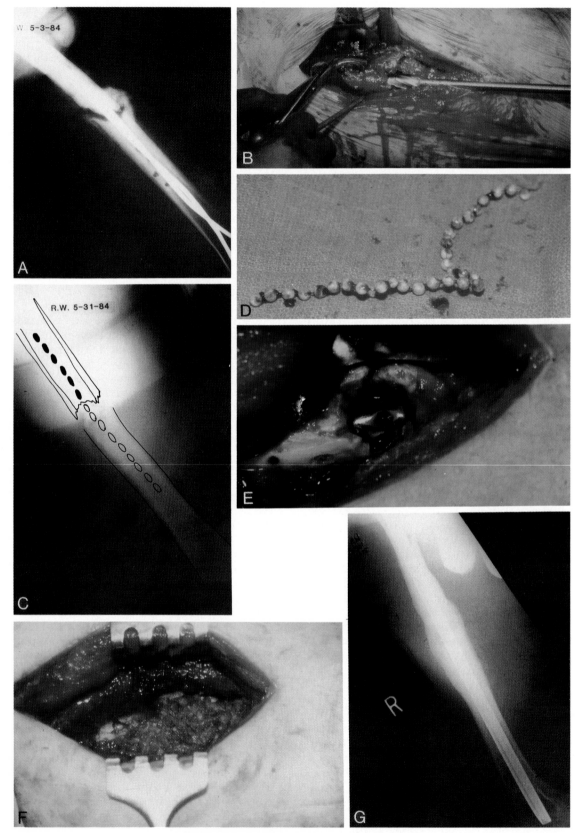

FIGURE 14–3 *See legend on opposite page*

teoporotic, either from disease or from prolonged immobilization, nailing also provides better stable fixation in appropriate sites than do plating or external fixation devices. The upper segment of the shaft of the femur and the subtrochanteric area is well stabilized by a combination of intramedullary rod insertion and nail fixation of the head and neck, such as with the Zickel nail; the lower third of the femur is stabilized by locking nails.

Skeletal Traction

There is no place for skeletal traction as a definitive treatment for infected nonunion. Skeletal traction is indicated as a temporary measure for immobilization, for 5 to 7 days, in patients with a florid local infection or with bacteremia or septicemia. There are three main disadvantages of skeletal traction:

1. It does not provide enough stability for bone union to occur in an infected fracture.

2. Frequent dressing changes, either at the bedside or in the operating room, are difficult because not enough stability is provided to remove the pain. Also, there is the inconvenience of getting the patient in and out of traction.

3. It is difficult to maintain good alignment.

Skeletal traction should be short-lived and must be replaced with external fixation, plating, or an intramedullary device.

CARE OF THE WOUND

Primary closure after initial debridement and sequestrectomy is not recommended in infected nonunion, even with a closed suction irrigation system, no matter how minor the infection appears to be. The wound must be packed open with moist dressings soaked with antibiotic solution or plain normal saline solution. Our practice is to bring the patient back to the operating room in 24 to 36 hours for change of dressings and further debridement of dead tissue and dead bone, if present. This is followed by daily dressing of the wound at the bedside and irrigation with normal saline solution or 0.1 percent bacitracin-polymixin solution. If early granulation tissue has developed and the infection is definitely under control, secondary closure may be performed, using direct suture without tension; hemovac suction, usually without irrigation, may be used. Suction irrigation systems may be instituted for 3 to 5 days if there is a large potential cavity. Prolonged use of an irrigation system could lead to a secondary superinfection, particularly of gram-negative bacteria, that is more difficult to treat than the original infection.

CLOSED SUCTION AND IRRIGATION

Early reports by Goldman and colleagues[18] in 1960, and McElvenny[19] in 1961, of continuous or intermittent closed suction irrigation treatment in conjunction with debridement showed a high success rate of cure in 17 cases of osteomyelitis. However, later reports by various investigators[20-25] revealed an incidence of recurrent drainage ranging from 17 to 52 percent. The majority of the studies were of osteomyelitis with healed fractures. Kelly and co-authors[26] reported a 34.8 percent failure rate in 23 cases of nonunion treated with debridement, antibiotics, and closed suction irrigation system, compared with 19 percent in 21 infected nonunited fractures treated in the same manner but without a closed suction irrigation system.

Installation of an open irrigation system for 1 to 4 weeks, depending on the severity of the infection, has been advocated by Meyer and co-workers.[11] According to these workers, the principles of treatment in 64 cases of infected nonunion consisted of (1) radical debridement

---

FIGURE 14-3. Infected nonunion of the midshaft left femur.

A, Draining sinus, 10 months following Ender nailing of Type II open fracture of femur, Anteroposterior (AP) x-rays showed definite gap between fracture ends with sclerosis.

B, Ender nails were removed. Medullary reaming was done proximally and distally.

C, Tobramycin beads were inserted as shown in x-rays. The patient was treated temporarily in traction.

D, Antibiotic beads were removed. Cultures were taken proximally and distally.

E, An intramedullary nail was inserted for fracture stability. The wound was left open.

F, Cancellous bone was treated, and the wound was closed in 5 days.

G, Thirteen months following nailing and grafting, the fracture healed completely without recurrence of sepsis.

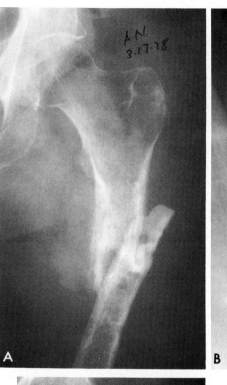

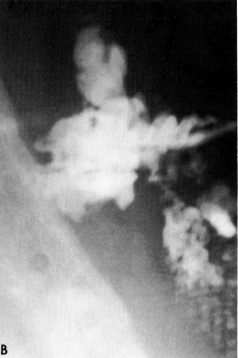

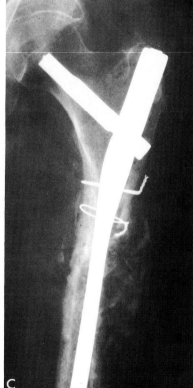

FIGURE 14–4. Infected nonunion and draining sinus tract of the proximal femur, of 2 years' duration, with severe osteoporosis and good soft tissue coverage. The patient was a 58-year-old woman who had undergone open reduction and plating of the left femur. Culture revealed coagulase-positive *Staphylococcus.* She had undergone two plating procedures and 6 months of traction, followed by a spica cast for 6 months.

A, Anteroposterior (AP) x-ray showed nonunion of a fracture of the upper third of the femur, with a sequestrum and marked sclerosis of the bone end. Diffuse severe osteoporosis was present.

B, Sinogram showed widespread soft tissue involvement, extending down to the site of nonunion and the sequestrum.

C, Extensive debridement and sequestrectomy were done. Stable internal fixation was achieved with a Zickel nail. The wound was left open for 7 days, after which cancellous bone grafting and delayed closure were performed. Suction was used for 3 days.

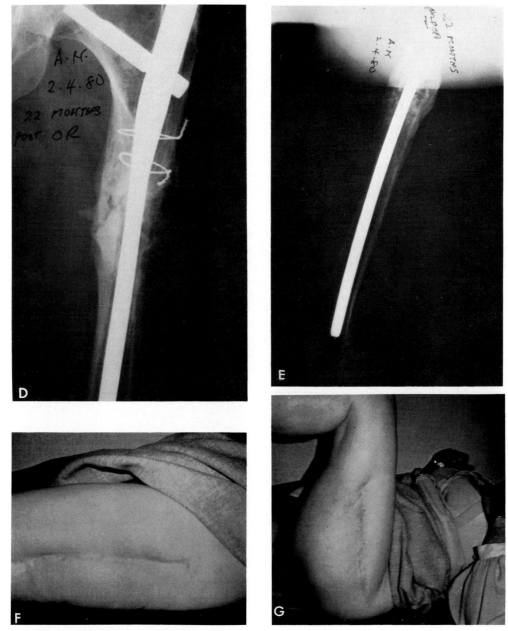

FIGURE 14–4 *Continued*

D, E, AP and lateral x-rays showed healed fracture 22 months later.

F, G, The wound has healed completely, and the patient has been walking without support. The left femur is ¾ inch shorter than the right.

(From Gustilo RB, ed: Management of infected nonunion. In Management of Open Fractures and Their Complications, Vol IV. Philadelphia, WB Saunders Co, 1982, pp 168–170.)

and sequestrectomy, (2) achievement of stability by plating or an external fixation device and occasionally by intramedullary nailing, (3) leaving the wound open, (4) no antibiotics and (5) an open irrigation system. The solution used was 1.0 mg/liter of neomycin-polymixin-bacitracin solution for 4 to 5 days, followed afterward by Ringer's lactate solution. Irrigation was discontinued when a layer of granulation tissue at the base of the wound and a minimal amount of persistent drainage were present. The authors[11] reported union in 53 of

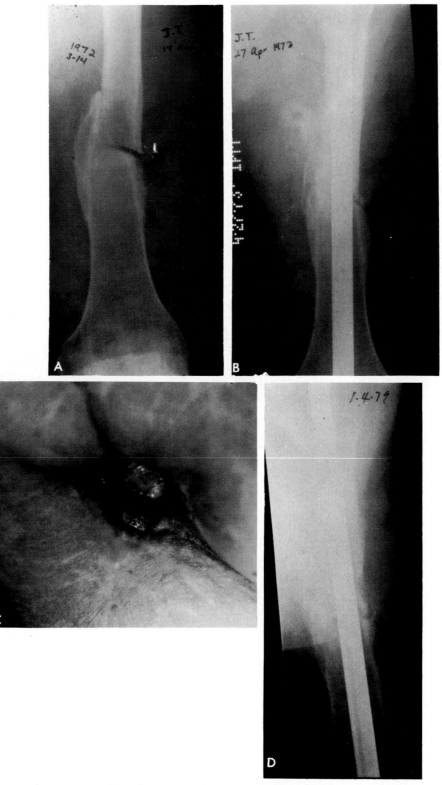

FIGURE 14–5. Infected nonunion of the right femur, with a draining sinus and a loose nail, in a 78-year-old man. Culture revealed coagulase-positive *Staphylococcus*.

A, Draining sinus of the distal third of the right femur; history of chronic osteomyelitis in the distal femur since 1968.

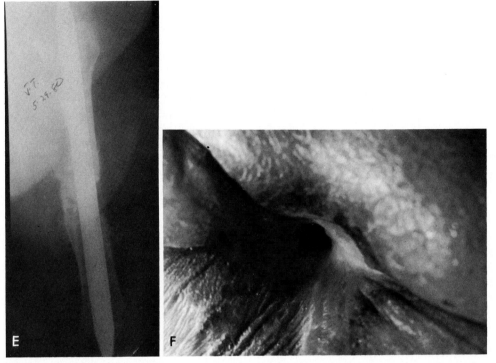

FIGURE 14–5 *Continued*

B, Fracture of the distal third of the right femur following a car accident in 1973. Intramedullary nailing and primary closure were performed, and suction irrigation was set up. The patient was hospitalized for eight weeks. Drainage had stopped for 5 years.

C, D, Recurrent drainage and pain for about a year. Anteroposterior (AP) and lateral x-rays show nonunion at the fracture site with sequestrum formation.

E, The loose 15-mm nail was removed, and a 19-mm nail inserted following reaming. The wound was left open. Two weeks later, cancellous bone grafting was done. The wound was allowed to heal by secondary intention.

F, Three months later, the wound showed granulation tissue covering most of the cancellous graft. Recurrent drainage was minimal. The patient was ambulatory without pain.

(From Gustilo RB, ed: Management of infected nonunion. In Management of Open Fractures and Their Complications, Vol IV. Philadelphia, WB Saunders Co, 1982, pp 180–181.)

57 cases of infected nonunion with 5 to 21 years of follow-up, persistent drainage in four, amputation in two, and death in two.

The question is: What are the indications for closed suction irrigation system at present? Which is better — continuous use of an irrigation system or intermittent use with pressure employed three to four times per day?

The indications for a closed suction irrigation system are limited, and one must adhere to the principles closely. The indications are (1) a large potential space or cavity after skin closure and (2) anticipation of a large amount of drainage or bleeding when the wound is closed.

The irrigation system must be used for a short time, 3 to 5 days, not 3 to 4 weeks as advocated by many, to prevent superinfection

with gram-negative organisms. Jergesen and Jawetz[24] advocated a system of intermittent pressure suction irrigation with a single tube rather than the continuous flow system advocated by many others.[20-22] There are, however, no comparative studies to show which system is better. The use of local antibiotic beads precludes continued usage of a suction irrigation system for local antibiotic delivery without the complication of superinfection. We have not used the suction irrigation method for at least 5 years.

Papineau Procedure

The Papineau procedure is indicated in cases of infected nonunion with inadequate soft tissue coverage and loss of bone. It is performed in three stages, in accordance with the following principles:

1. Excision of infected soft tissue and cicatrix; sequestrectomy, including, if indicated, removal of bone ends, resulting in bone loss and instability; stabilization of the fracture site.
2. Cancellous bone grafting.
3. Skin grafting if necessary.
4. Appropriate and prolonged antibiotic therapy.

The removal of devitalized, necrotic, and infected soft tissue, as well as of sequestra, must be thorough and complete to ensure that a vascular environment has been achieved. Either an internal or an external fixation device must be applied to achieve stability of the fracture. My preferred devices for stabilization are (1) an external fixation device, (2) an intramedullary nail, if stability can be achieved, and (3) plating. The introduction of locking nails has extended the indications of intramedullary nails in the stabilization of infected nonunion.

The wound must be covered with healthy granulation tissue as an essential prerequisite to cancellous bone grafting. The iliac crest is the preferred donor site, for it provides enough bone to cover the whole cavity or large gaps between bone ends. Some have used the greater trochanter, the proximal tibia, or the distal femur as donor sites, but usually they provide insufficient cancellous bone. The cavity must be filled up to the skin level with cancellous bone.

CANCELLOUS BONE GRAFTING

Early cancellous bone grafting is recommended when there is no evidence of purulent drainage and when early or good granulation has occurred.

Cancellous bone grafting can be performed as early as 5 to 10 days after initial debridement and irrigation and may be used in conjunction with internal fixation. The wound is left open, and 5 to 10 days later it can be closed without tension. However, suction may be inserted at the time of closure without an irrigation set-up.

In infected nonunion with a large cavity or bone defect and inadequate soft tissue coverage and inability to close the skin directly, with or without bony continuity, the operation described by Papineau and colleagues may be performed.[27] They achieved 93 percent good to excellent results in 39 cases of chronic osteomyelitis treated with open excision and radial saucerization followed by cancellous bone grafting on granulation tissue.

Wound Care

Dressings are not changed after cancellous bone grafting until the fourth or fifth postoperative day. They are changed every day thereafter, and the area is soaked with normal saline solution. Care should be taken during the removal of dressings, particularly during the first 7 to 10 days, in order to avoid removing cancellous bone pieces that are still mobile. At the end of 2 to 3 weeks, usually the graft is infiltrated with early granulation tissue from the wound periphery and the underlying surface of the graft, making the graft then difficult to remove. At that time, the wound appears brown or black, which is the normal appearance. With frequent dressings, it becomes covered with red granulation tissue.

Skin Closure

Closure of the wound can be achieved by either split-thickness skin grafts over the granulation tissue or local rotational or free vascularized muscle flap. Ambulation is started in 4 to 6 weeks, but weight bearing is not allowed until the fracture is completely healed, which takes 8 to 9 months. X-rays taken in anteroposterior, lateral, and oblique projections must show complete healing of the fracture with corticalization of the cancellous bone.

Posterolateral Bone Grafting

In infected nonunion of the tibia with indolent ulceration or draining sinus anteriorly, usually with poor skin, posterolateral bone grafting and cast immobilization are recommended. Patzakis[28] reported over 90 percent success rate of union with cessation of drainage anteriorly. Usually, the patient is in a cast for 4 to 6 months. The other alternative is external fixation for immobilization and posterolateral bone grafting.

ANTIBIOTIC THERAPY

Several cultures and smears must be taken at the very depth of the wound, including the intramedullary canal, at the time of surgery. Interpretation of bacteria from the cultures taken from the sinus tract is misleading in identifying the real infecting organisms. Only when cultures have been taken from the depth of the wound can treatment with antibiotics be started. Before the results of the culture are known, antibiotic treatment, usually with cephalosporins, may be begun immediately, during surgery, and after surgery.

In general, cephalosporins are effective against gram-positive and a number of gram-negative bacteria, except *Pseudomonas*. The usual dose is 6 to 12 gm, depending on the type of cephalosporin and the severity of the infection. When the infection is caused by a gram-positive bacterium (coagulase-positive *Staphylococcus*) that is sensitive to penicillin, penicillin is the drug of choice (10,000,000 to 12,000,000 units daily). Seventy percent of coagulase-positive *Staphylococcus* in cases of infected nonunion are resistant to penicillin. Synthetic penicillin, such as oxacillin and sodium methicillin (Staphcillin) is the drug of choice in 6- to 12-gm doses. When culture and sensitivity results are reported, the antibiotic therapy must be changed accordingly. Appropriate massive antibiotics are given intravenously for 4 to 6 weeks and then orally for 3 to 6 months.

In wounds that have been left open for a long time, superinfection with gram-negative rods or mixed infection with gram-negative rods and coagulase-positive *Staphylococcus* presents a very difficult problem.[1, 29] Usually, these organisms are sensitive only to aminoglycosides, which have potential nephrotoxic and ototoxic complications. The difficulty in the management of infection with gram-negative rods, either alone or in a mixed infection with coagulase-positive *Staphylococcus*, has been shown by Kelly and colleagues,[1] who reported a failure rate of 28 percent, in contrast to a 100 percent success rate in the treatment of pure gram-positive infection. The patient, therefore, is usually given a program of aminoglycoside therapy for 10 days during the initial debridement and cancellous bone grafting. When the wound is closed, the patient is given a second course of aminoglycoside therapy for another 10 days. Daily serum creatinine levels, as well as the blood level of aminoglycosides, are monitored in order to determine effectiveness as well as to check toxicity level. Prolonged antibiotic therapy over 6 weeks in infection is of questionable value in the treatment of infected nonunion.

Local Antibiotic Bead Therapy

The release of gentamicin from polymethylmethacrylate beads in high concentration and its penetration to surrounding tissues including cortical and cancellous bone, as shown by Wahlig[30] and Hoff[31] and their associates, leads to a superior delivery of local antibiotic therapy, particularly aminoglycosides. We use tobramycin beads — 6 mm in diameter, 60 to 90[6] in number, and placed inside the intramedullary canal and wound area following sequestrectomy and intramedullary reaming. The dose is 1.2 gm of tobramycin powder in 20 gm of bone cement. The antibiotic beads are left in place for 2 to 3 weeks and removed when cancellous bone grafting or intramedullary nailing is done. The experience in the United States is still limited. However, this method of delivering aminoglycosides at very high concentrations at the infected fracture site at very high concentrations without toxicity is undergoing extensive clinical trial in our institution.

SUMMARY

The prerequisites for a satisfactory outcome in the management of an infected nonunion are as follows:

1. Radical excision of soft tissue and dead bone.
2. Achievement of fracture stability.
3. Early and massive cancellous bone graft overlying early granulation tissue.
4. Daily dressing change after the fourth or fifth, with use of normal saline solution to prevent accumulation of purulent material.
5. Non–weight bearing until the soft tissue has healed.
6. Skin coverage by skin graft overlying granulation tissue or healing by secondary intention.
7. Prolonged non–weight bearing until the fracture is completely healed and the cancellous graft has been incorporated with cortical bone.
8. Appropriate antibiotic therapy and antibiotic beads.

References

1. Kelly PJ, Wilkowski CJ, Washington JA II: Comparison of gram-negative bacillary and staphylococcal osteomyelitis of the femur and tibia. Clin Orthop 96:70, 1973.
2. Gustilo RB: Use of antimicrobials in the management of open fractures. Arch Surg 114:805, 1979.
3. Gustilo RB, Gruninger R, Davis T: Classification of

Type III (severe) open fractures relative to treatment and results. Orthopedics 10:1781, 1987.

4. Lidgren L, Torholm C: Intramedullary reaming in chronic diaphyseal osteomyelitis: a preliminary report. Clin Orthop 151:215–221, 1980.

5. Rittmann WW, Perren SM: Corticale Knochenheilung nach Osteosynthese und Infektion. Biomechanik und Biologie. Berlin, Springer-Verlag, 1974.

6. Friedrich B, Klaue P: Mechanical stability and posttraumatic osteitis: an experimental evaluation of the relation between infection of bone and internal fixation. Injury 9:23, 1977.

7. Gristina AG, Rovere GD: An in vitro study of the effects of metals used in internal fixation on bacterial growth and dissemination. J Bone Joint Surg 58A:453, 1976.

8. Green SA, and Dlabal TA: The open bone graft for septic nonunion. Clin Orthop 180:117–124, 1983.

9. Lifeso RM, Al-Saati F: The treatment of infected and uninfected nonunion. J Bone Joint Surg 66B:573–579, 1984.

10. Watson-Jones R: Fractures and Joint Injuries, Vol I. Principles of Fracture Treatment. Edinburgh, E. & S. Livingstone, Ltd., 1952, p 32.

11. Meyer S, Weiland AJ, Willenegger H: The treatment of infected nonunion of fractures of long bones. J Bone Joint Surg 57A:836, 1975.

12. Mueller ME, Thomas RJ: Treatment of nonunion in fractures of long bones. Clin Orthop 138:141, 1979.

13. Rosen H: Compression treatment of long bone pseudoarthroses. Clin Orthop 138:154, 1979.

14. Macausland WR Jr, Eaton RG: Sepsis following fixation of fractures of the femur. J Bone Joint Surg 45A:1647, 1963.

15. Kostuik JP, Harrington IJ: Treatment of infected ununited femoral shaft fractures. Clin Orthop 108:90, 1975.

16. Lottes JO: Medullary nailing of infected fractures of the tibia. J Bone Joint Surg 45A:543, 1963.

17. Lottes JO: Medullary nailing of the tibia with the triflange nail. Clin Orthop 105:253, 1974.

18. Goldman MD, Johnson RK, Grossberg NM: A new approach to chronic osteomyelitis. Am J Orthop 2:63, 1960.

19. McElvenny RT: Circulation and suction, Part II. Am J Orthop 3:154, 1961.

20. Clawson DK, Davis FJ, Hansen ST Jr: Treatment of chronic osteomyelitis with emphasis on closed suction-irrigation technique. Clin Orthop 96:88, 1973.

21. Compere EL, Metzger WI, Mitra RN: The treatment of pyogenic bone and joint infections by closed irrigation (circulation) with a nontoxic detergent and one or more antibiotics. J Bone Joint Surg 49A:614, 1967.

22. Dombrowski ET, Dunn AW: Treatment of osteomyelitis by debridement and closed wound irrigation-section. Clin Orthop 43:215, 1965.

23. Horwitz T: Surgical treatment of chronic osteomyelitis complicating fractures. Clin Orthop 96:118, 1973.

24. Jergesen F, Jawetz E: Pyogenic infections in orthopedic surgery: combined antibiotic and closed wound treatment. Am J Surg 106:152, 1963.

25. Lawyer RO Jr, Eyring EJ: Intermittent closed suction-irrigation treatment of osteomyelitis. Clin Orthop 8:80, 1972.

26. Kelly PJ, Martin WJ, Coventry MB: Chronic osteomyelitis. II. Treatment with closed irrigation and suction. JAMA 213:1843, 1970.

27. Papineau LJ, Alfageme A, Dalcourt JP, et al: Ostéomyélite chronique: excision et greffe de spongieux a l'air libre aprés mises a plat extensives. Int Orthop 3:165, 1979.

28. Patzakis MJ: Personal communication. University of California, Los Angeles.

29. Fitzgerald RH, Ruttle PE, Arnold PG, Kelly PJ, Irons GB: Local muscle flaps in the treatment of chronic osteomyelitis. J Bone Joint Surg 67A:175–185, 1985.

30. Wahlig H, Dingeldein E, Bergmann R, Reuss K: The release of gentamicin from polymethylmethacrylate beads: an experimental and pharmacokinetic study. J Bone Joint Surg 60B:270–275, 1978.

31. Hoff SF, Fitzgerald RH, Kelly PJ: The depot administration of penicillin G and gentamicin in acrylic bone cement. J Bone Joint Surg 63A:798–804, 1981.

CHAPTER

15

Management of Chronic Osteomyelitis

INTRODUCTION

Chronic osteomyelitis challenges every orthopedic surgeon because it is an infection that is difficult to treat and to eradicate completely and indefinitely. It involves repeated surgery, expensive antibiotic therapy, and prolonged hospitalization. The changes during the last decade in the treatment of chronic osteomyelitis (healed fracture) that have affected the outcome of success or failure include the following:

1. Change of bacterial flora from gram-positive to gram-negative or mixed infection or anaerobic infection.

2. Good surgical technique in performing osteomyelitis surgery with removal of the bone and infected soft tissues.

3. Sophisticated wound coverage technique — free flaps, local flaps, and so forth.

4. Aggressive and early cancellous bone grafting.

5. Combined orthopedic and infectious disease consultant approach to monitor microbiologic procedures for bacterial identification and to supervise prolonged antibiotic therapy.

DIAGNOSIS

Oftentimes the diagnosis of chronic osteomyelitis is easy. Usually, there is a history of an open fracture, an open reduction and internal fixation of an open or closed fracture, or hematogenous osteomyelitis. The patient may tell the physician that at one time the bone became infected, that there was purulent drainage, and that antibiotic therapy was given for a time. The patient may present with a draining sinus, either intermittently or chronically. There may be recurrent redness and swelling followed by spontaneous drainage or apparent regression with oral antibiotic therapy. Oftentimes, there is a history of at least two or three surgical procedures. Radiographs (anteroposterior, lateral, and oblique) of the extremities are often confirmatory, revealing periosteal elevation, sequestrum formation, lysis, or bone defect. Sinograms usually show extension of the sinus tract and to some degree the extent of the infection. We recommend bone scanning using three-phase technetium 99m (^{99m}Tc) and, if results are positive, following with gallium. This will help in making the diagnosis in case of a negative plain radiograph but strong clinical evidence of osteomyelitis. The use of indium 111 or magnetic resonance imaging (MRI) is very useful in difficult diagnostic problems. The latter examination is particularly useful in determining intramedullary extent of osteomyelitis.

TREATMENT

The goals of treatment of chronic osteomyelitis are (1) to eradicate the infection by achieving a viable and vascular environment, (2) to prevent recurrences, and (3) to achieve a normal functioning limb if possible.

The current concepts of treatment include:

1. Radical surgery of bone and soft tissue.

2. Proper identification of the bacteria followed by appropriate massive and prolonged antibiotic therapy for 6 weeks.

3. Local antibiotic beads.

4. Appropriate and timely wound coverage.

5. Cancellous bone grafting to fill large defects.

From the Department of Orthopaedic Surgery, Hennepin County Medical Center, Minneapolis, Minnesota.

6. Early rehabilitation of the involved extremity. An early isometric and active exercise program is started in the involved joint above and below the involved bone.

7. Deciding on early amputation.

Figure 15–1 illustrates concepts of management.

Radical Surgery

Radical excision of the sinus tract and avascular scarred and infected soft tissue is performed to produce active bleeding in the area of the margins surrounding the fracture site. Excision sometimes involves skin, subcutaneous tissue, fascia and muscles, and intervening scar tissue between the fracture ends. The longitudinal incision must be generous to accomplish complete debridement. Viable skin should be left in place. Apprehension over not being able to close the skin should not and must not be a determining factor during the excision of infected and scarred tissues.

Removal of necrotic bone and sequestrum is often difficult to achieve in chronic osteomyelitis because of the surgeon's inability to differentiate between normal and dead bone. Also, one becomes apprehensive about removing too much bone and creating marked instability or loss of bone continuity. Dead bone must be removed with sharp rongeurs or osteotomes. Predrilling oftentimes helps to prevent fracturing the shaft when using osteotomes on hard, sclerotic bone. The intramedullary canal must be curetted to remove necrotic debris inside the canal. At intervals, copious irrigation by jet lavage, with bacitracin-polymyxin solution or normal saline solution, is essential.

Intramedullary Reaming (Fig. 15–2)

In chronic diaphyseal osteomyelitis, there is marked sclerosis and long segmental avascular bone. It is very difficult to determine the extent of endosteal or intramedullary extension of the infection. Lidgren and Torholm,[1] in justifying intramedullary reaming in chronic osteomyelitis, believe it diminishes interosseous pressure and revascularizes the bone, thereby improving the endosteal circulation. They obtained satisfactory results in 16 of 18 cases. We have been reaming 2 mm over size the measured intramedullary canal either from above or through the open diaphyseal segment where sequestrectomy has been performed or proximally, as done in closed nailing. Bleeding bone surface and bleeding soft tissue around and at the fracture site must be obtained. Repeat debridement under general anesthesia is mandatory, in 2 to 3 days, to ensure that complete removal of dead bone and infected tissue has been accomplished. Our preliminary results were encouraging, at 18 to 24 months follow-up, with 80 percent cessation of drainage.

Antibiotic Therapy

Several cultures and smears must be taken at the very depth of the wound, including the intramedullary canal, at the time of surgery. Interpretation of bacteria from the cultures taken from the sinus tract is misleading in identifying the real infecting organisms. Only when cultures have been taken from the depth of the wound can treatment with antibiotics be started. Before the results of the culture are known, antibiotic treatment, usually with cephalosporins, may be begun immediately, during and after surgery.

In general, cephalosporins are effective against gram-positive and a number of gram-negative bacteria, except *Pseudomonas.* The usual dose is 6 to 12 gm, depending on the type of cephalosporin and the severity of the infection. When the infection is caused by a gram-positive bacterium (coagulase-positive *Staphylococcus*) that is sensitive to penicillin, penicillin is the drug of choice, 10 to 12 million units daily being given. Seventy percent of coagulase-positive *Staphylococcus* in cases of chronic osteomyelitis is resistant to penicillin. Synthetic penicillin, such as oxacillin and sodium methicillin (Staphcillin) is the drug of choice in 6- to 12-gm doses, or vancomycin, 750 to 1000 mg every 12 hours. When culture and sensitivity results are reported, the antibiotic therapy must be changed accordingly. Appropriate massive antibiotics are given intravenously for 4 to 6 weeks. Oral antibiotics are generally not recommended.

In wounds that have been left open for a long time, or in chronic draining sinus, particularly with soft tissue defect, gram-negative rods or mixed infection with gram-negative rods and coagulase-positive *Staphylococcus* is common and presents a very difficult problem. Fitzgerald and associates[2] reported *Pseudomonas* as the most common causal organism in 42 chronic osteomyelitis cases present for at least 2 years after treatment. Usually, these

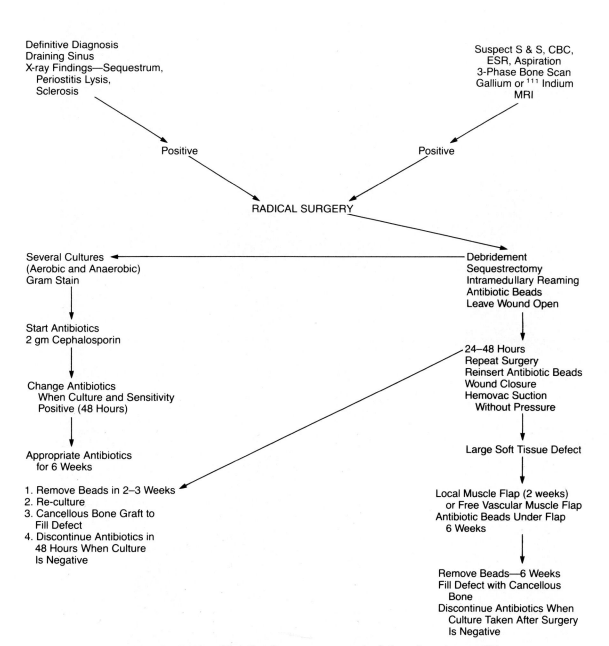

FIGURE 15–1. Algorithm for the management of chronic osteomyelitis.

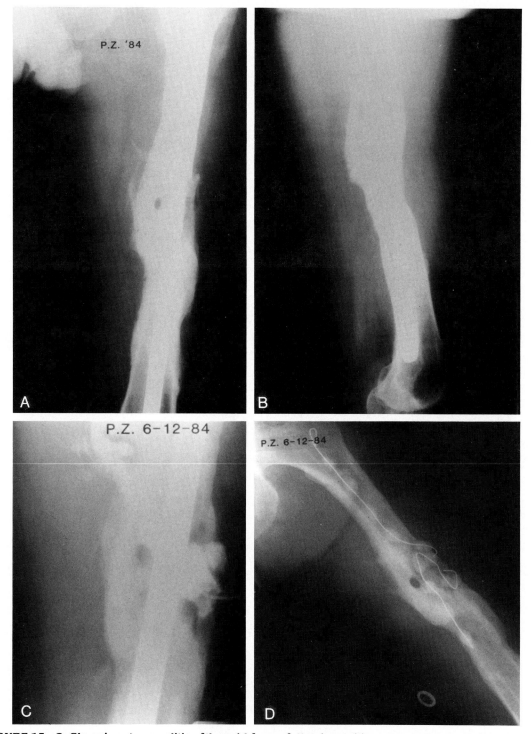

FIGURE 15 – 2. Chronic osteomyelitis of the mid-femur following nailing. *A, B,* Anteroposterior (AP) and lateral x-rays showed healed fracture with intramedullary nail.

C, Sinogram showed extension of infection inside canal.

D, The intramedullary nail was removed, and the entire medullary canal was reamed to bleeding bone. Tobramycin beads were inserted inside the intramedullary canal. The fracture was healed.

E, F, Tobramycin beads were removed after 2 weeks. The wound appeared clean and granulating. The cavity was filled with autogenous cancellous bone.

G, H, Follow-up x-rays at 2 years showed no evidence of recurrent sepsis with healed fracture. The patient is ambulating without support.

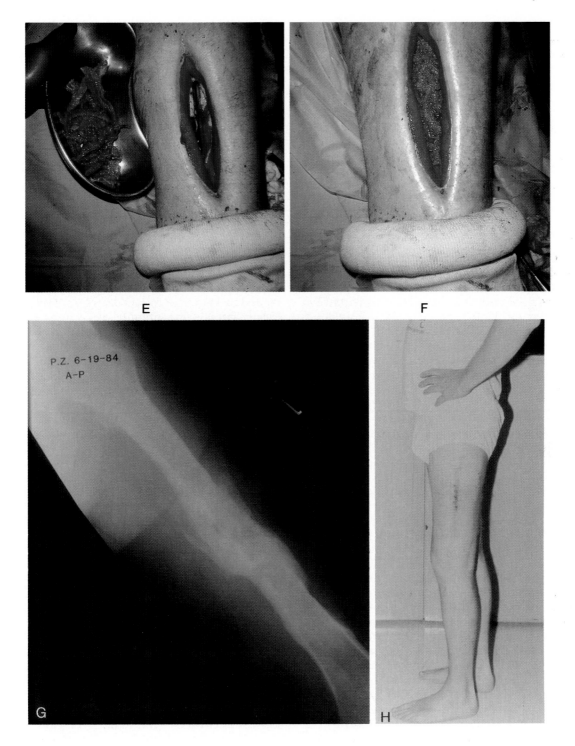

organisms are sensitive only to aminoglycosides, which have potential nephrotoxic and ototoxic complications. The difficulty in the management of infection with gram-negative rods, either alone or in a mixed infection with coagulase-positive *Staphylococcus,* has been shown by Kelly and colleagues,[3] who reported a failure rate of 28 percent, in contrast to a 100 percent success rate in the treatment of pure gram-positive infections. The patient, therefore, is usually given a program of aminoglycoside therapy for 10 days during the initial debridement and cancellous bone grafting. When the wound is closed, the patient is given a second course of aminoglycoside therapy for another 10 days. Daily serum creatinine levels, as well as the blood level of aminoglycosides, are monitored in order to determine the effectiveness as well as to check toxicity level. Prolonged antibiotic therapy in chronic osteomyelitis over 4 to 6 weeks is controversial. There is no evidence in the literature to indicate that prolonged antibiotic treatment of over 4 to 6 weeks in chronic osteomyelitis is beneficial or has improved long-term results.

LOCAL ANTIBIOTIC BEADS

The release of gentamicin from polymethylmethacrylate beads in high concentration and its penetration to surrounding tissues, including cortical and cancellous bone as shown by Wahlig[4] and Hoff[5] and their co-authors, lend to a superior delivery of antibiotic therapy, particularly aminoglycosides. The use of local antibiotic beads obviates the possible toxicity of prolonged parenteral aminoglycoside therapy and expense. We use tobramycin beads (6 mm in diameter and 60 to 90 in number) placed inside the intramedullary canal and wound area. The dose is 1.2 gm of tobramycin powder in 20 gm of bone cement. The antibiotic beads are left in place for 4 to 6 weeks and removed when cancellous bone grafting is done.

Appropriate and Timely Wound Coverage

We do not recommend primary wound closure after initial debridement, sequestrectomy, or reaming the diaphysis in chronic osteomyelitis. The wound must be packed open with moist dressings soaked with antibiotic solution or plain normal saline solution or packed with antibiotic beads (our choice). Our practice is to bring the patient back to the operating room in 24 to 48 hours for change of dressings and further debridement of dead tissue and dead bone if present. At that time, if the wound looks clean, tobramycin beads (90 to 120) are reinserted and the wound is closed in one layer without tension, with hemovac suction, but no pressure. The suction is in place for excess drainage or hematoma. The rationale is to avoid suctioning hematoma with high concentrations of antibiotics. If excessive drainage continues for 7 to 10 days after

wound closure, the wound is reopened, recultured, redebrided, irrigated, and repacked with a new batch of tobramycin beads. If free flap coverage is required, this is accomplished at 7 to 14 days with antibiotic beads underneath the flap. The use of local muscle flaps in the treatment of chronic osteomyelitis was successful in 93 percent in eradicating the infectious process, as reported by Fitzgerald and colleagues.[2] Our current practice is to leave tobramycin beads underneath the flaps for 6 weeks and then replace them with cancellous bone if there is a large defect to be filled.

Closure of the wound can be achieved by either split-thickness skin grafts over the granulation tissue or local rotational or cross-leg flap. Minimal weight bearing is started in 4 to 6 weeks, but full weight bearing is not allowed until the fracture is completely healed, which takes 8 to 9 months. X-rays taken in anteroposterior, lateral, and oblique projections must show complete healing of the fracture with corticalization of the cancellous bone. Our choice is to provide free flap coverage, followed 6 weeks later by cancellous bone grafting. During that period of time, the patient is receiving parenteral antibiotics and grafting and the beads are removed. Cancellous bone is used to fill the defect. Cultures are taken at the time of bone grafting, and parenteral antibiotics are continued postoperatively for 5 days until culture results are negative and the wound is healing well.

Cancellous Bone Grafting to Fill Large Defects

Early cancellous bone grafting is recommended when there is no evidence of purulent drainage and when early or good granulation has occurred.

Cancellous bone grafting can be performed as early as 5 to 10 days after initial debridement and irrigation. The wound is left open, and 5 to 10 days later it can be closed without tension.

In chronic osteomyelitis with inadequate soft tissue coverage and inability to close the skin directly, with bony continuity, the operation as described by Papineau and associates[6] is the other alternative of treatment. They achieved 93 percent good to excellent results in 39 cases of chronic osteomyelitis treated with open excision and radial saucerization followed by cancellous bone grafting on granulation tissue.

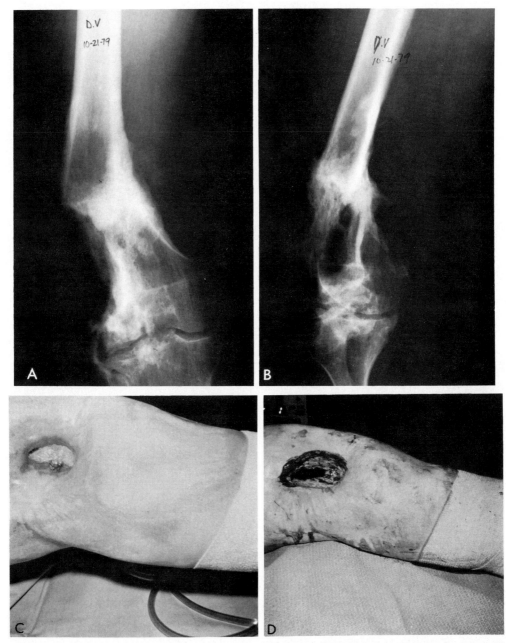

FIGURE 15–3. Chronic osteomyelitis of 10 years' duration, following treatment of a Type III open supracondylar fracture with vascular injury in a 31-year-old man. Healed fracture, chronic draining sinus, inadequate soft tissue coverage. Culture revealed *Pseudomonas aeruginosa.*

A, B, Anteroposterior (AP) and lateral x-rays showed complete healing of the fracture. However, there is a large area of lucency with a sequestrum at the supracondylar area. Note the large concavity defect.

C, Large, open draining cavity with sinus tract formation. Culture revealed *P. aeruginosa,* sensitive to aminoglycoside.

D, Radical debridement of scarred tissue and dead bone, sequestrectomy, and copious irrigation were performed. The patient was given gentamicin intravenously for 10 days.

Illustration continued on following page

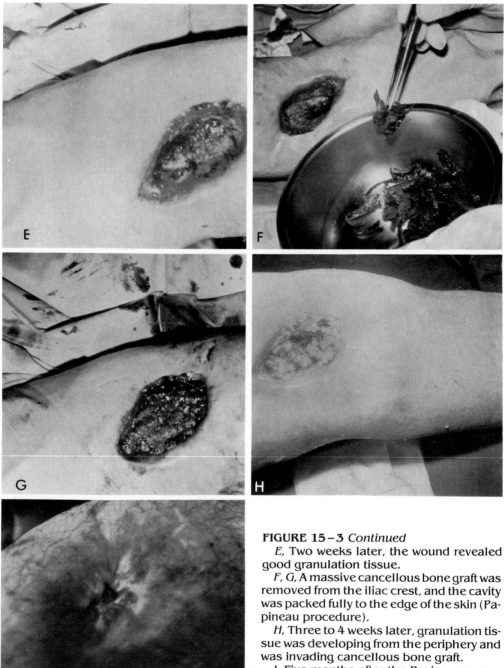

FIGURE 15–3 *Continued*

E, Two weeks later, the wound revealed good granulation tissue.

F, G, A massive cancellous bone graft was removed from the iliac crest, and the cavity was packed fully to the edge of the skin (Papineau procedure).

H, Three to 4 weeks later, granulation tissue was developing from the periphery and was invading cancellous bone graft.

I, Five months after the Papineau procedure, the wound was almost completely covered, with epithelialization taking place.

PAPINEAU PROCEDURE (Fig. 15–3)

The Papineau procedure is indicated in cases of infected nonunion with inadequate soft tissue coverage and loss of bone. It is performed in three stages, in accordance with the following principles:

1. Excision of infected soft tissue and cicatrix; sequestrectomy, including, if indicated, removal of bone ends, resulting in bone loss and instability.

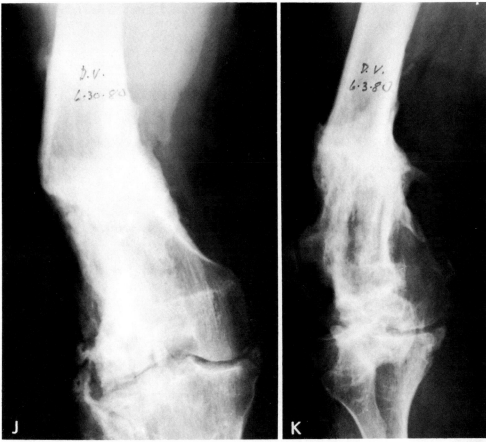

FIGURE 15-3 *Continued*

J, K, AP and lateral x-rays show sclerosis and filling of the cavity with bone. The patient had no recurrent drainage or pain.

L, Fifteen months after grafting, wound completely epithelialized and healed.

(From Gustilo RB, ed: Management of infected nonunion. In Management of Open Fractures and Their Complications, Vol IV. Philadelphia, WB Saunders Co, 1982, pp 174–176.)

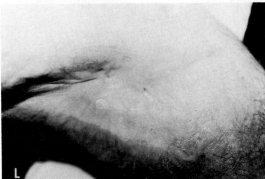

2. Stabilization of the fracture if not united.

3. Cancellous bone grafting.

4. Skin grafting if necessary.

5. Appropriate and prolonged antibiotic therapy.

The removal of devitalized, necrotic, and infected soft tissue, as well as sequestra, must be thorough and complete to ensure that a vascular environment has been achieved. Either an internal or an external fixation device must be applied to achieve stability of the fracture. My preference of devices for stabilization is (1) external fixation devices; (2) intramedullary nailing, if stability can be achieved; and (3) plate.

The wound must be covered with healthy granulation tissue as an essential prerequisite to cancellous bone grafting. The iliac crest is the preferred donor site, for it provides enough bone to cover the whole cavity or large gaps between bone ends. Some have used the greater trochanter, the proximal tibia, or the distal femur as donor sites, but usually they provide insufficient cancellous bone. The cavity must be filled up to the skin level with cancellous bone.

WOUND CARE

Dressings are not changed after cancellous bone grafting until the fourth or fifth postoperative day; they are changed every day thereafter, and the area is soaked with normal saline solution. Care should be taken during the removal of dressings, particularly during the first 7 to 10 days, in order to avoid removing the cancellous bone pieces that are still mobile. At the end of 2 to 3 weeks, usually, the graft is infiltrated with early granulation tissue from the wound periphery and the underlying surface of the graft, making the graft then difficult to remove. At that time, the wound appears brown or black, which is the normal appearance. With frequent dressings, it becomes covered with red granulation tissue.

Suction Irrigation System

The majority of studies[7-12] have involved osteomyelitis with healed fractures. Kelly and colleagues[13] reported a 34.8 percent failure rate in 23 cases of nonunion treated with debridement, antibiotics, and closed suction irrigation system, compared with 19 percent in 21 infected nonunited fractures treated in the same manner but without a closed suction irrigation system. Installation of an open irrigation system for 1 to 4 weeks, depending on the severity of the infection, has been advocated by Meyer and co-workers.[14] According to these workers, the principles of treatment in 64 cases of infected nonunion consisted of (1) radical debridement and sequestrectomy, (2) achievement of stability by plating or an external fixation device and occasionally by intramedullary nailing, (3) leaving the wound open, (4) no antibiotics, and (5) an open irrigation system. The solution used was 1.0 mg/liter of neomycin-polymyxin-bacitracin for 4 to 5 days, followed afterwards by Ringer's lactate solution. Irrigation was discontinued when there was a layer of granulation tissue at the base of the wound and a minimal amount of persistent drainage. The authors reported union in 53 of 57 cases of infected nonunion with 5 to 21 years of follow-up, persistent drainage in four, amputation in two, and death in two. The question is: What are the indications for closed suction irrigation system? Which is better — continuous use of an irriga-

tion system or intermittent use with pressure employed three to four times per day?

The indications for closed suction irrigation system are limited, and one must adhere to their principles closely. The indications are (1) a large potential space or cavity after skin closure and (2) anticipation of a large amount of drainage or bleeding when the wound is closed.

The irrigation system must be used for a short time, 3 to 5 days, not 3 to 4 weeks as advocated by many, to prevent superinfection with gram-negative organisms. Jergesen and Jawetz[15] and co-workers advocated a system of intermittent pressure suction irrigation with a single tube rather than the continuous flow system advocated by many others.[7-9, 16] There are, however, no comparative studies to show which system is better. The use of local antibiotic beads precludes the use of irrigation systems for antibiotic delivery.

Early Rehabilitation

An early isometric and active exercise program is started on day 1 in the involved joint above and below the involved bone.

Early Amputation

The patient must be apprised fully of the nature of the problem, the prolonged treatment, economic implications, and the permanent possibility of an amputation. The absolute indications for amputation are as follows:

1. When there is chronic, draining osteomyelitis of the tibia with an insensitive foot, particularly when below the knee amputation can be done.

2. When there is chronic, draining osteomyelitis with a large bone exposed; when there is a stiff foot; and when outer and free flap coverage is not possible because of arterial compromise.

3. When there have been repeated surgical procedures with failures and when the patient demands amputation.

SUMMARY

The key words for success in the treatment of chronic osteomyelitis are (1) radical surgery, (2) appropriate and massive parenteral and local antibiotics, (3) appropriate wound closure, and (4) cancellous bone grafting.

References

1. Lidgren L, Torholm C: Intramedullary reaming in chronic diaphyseal osteomyelitis: a preliminary report. Clin Orthop 151:215–221, 1980.
2. Fitzgerald RH, Ruttle PE, Arnold PG, Kelly PJ, Irons GB: Local muscle flaps in the treatment of chronic osteomyelitis. J Bone Joint Surg 67A:175–185, 1985.
3. Kelly PJ, Wilkowski CJ, Washington JA II: Comparison of gram-negative bacillary and staphylococcal osteomyelitis of the femur and tibia. Clin Orthop 96:70, 1973.
4. Wahlig H, Dingeldein E, Bergmann R, Reuss K: The release of gentamicin from polymethylmethacrylate beads: an experimental and pharmokinetic study. J Bone Joint Surg 60B:270–275, 1978.
5. Hoff SF, Fitzgerald RH, Kelly PJ: The depot administration of penicillin G and gentamicin in acrylic bone cement. J Bone Joint Surg 63A:798–804, 1981.
6. Papineau LJ, Alfageme A, Dalcourt JP, et al: Ostéomyélite chronique: excision et greffe de spongieux a l'air libre aprés mises a plat extensives. Int Orthop 3:165, 1979.
7. Clawson DK, Davis FJ, Hansen ST Jr: Treatment of chronic osteomyelitis with emphasis on closed suction-irrigation technique. Clin Orthop 96:88, 1973.
8. Compere EL, Metzger WI, Mitra RN: The treatment of pyogenic bone and joint infections by closed irrigation (circulation) with a nontoxic detergent and one or more antibiotics. J Bone Joint Surg 49A:614, 1967.
9. Dombrowski ET, Dunn AW: Treatment of osteomyelitis by debridement and closed wound irrigation-suction. Clin Orthop 43:215, 1965.
10. Goldman MD, Johnson RK, Grossberg NM: A new approach to chronic osteomyelitis. Am J Orthop 2:63, 1960.
11. Horwitz T: Surgical treatment of chronic osteomyelitis complicating fractures. Clin Orthop 96:118, 1973.
12. McElvenny RT: Circulation and suction. Part II. Am J Orthop 3:154, 1961.
13. Kelly PJ, Martin WJ, Coventry MB: Chronic osteomyelitis. II. Treatment with closed irrigation and suction. JAMA 213:1843, 1970.
14. Meyer S, Weiland AJ, Willenegger H: The treatment of infected nonunion of fractures of long bones. J Bone Joint Surg 57A:836, 1975.
15. Jergesen F, Jawetz E: Pyogenic infections in orthopedic surgery: combined antibiotic and closed wound treatment. Am J Surg 106:152, 1963.
16. Lawyer RO Jr, Eyring EJ: Intermittent closed suction-irrigation treatment of osteomyelitis. Clin Orthop 8:80, 1972.

Dean T. Tsukayama, M.D.
David R.P. Guay, Pharm.D.
Phillip K. Peterson, M.D.

CHAPTER

16

Antibiotic Therapy of Chronic Osteomyelitis

INTRODUCTION

Chronic osteomyelitis is a debilitating disease associated clinically with pain, draining sinus tracts, and functional impairment. Left untreated, the infection can lead to skeletal instability and pathologic fracture, which may necessitate amputation. Prolonged disease has been associated with the development of local neoplasm and systemic amyloidosis. Thus, it is clear that chronic osteomyelitis, although it does not have a fulminant life-threatening presentation, must be treated expeditiously and effectively in order to give symptomatic relief to the patient as well as to avoid the sequelae of ongoing disease.

Unfortunately, the treatment of chronic osteomyelitis, which consists primarily of surgical debridement and antibiotic administration, is unsuccessful in 20 to 40 percent of cases.[1-4] These disappointing results continue to be observed in clinical trials utilizing potent antibiotics appropriately selected on the basis of in vitro susceptibility tests. Although the reasons for this are not entirely clear, several mechanisms have been proposed to explain the discrepancy between in vitro activity and lack of clinical efficacy (Table 16–1).

Despite adequate blood levels, poor antibiotic penetration into the site of infection can result from the relative avascularity of the local environment, fibrous scarring, and sequestered foci of bacteria. For example, in a study of cefamandole, there was no detectable antibiotic in the necrotic bone of seven patients with chronic osteomyelitis despite adequate serum concentrations.[5] Antibiotics may also encounter local conditions that adversely affect their activity. Animal models have shown that areas of chronic bone infection are relatively anaerobic[6, 7]; in such an environment the effectiveness of some antibiotics, especially aminoglycosides[8] and possibly vancomycin,[9] may be decreased. Polymorphonuclear leukocyte function is also impaired under anaerobic conditions.[7] With chronic infection, bacteria in a stationary phase of growth may exhibit altered susceptibility to antibiotics, which ordinarily are bactericidal under conditions that support bacterial growth.[10] Cell wall–deficient variants have also been described in chronic osteomyelitis,[11, 12] which can be characterized by susceptibility patterns that are different from their parent strains. Several bacterial pathogens, including some *Staphylococcus aureus* strains, have the ability to exist intracellularly, where they are protected from the action of many antibiotics. Gristina and Costerton[13] and Gristina and co-workers[13, 14] have shown that many bacteria produce a "glycocalyx," an exopolysaccharide biofilm that surrounds microcolonies of bacteria, and these investigators suggest that this material protects the bacteria from phagocytic cells and antimicrobial agents.

Given these many potential obstacles to success with antibiotic therapy, it is not surprising that the generally accepted recommendation for antimicrobial therapy in chronic osteomyelitis calls for intravenous administration of high doses of antibiotic for a prolonged period of time, usually 4 to 6 weeks. Evidence supporting this duration of therapy is limited, but includes a review of 99 cases of acute osteo-

From the Musculoskeletal Sepsis and Drug Evaluation Units, Hennepin County Medical Center and Metropolitan Medical Center, and the University of Minnesota Medical School and School of Pharmacy, Minneapolis, Minnesota.

TABLE 16–1. Factors That May Adversely Affect Antimicrobial Therapy in Chronic Osteomyelitis

Inadequate antibiotic levels at the site of infection
Anaerobic environment
Stationary growth phase of bacteria
Cell wall–deficient variants
Intracellular bacteria
Protective biofilm produced by bacteria

myelitis by Dich and colleagues,[15] who found a relapse rate of 19 percent in patients receiving antibiotic therapy for less than 3 weeks, in contrast to a relapse rate of only 2 percent in patients receiving therapy for more than 3 weeks. Also, in an animal study of chronic osteomyelitis, eradication of bacteria from bone was significantly greater at 4 weeks than at 2 weeks.[16] On the other hand, extended intravenous therapy for 3 months or longer does not appear to improve the outcome.[17]

The choice of antibiotic(s) is directed by the results of cultures (aerobic and anaerobic) and susceptibility data derived from isolates recovered from the infected bone. Cultures taken from superficial draining sinuses are often misleading.[18] Empiric therapy without bone culture is not advisable because of the large number of potential pathogens and the frequency of polymicrobial infections. Further considerations in choosing antibiotics are the potential for adverse side effects and cost. Because of the prolonged duration of therapy required, agents with a low risk of serious toxicity and with low cost should be used if possible.

The in vitro activities and pharmacologic features of the antibacterial agents most commonly used in the treatment of chronic osteomyelitis are summarized in Tables 16–2 and 16–3. The following sections of this chapter deal primarily with newer approaches to the treatment of the major groups of bacterial pathogens causing chronic osteomyelitis. Mycobacterial and fungal infections are discussed elsewhere in this book.

STAPHYLOCOCCAL OSTEOMYELITIS

S. aureus is the most frequently cultured pathogen in patients with osteomyelitis.[1, 4] Staphylococcal osteomyelitis can occur secondary to fractures, a contiguous focus of infection, in association with prosthetic hardware, or following hematogenous seeding. As a result of the high frequency of penicillin re-

sistance among S. aureus strains, the antimicrobial therapy of choice is usually a penicillinase-resistant semisynthetic penicillin, such as nafcillin or oxacillin, or a first-generation cephalosporin, such as cefazolin. Alternative antimicrobial agents can also be used, especially for patients with a history of penicillin allergy. Vancomycin is an effective anti-staphylococcal agent with a low incidence of serious side effects when serum concentrations are monitored appropriately.[19]

Clindamycin has been well studied in the treatment of acute staphylococcal osteomyelitis in children[20, 21] and has been shown to be an effective antibiotic with excellent bone penetration. Animal studies have also shown clindamycin to be effective therapy for chronic osteomyelitis,[16] but clinical data regarding the efficacy and safety of this agent in the therapy of chronic osteomyelitis in adults are lacking. Use of clindamycin should be based on in vitro sensitivity data, and the development of antibiotic associated colitis should be watched for carefully.

Third-generation cephalosporins have also been found to be clinically effective against staphylococcal osteomyelitis, although these agents are less active in vitro against S. aureus than are the first-generation cephalosporins.[22] Their use in the treatment of S. aureus osteomyelitis is most appropriate when S. aureus is part of a polymicrobial infection involving susceptible gram-negative bacilli, which can then be treated with a third-generation cephalosporin as a single agent. Imipenem and ticarcillin-clavulanic acid are other broad-spectrum antibiotics with activity against S. aureus.

Methicillin-resistant S. aureus (MRSA), which has emerged as an important pathogen in many geographic areas, is not sensitive to the action of either semisynthetic penicillins or any of the cephalosporins. Vancomycin is the therapy of choice for all MRSA infections, including osteomyelitis.[23] Staphylococci that are resistant to vancomycin have not yet been reported. Trimethoprim-sulfamethoxazole[24] and ciprofloxacin[25] are potentially useful alternative agents; however, MRSA is not uniformly susceptible to either antibiotic and clinical experience with any agent other than vancomycin in the treatment of MRSA infections is limited. Teicoplanin[25] is a promising new investigational agent with a spectrum of activity similar to that of vancomycin and with a prolonged half-life.

Coagulase-negative staphylococci can also cause osteomyelitis, most often in association

TABLE 16–2. Overview of the Clinically Relevant in Vitro Activity of the Major Antimicrobial Agents Useful in Treating Chronic Osteomyelitis*

Agent	STREPTOCOCCI†	ENTEROCOCCI	STAPHYLOCOCCI‡	GNB	PSEUDOMONAS AERUGINOSA	BACTEROIDES
Penicillins						
Penicillin G	+++	+++	0	0	0	0
Penicillin V	+++	0	0	0	0	0
Ampicillin	+++	+++	0	+	0	0
Amoxicillin + clavulanic acid	+++	0	+++	++	0	+
Oxacillin	++	0	+++	0	0	0
Ticarcillin	++	0	0	++	++	±
Ticarcillin + clavulanic acid	++	0	++	+++	++	++
Piperacillin	++	+++	0	+++	+++	++
Cephalosporins						
Cefazolin	++	0	+++	+	0	0
Cefonicid	++	0	++	+	0	0
Cefoxitin	+	0	+	++	0	++
Cefamandole	+	0	+	++	0	0
Cefotaxime	+	0	+	+++	±	±
Ceftriaxone	+	0	+	+++	0	0
Ceftazidime	+	0	+	+++	+++	0
Aztreonam	0	0	0	+++	+++	0
Imipenem-cilastatin	+++	+	+++	+++	+++	+++
Aminoglycosides (G, T, N, A)	0	0§	±	+++	+++	0
Chloramphenicol	+++	++	+	+	0	+++
Clindamycin	+++	0	+++	0	0	+++
Metronidazole	0	0	0	0	0	+++
Rifampin#	+++	++	+++	±	0	0
Trimethoprim-sulfamethoxazole	++	±	++	+++	0	0
Vancomycin	+++	+++	+++	0	0	0

* Number of plus signs (+) indicates relative percentage of susceptible strains.

† Excluding enterococci

‡ Must distinguish between methicillin- or oxacillin-sensitive and resistant isolates. Only agents active against resistant organisms are vancomycin ± rifampin (possibly trimethoprim-sulfamethoxazole).

§ Synergistic activity when used in combination with penicillin, ampicillin, or vancomycin.

As a result of rapid emergence of resistance, rifampin should be used only in combination with penicillinase-resistant penicillin (oxacillin), cefazolin, or vancomycin for treatment of staphylococcal infections unresponsive to these agents used alone.

Abbreviations: G = Gentamicin; T = tobramicin; N = netilmicin; A = amikacin; GNB = gram-negative bacteria.

with prosthetic material. Therapy is similar to that of *S. aureus*, although methicillin resistance is more frequently encountered. When prosthetic material is involved, its removal is usually necessary as well, except when the infection occurs early in the postoperative period after implantation of the prosthetic device.

Combination antimicrobial therapy for staphylococcal osteomyelitis has been attempted as a means of improving the success rate of treatment. Rifampin in addition to either an anti-staphylococcal penicillin or vancomycin has been most extensively studied. Clinical trials[26-28] suggest that combination therapy may be useful, although a clear benefit has never been demonstrated. One animal study[9] has shown a significant benefit of vancomycin plus rifampin versus vancomycin alone. In vitro testing for synergy has yielded conflicting results,[26, 29] with some studies paradoxically showing antagonism between rifampin and other anti-staphylococcal agents. The clinical significance of these findings is unclear at this time.

There is growing experience with oral antibiotic treatment of staphylococcal osteomyelitis. Most trials have been carried out in children with acute hematogenous osteomyelitis, and cure rates of greater than 90 percent have been reported.[30, 31] Anti-staphylococcal penicillins, first-generation cephalosporins, and

TABLE 16–3. Overview of the Clinical Pharmacology of the Major Antimicrobial Agents Useful in Treating Chronic Osteomyelitis

Agent	Serum Half-Life* (Hours)	Adjust Dose R(H)†	Dose Interval (Hours) M/S‡	Bone Penetration§	Reviews, Symposia#
Penicillins					
Penicillin G	0.5	+(0)	4–6/2–4	<20	66
Penicillin V	0.75	+(0)	6/6	ND	66
Ampicillin	1.25	+(0)	6/4–6	ND	66
Amoxicillin + clavulanic acid	1/1¶	+(0)	8/8	ND	67
Oxacillin	0.5	0(0)	6/4–6	ND	68
Ticarcillin	1.2	+(0)	4/4	ND	69
Ticarcillin + clavulanic acid	1.2/1.2¶	+(0)	6–8/4–6	ND	70
Piperacillin	1.0	+(0)	6/4	33	66, 71
Cephalosporins					
Cefazolin	1.4	+(0)	8–12/6	19.6(<6–37.5)	72
Cefonicid	4.5	+(0)	24/24	12	73
Cefoxitin	0.8	+(0)	4–8/4–6	13.3(5–20.6)	74
Cefamandole	0.6	+(0)	4–8/4–6	13.7(13–14.3)	74
Cefotaxime	1.1	±(0)	6–8/4–6	30.8(6–99)	75
Ceftriaxone	5.8–8.7	R+H**	24/12	6.7	76
Ceftazidime	1.8	+(0)	8/8	47.5(40–55)	77
Aztreonam	1.5–2	+(±)	8–12/6–8	41.8	78, 79
Imipenem-cilastatin	1/1¶	+(0)	6–8/6	ND	80
Aminoglycosides (G, T, N, A)	2	+(0)	variable††	30(G)	81, 82, 83
Chloramphenicol	4	0(+)	6/6	ND	84, 85
Clindamycin	2–4	±(+)	6–8/6	38.1(21.4–49)	86
Metronidazole	7–8	0(+)	6–8/6–8	75	87
Rifampin	1.5–5	0(+)	12–24/12	20(0–41)	88, 89
Trimethoprim-sulfamethoxazole	13/12¶	+(0)	6–12/6–12	ND	90
Vancomycin	4–8	+(0)	variable††	ND	91, 92

* Values are shown for adults with normal renal function.

† Dosage adjustment necessary in presence of renal (R) or hepatic (H) impairment.

‡ Dosage interval for mild to moderate (M) and severe (S) infections.

§ Penetration expressed as percentage ratio of bone:serum concentration; parentheses indicate range where reported.

Numbers refer to references at the end of this chapter.

¶ Half-lives of the two components of the antimicrobial combination, respectively.

** Dosage adjustment only necessary for combined severe renal and hepatic impairment.

†† Dosage regimen adjusted using nomograms or individualized pharmacokinetics parameters to achieve peaks (postdose) concentrations of 5–10 (G, T, N), 20–30 (A) or 20–40 (vancomycin) mg/L and trough (predose) concentrations of <2 (G, T, N) or 5–10 (A and vancomycin) mg/L.

Abbreviations: G = Gentamicin, T = tobracin, N = netilmicin, A = amikacin; ND = no data.

clindamycin were used. There are also studies reporting success in treatment of chronic osteomyelitis in adults with oral penicillins. In 1976 Bell[32] reported that 19 patients treated with a high dose (5 gm/day) of cloxacillin or penicillin remained free of disease at follow-up 7 to 9 years after initiation of therapy. Eight of these patients received antibiotics for greater than 1 year, and four were still receiving an antibiotic at the time of follow-up. A similar study by Hedstrom evaluated 41 patients with chronic staphylococcal osteomyelitis treated with cloxacillin (0.5 to 1 gm, five to six times a day) for at least 6 months. The initial response rate, 4 to 33 months after termination of treatment, was 90 percent.[33] However, on subsequent follow-up 18 to 60 months after the end of treatment, the recurrence rate increased to 29 percent,[34] underscoring the importance of long-term observation in assessing any therapy for chronic osteomyelitis. A third study[35] reported a 71 percent success rate in 14 patients treated with dicloxacillin after 0.5 to 2.5 years of follow-up, but cautioned that patients should be monitored closely for hepatic or hematologic toxicity. Oral cephalosporins[31] (cephalexin, cephadrine, cefaclor, and cefadroxil) appear to be effective in acute osteomyelitis in children when used in high doses (100 mg/kg/day), but their activity against *S. aureus* is only one-tenth that of cefazolin or cephalothin[22] and may fail to achieve adequate tissue concentration when given in conventional doses (500 mg orally every 6 hours).[36] Oral clindamycin[31] has also been found to be effective in the treatment of acute osteomyelitis caused by *S. aureus.* In a study of 29 children,[21] no diarrhea or manifestations of enterocolitis were found despite high doses (25 mg/kg/day) for periods of up to 9 weeks.

In summary, it would appear that oral antibiotics in high doses can be used in the treatment of chronic staphylococcal osteomyelitis with a reasonable expectation of success. However, the duration of therapy required is unknown, and consideration of compliance, side effects, and toxicity must be carefully weighed against the convenience of oral therapy. There are insufficient data to comment on the efficacy of oral therapy in chronic osteomyelitis caused by other organisms; however, in theory, if adequate antibiotic levels can be attained, oral therapy should be an acceptable alternative to parenteral antibiotics.

GRAM-NEGATIVE OSTEOMYELITIS

Facultative gram-negative bacilli (GNB) are frequently cultured from bone infections associated with fractures, contiguous foci of infection such as pressure sores, ulcers associated with vascular insufficiency, and prosthetic devices.[2, 37] Gram-negative bacillary osteomyelitis resulting from hematogenous seeding is rare except in the setting of intravenous drug abuse, vertebral osteomyelitis, or hemoglobinopathies. Treatment results from two studies[38, 39] suggest that GNB osteomyelitis and mixed infections including GNB may be more difficult to cure than staphylococcal osteomyelitis. Aminoglycosides are often used as part of an antibiotic regimen that includes a beta-lactam agent but, when used alone, may have a high failure rate. In one series of 60 patients with GNB osteomyelitis treated with amikacin, there was a 42 percent failure rate after limited follow-up.[38] This may be due to the decreased effectiveness of aminoglycosides in an anaerobic environment. Prolonged treatment with aminoglycosides also places patients at significant risk for ototoxicity and nephrotoxicity. The use of aminoglycoside-impregnated cement beads has obviated these serious complications (see Chapter 8).

The third-generation cephalosporins are potentially an attractive alternative to aminoglycoside therapy. They are very active against most GNB,[22] are associated with a low incidence of serious side effects, and in clinical trials have been reported to control infection in 80 percent of cases.[4] A potential problem is the development of resistance during therapy, which thus far seems to occur at a rate of approximately 5 percent[4] and is most often reported with *Pseudomonas aeruginosa.* Among the third-generation cephalosporins, ceftazidime is notable for its superior activity against *P. aeruginosa,*[40] and ceftriaxone is unique for its prolonged half-life,[41] which permits once-a-day administration of the antibiotic.

Penicillins with substantial activity against GNB include ticarcillin, piperacillin, mezlocillin, and azlocillin, which are used primarily as anti-pseudomonal agents, and the new combination antibiotics, ticarcillin-clavulanic acid[42] and amoxicillin-clavulanic acid. Clavulanic acid, a beta-lactamase inhibitor, expands the spectrum of activity of these combination agents to include *S. aureus* and many anaerobes as well as improving the activity against many Enterobacteriaceae. Other penicillin-like agents with activity against GNB are imipenem,[43] which has the broadest spectrum of activity of any antibiotic currently available, and aztreonam,[44] which is effective against GNB but not against anaerobes or gram-positive organisms.

A number of new antibiotics of the quinolone group have been introduced into clinical trials. Of these, ciprofloxacin has been best studied as therapy for osteomyelitis[45, 46] and may become the first orally administered agent available for the treatment of GNB osteomyelitis, including *P. aeruginosa.*[47] As noted with the third-generation cephalosporins, development of resistance on single-agent therapy with any of the newer antibiotics is a potential problem,[48] but the frequency with which this occurs is not yet known.

ANAEROBIC OSTEOMYELITIS

With greater clinical awareness and advances in culture techniques, the reported incidence of anaerobic osteomyelitis has risen from 2 percent in 1970[1] to 20 percent or greater in more recent series.[49, 50] Anaerobes are often cultured as part of a mixed flora and are seen in the clinical setting of trauma, prosthetic devices, diabetic foot infections, decubitus ulcers, and human bites. Although a variety of anaerobic organisms can be found,

Bacteroides species and peptostreptococci appear to be isolated most frequently. Hall and associates[49] reported a failure rate of 61.5 percent, three times higher in mixed aerobic-anaerobic osteomyelitis than in aerobic osteomyelitis, suggesting that the presence of anaerobes may adversely affect prognosis in bone infections. Penicillin, clindamycin, metronidazole, and chloramphenicol are the antibiotics most often used in the treatment of anaerobic infections, but each may be ineffective under certain circumstances. Although often effective in the treatment of infections caused by anaerobic gram-positive cocci and bacilli, penicillin is generally ineffective against the *Bacteroides species.*[51] Clindamycin has variable activity against some *Clostridium species* and anaerobic gram-positive cocci,[52] whereas metronidazole is not reliably active against anaerobic gram-positive cocci, *Actinomyces,* and anaerobic gram-positive non–spore-forming bacilli.[53] Chloramphenicol is a very effective antibiotic against anaerobes but should probably be considered a second-line agent because of the potential for toxicity with long-term treatment. Several newer agents may also be useful in the treatment of anaerobic osteomyelitis, including two second-generation cephalosporins, cefoxitin and cefotetan, and several extended spectrum penicillins such as piperacillin, mezlocillin, ticarcillin-clavulanic acid, and imipenem.

STREPTOCOCCAL INFECTIONS

Streptococcal organisms are infrequently cultured as the sole pathogen in chronic osteomyelitis[54–56] but are commonly found as part of a polymicrobial infection.[57] The most commonly isolated streptococci include group A, group B, group G, *Streptococcus viridans,* enterococci, and pneumococci. Infection of prosthetic joints by *S. viridans* following dental procedures has been described,[58] although osteomyelitis secondary to streptoccocal bacteremia appears to be rare.[1] The treatment of choice for streptococcal infections is penicillin G (or ampicillin in the case of enterococci). Effective alternative agents include other penicillin agents, cephalosporins (not for enterococci), and vancomycin.

Enterococci are characterized by a markedly different susceptibility to antibiotics compared with other streptococci, showing greater resistance in almost all instances. Penicillin, ampicillin, piperacillin, mezlocillin, imipenem, and vancomycin show the best in vitro activity, but killing of organisms (bactericidal activity) requires the addition of an aminoglycoside to which enterococci are relatively susceptible (minimal inhibitory concentration [MIC] <2000 gm/ml).[59] Combination therapy, including an aminoglycoside, is recommended for enterococcal endocarditis,[60] but there are no studies comparing combination therapy versus single-agent therapy in the treatment of enterococcal osteomyelitis.

OUTPATIENT INTRAVENOUS ANTIBIOTIC THERAPY

The emergence of prospective payment reimbursement schemes in the United States, as evidenced by the recent implementation of diagnosis-related groups (DRGs), has demanded a reconsideration of usual and customary medical practices. The movement toward outpatient delivery of parenteral antibiotics has met with a receptive audience among university and community hospitals and patients. Hospital-based and commercial enterprises have appeared throughout the United States in the face of heightened public awareness of escalating health care costs, the pressures of DRGs, and an anticipated market of over $16 billion in 1990 for home parenterals.[61]

Chronic osteomyelitis is eminently suitable for this form of therapy when oral antibiotics cannot be used. Current therapeutic guidelines (as discussed elsewhere in this chapter) include a minimum of 4 to 6 weeks of antibiotic therapy. With a DRG allocation of only 14 days for osteomyelitis, the potential economic impact of outpatient intravenous (IV) therapy is enormous. In addition, a majority of the adult and pediatric patients included in studies examining the efficacy, safety, and cost-effectiveness of this form of antibiotic therapy were treated for osteomyelitis or joint infections.[62–64]

Regardless of whether a hospital-based or commercial enterprise is chosen to provide this service to the patient with osteomyelitis, careful attention must be paid to patient selection, education, and follow-up. A team approach encompassing physicians, nurses, and pharmacists is mandatory for safe and effective therapy. Home intravenous therapy standards of practice must be followed closely. In most programs, an assessment of patient suitability is a joint decision of the team members. If the patient is accepted into the program, a specially trained nurse teaches the patient (and one or more family members, if possible) the technique of IV antibiotic self-administration. Patients are taught to maintain IV heparinized cannulas. Antibiotics are scheduled so as to interfere with sleep and other activities as little as possible. In this regard, the newer prolonged half-life cephalosporins such as ceftriaxone, which must be administered only once or twice a day, may prove advantageous. The pharmacist prepares the prepackaged antibiotics and teaches the patient about adverse drug reactions. Upon successful completion of the training program, the patient is readied for discharge, receiving a 48- to 72-hour supply of antibiotics, miscellaneous supplies for IV administration, and written instructions regarding procedures for drug infiltration, cannula-associated phlebitis, or other emergencies. Some programs provide for outpatient clinic visits every 48 to 72 hours for changing the cannula site and collection of new supplies; other programs utilize home care nursing visits for the above procedures. Laboratory tests are tailored to the agent being administered, but routine tests should be obtained at least weekly.

In general, adverse reactions occur no more frequently with outpatient therapy than in an inpatient setting, including IV access problems. Cost savings may be considerable, up to $5000 per patient per treatment course. However, clinicians should be cognizant of the potential pitfalls of outpatient IV therapy as discussed in detail by Goldenberg.[65] Potential problems may be encountered in patient selection, antibiotic selection, medicolegal considerations, political issues, and financial problems. With regard to the last item, there exists a wide variability in reimbursement procedures despite the cost savings of this therapy. This ranges from no reimbursement from Medicare at present to full coverage by some private third-party insurers. Although the implementation of outpatient antibiotic therapy has proved to be extremely useful in the management of osteomyelitis, it cannot be considered a panacea for rising costs and several problems remain to be worked out with this relatively new mode of therapy.

SUMMARY

Recent advances have been made in the antimicrobial therapy of chronic osteomyelitis.

Third-generation cephalosporins offer a less toxic alternative to aminoglycosides in the therapy of osteomyelitis caused by gram-negative bacilli. Antibiotics such as imipenem and ticarcillin-clavulanic acid, with potent activity against many of the bacteria frequently encountered in chronic osteomyelitis, may be useful as single-agent therapy in polymicrobial infections, allowing home IV therapy to become a practical alternative in many cases and reducing the expense of therapy. The new quinolones, such as ciprofloxacin, may allow oral therapy of gram-negative osteomyelitis for the first time, and agents with prolonged half-lives, such as ceftriaxone and teicoplanin, may significantly reduce the cost of therapy. However, it is doubtful that improved antimicrobial agents alone will significantly impact on the overall cure rate of chronic osteomyelitis. Without parallel advances in surgical management, more effective delivery of antibiotics to the site of infection, and a better understanding of the factors responsible for the persistence of chronic bone infection, we can anticipate continued therapeutic failure in a substantial proportion of patients with chronic osteomyelitis.

References

1. Waldvogel FA, Medoff G, Swartz MN: Osteomyelitis: a review of clinical features, therapeutic considerations and unusual aspects. N Engl J Med 282:198–206, 260–266, 316–322, 1970.
2. Meyers BR, Berson BL, Gilbert M, Hirschman SZ: Clinical patterns of osteomyelitis due to gram-negative bacteria. Arch Intern Med 131:228–233, 1973.
3. Kelly PJ, Martin WJ, Coventry MB: Chronic osteomyelitis. II. Treatment with closed irrigation and suction. JAMA 213:1843–1848, 1970.
4. Gentry LO: Role for newer beta-lactam antibiotics in treatment of osteomyelitis. Am J Med 78(Suppl 6A):134–139, 1985.
5. Perry H, Ritterbusch JK, Burdge RE, Perry CR: Cefamandole levels in serum and necrotic bone. Clin Orthop 199:280–283, 1985.
6. Niinkowski J, Hunt TK: Oxygen tensions in healing bone. Surg Gynecol Obstet 134:746–750, 1972.
7. Mader JT, Brown GL, Guckian JC, Wells CH, Reinarz JA: A mechanism for the amelioration by hyperbaric oxygen of experimental staphylococcal osteomyelitis in rabbits. J Infect Dis 142:915–922, 1980.
8. Verklin RM, Mandell GL: Alteration of effectiveness of antibiotics by anaerobiasis. J Lab Clin Med 8:65–71, 1977.
9. Norden CW, Shaffer M: Treatment of experimental chronic osteomyelitis due to *Staphylococcus aureus* with vancomycin and rifampin. J Infect Dis 147:352–357, 1983.
10. Kim KS, Anthony BF: Importance of bactericidal growth phase in determining minimal bactericidal

concentrations of penicillins and methicillin. Antimicrob Agents Chemother 19:1075–1077, 1981.

11. Gordon SL, Greer RB, Craig CP: Recurrent osteomyelitis: report of four cases culturing L-form variants of staphylococci. J Bone Joint Surg 53-A:1150–1156, 1971.

12. Rosner R: Isolation of protoplasts of *Staphylococcus aureus* from a case of recurrent acute osteomyelitis. Am J Clin Pathol 50:385–390, 1968.

13. Gristina AG, Costerton JW: Bacterial adherence and the glycocalyx and their role in musculoskeletal infection. Orthop Clin North Am 15:517–536, 1984.

14. Gristina AG, Oga M, Webb LX, Hobgood CD: Adherent bacterial colonization in the pathogenesis of osteomyelitis. Science 228:990–993, 1985.

15. Dich VQ, Nelson JD, Haltalin KC: Osteomyelitis in infants and children. Am J Dis Child 129:1273–1278, 1975.

16. Norden CW, Shinners E, Niederriter K: Clindamycin treatment of experimental chronic osteomyelitis due to *Staphylococcus aureus*. J Infect Dis 153:956–959, 1986.

17. Wagner DK, Collier BD, Rytel NW: Long-term intravenous antibiotic therapy in chronic osteomyelitis. Arch Intern Med 145:1073–1078, 1985.

18. Mackowiak PA, Jones SR, Smith JW: Diagnostic value of sinus-tract cultures in chronic osteomyelitis. JAMA 239:2772–2775, 1978.

19. Fekety R: Vancomycin. Med Clin North Am 66:175–181, 1982.

20. Kaplan SL, Mason EO, Feigin RD: Clindamycin versus nafcillin or methicillin in the treatment of *Staphylococcus aureus* osteomyelitis in children. South Med J 75:138–142, 1982.

21. Rodriguez W, Ross S, Khan W, McKay D, Moskowitz P: Clindamycin in the treatment of osteomyelitis in children. Am J Dis Child 131:1088–1093, 1977.

22. Neu HC: Cephalosporin antibiotics as applied in surgery of bones and joints. Clin Orthop 190:50–64, 1984.

23. Sheftel TG, Mader JT, Pennick JJ, Cierny G: Methicillin-resistant *Staphylococcus aureus* osteomyelitis. Clin Orthop 198:231–239, 1985.

24. Markowitz N, Saravolatz L, Pohlod D, Salo S, Quinn E, Somerville M, del Busto R, Cardenas R, Rathod M, Fisher E: Comparative efficacy and toxicity of trimethoprim-sulfamethoxazole versus vancomycin in the therapy of serious *S. aureus* infections. Proceedings of the 23rd Interscience Conference on Antimicrobial Agents and Chemotherapy. Washington DC, American Society for Microbiology, 1983, p 201.

25. Del Bene VE, John JF, Twitty JA, Lewis JW: Antistaphylococcal activity of teicoplanin, vancomycin, and other antimicrobial agents: the significance of methicillin resistance. J Infect Dis 154:349–352, 1986.

26. Van der Auwera P, Meunier-Carpentier F, Klastersky J: Clinical study of combination therapy with oxacillin and rifampin for staphylococal infections. Rev Infect Dis 5:S515–522, 1983.

27. Norden CW, Fierer J, Bryand RE: Chronic staphylococcal osteomyelitis: treatment with regimens containing rifampin. Rev Infect Dis 5:S495–501, 1983.

28. Van der Auwera P, Klastersky J, Thys JP, Meunier-Carpentier F, Legrand JL: Double blind, placebo-controlled study of oxacillin combined with rifampin in the treatment of staphylococcal infections. Antimicrob Agents Chemother 27:615–618, 1985.

29. Varaldo PE, Debbia E, Schito GC: In vitro activities of rifampentine and rifampin, alone and in combination with six other antibiotics, against methicillin-susceptible and methicillin-resistant staphylococci of different species. Antimicrob Agents Chemother 27:615–618, 1985.

30. Tetzlaff TR, McCracken GH, Nelson JD: Oral antibiotic therapy for skeletal infections of children. J Pediatr 92:485–490, 1978.

31. Conrad DA, Marks MI: Oral therapy for orthopedic infections in children and adults. Orthopedics 7:1585–1591, 1984.

32. Bell SM: Further observations on the value of oral penicillins in chronic staphylococcal osteomyelitis. Med J Aust 2:591–593, 1976.

33. Hedstrom SA: General and local antibiotic treatment of chronic osteomyelitis. Scand J Infect Dis 1:175–180, 1969.

34. Hedstrom SA: The prognosis of chronic staphylococcal osteomyelitis after long-term antibiotic treatment. Scand J Infect Dis 6:33–38, 1974.

35. Hodgin UG: Antibiotics in the treatment of chronic staphylococcal osteomyelitis. South Med J 68:817–823, 1975.

36. Sattor MA, Barrett SP, Cawley MID: Concentrations of some antibiotics in synovial fluid after oral administration, with special references to anti-staphylococal activity. Ann Rheum Dis 42:67–74, 1983.

37. Sugarman B, Hawes S, Musher DM, Klima M, Young EJ, Pircher F: Osteomyelitis beneath pressure sores. Arch Intern Med 143:683–688, 1983.

38. Schurman DJ, Wheeler R: Gram negative bone and joint infection. Clin Orthop 134:268–274, 1978.

39. Kelly PJ, Wilkowski CJ, Washington JA: Comparison of gram-negative bacillary and staphylococcal osteomyelitis of the femur and tibia. Clin Othop 96:70–75, 1973.

40. Neu HC, Labthavikul P: Antimicrobial activity and beta-lactamase stability of ceftazidime, an aminothiazolyl cephalosporin potentially active against *Pseudomonas aeruginosa*. Antimicrob Agents Chemother 21:11–18, 1982.

41. Patel IN, Kaplan SA: Pharmacokinetic profile of ceftriaxone in man. Am J Med 77(4C):17–25, 1984.

42. Johnson CC, Reinhardt JF, Wallace SL, Terpenning MS, Helsel CL, Mulligan ME, Finegold SM, George WL: Safety and efficacy of ticarcillin plus clavulanic acid in the treatment of infections of soft tissue, bone, and joint. Am J Med 79 (Suppl 5B):136–140, 1985.

43. MacGregor RR, Gentry LO: Imipenem/cilastin in the treatment of osteomyelitis. Am J Med 78 (Suppl 6A):100–103, 1985.

44. Romero-Vivas J, Rodriguez-Creixems M, Bouza E, Hellin T, Guerroro A, Martinez-Beltran J, delaTorre MG: Evaluation of aztreonam in the treatment of severe bacterial infections. Antimicrob Agents Chemother 28:222–226, 1985.

45. Fong IW, Ledbetter WH, Vandenbroucker AC, Simbul M, Rahm V: Ciprofloxacin concentrations in bone and muscle after oral dosing. Antimicrob Agents Chemother 29:405–408, 1986.

46. Norden CW, Shinners E: Ciprofloxacin as therapy for experimental osteomyelitis caused by *Pseudomonas aeruginosa*. J Infect Dis 151:291–294, 1985.

47. Eron LJ, Harvey L, Hixon DL, Poretz DM: Ciprofloxacin therapy of infections caused by *Pseudomonas aeruginosa* and other resistant bacteria. Antimicrob Agents Chemother 27:308–310, 1985.

48. Gentry LO, Macho V, Lind R, Heilman A: Ticarcillin plus clavulanic acid (Timentin) therapy for osteomyelitis. Am J Med 79 (Suppl 5B):116–121, 1985.

49. Hall BB, Fitzgerald RH, Rosenblatt JE: Anaerobic osteomyelitis. J Bone Joint Surg 65A:30–35, 1983.

50. Lewis RP, Sutter VL, Finegold SM: Bone infections involving anaerobic bacteria. Medicine 57:279–305, 1978.

51. Cunha BA: The use of penicillins in orthopaedic surgery. Clin Orthop 190:36–48, 1984.

52. Steigbigel NH: Erythromycin, lincomycin, and clindamycin. In Mandell GL, Douglas RG, Bennett JE, eds: Principles and Practice of Infectious Diseases. New York, John Wiley & Sons, Inc, 1985, pp 224–231.

53. Brogden RN, Heel RC, Speight TM, Avery GS: Metronidazole in anaerobic infections: a review of its activity, pharmacokinetics and therapeutic use. Drugs 16:387–417, 1978.

54. Gordon DM, Oster CN: Hematogenous group B streptococcal osteomyelitis in an adult. South Med J 77:643–645, 1984.

55. Ribner BS, Freimer EH: Osteomyelitis caused by viridans streptococci. Arch Intern Med 142:1739, 1982.

56. Hadari I, Dugan R, Gedalia P, Jeanine N, Moses S: Pneumococcal osteomyelitis. Clin Pediatr 24:143–145, 1985.

57. Pichiero ME, Friesen HA: Polymicrobial osteomyelitis: report of three cases and review of the literature. Rev Infect Dis 4:86–96, 1982.

58. Lindqvist C, Slatis P: Dental bacteremia: a neglected cause of arthroplasty infection? Acta Orthop Scand 56:506–508, 1985.

59. Musher DM: *Streptococcus faecalis* and other group D streptococci. In Mandell GL, Douglas RG, Bennett JE, eds: Principles and Practice of Infectious Diseases. New York, John Wiley & Sons, Inc, 1985, pp 1152–1155.

60. Sande MA, Scheld WM: Combination antibiotic therapy of bacterial endocarditis. Ann Intern Med 92:390–395, 1980.

61. Eron LJ: Intravenous antibiotic administration in outpatient settings. Infect Dis, January 1984, pp 4–11.

62. Stiver HG, Telford GO, Mossey JM, Cote DD, Van Middlesworth EJ, Trosky SK, McKay NC, Mossey WL: Intravenous antibiotic therapy at home. Ann Intern Med 9:690–693, 1978.

63. Rehm SJ, Weinstein AJ: Home intravenous antibiotic therapy: a team approach. Ann Intern Med 99:388–392, 1983.

64. Kind AC, Williams DN, Gibson J: Outpatient intravenous antibiotic therapy. Postgrad Med 77:105–111, 1985.

65. Goldenberg RI: Pitfalls in the delivery of outpatient intravenous therapy. Drug Intell Clin Pharm 19:293–296, 1985.

66. Wright AJ, Wilkowske CJ: The penicillins. Mayo Clin Proc 58:21–32, 1983.

67. Stein GE, Gurwith MJ: Amoxicillin-potassium clavulanate: a beta-lactamase-resistant antibiotic combination. Clin Pharm 3:591–599, 1984.

68. Neu HC: Antistaphylococcal penicillins. Med Clin North Am 66:51–60, 1982.

69. Neu HC: Carbenicillin and ticarcillin. Med Clin North Am 66:61–77, 1982.

70. Neu HC: Beta-lactamase inhibition: therapeutic advances. Am J Med 79(SB):1–196, 1985.

71. Drusano GL, Schimpff SC, Hewitt WL: The acylampicillins: mezlocillin, piperacillin, and azlocillin. Rev Infect Dis 6:13–32, 1984.

72. Quintiliani R, Nightingale CH: Cefazolin. Ann Intern Med 89:650–656, 1978.

73. Dudley MN, Quintiliani R, Nightingale CH: Review of cefonicid, a long-acting cephalosporin. Clin Pharm 3:23–32, 1984.

74. Sanders CV, Greenberg RN, Marier RL: Cefamandole and cefoxitin. Ann Intern Med 103:70–78, 1985.

75. Dudley M, Barriere SL: Cefotaxime: microbiology, pharmacology, and clinical use. Clin Pharm 1:114–124, 1982.

76. Beam TR Jr: Ceftriaxone: a beta-lactamase stable, broad-spectrum cephalosporin with an extended half-life. Pharmacotherapy 5:237–253, 1985.

77. Gentry LO: Antimicrobial activity, pharmacokinetics, therapeutic indications and adverse reactions of ceftazidime. Pharmacotherapy 5:254–267, 1985.

78. Guay DRP, Koskoletos C: Aztreonam, a new monobactam antimicrobial. Clin Pharm 4:516–526, 1985.

79. Acar JF, Neu HC: Gram-negative aerobic bacterial infections: a focus on directed therapy, with special reference to aztreonam. Rev Infect Dis 7 (Supp 4):S536–S843, 1985.

80. Pastel DA: Imipenem-cilastatin sodium, a broad-spectrum carbapenem antibiotic combination. Clin Pharm 5:719–736, 1986.

81. Burkle WS: Comparative evaluation of the aminoglycoside antibiotics for systemic use. Drug Intell Clin Pharm 15:847–862, 1981.

82. Guay DR: Netilmicin (Netromycin, Schering-Plough). Drug Intell Clin Pharm 17:83–91, 1983.

83. Meyer RD: Amikacin. Ann Intern Med 95:328–332, 1981.

84. Shalit I, Marks MI: Chloramphenicol in the 1980's. Drugs 28:281–291, 1984.

85. Ambrose PJ: Clinical pharmacokinetics of chloramphenicol and chloramphenicol succinate. Clin Pharmacokinet 9:222–238, 1984.

86. Dhawan VK, Thadepalli H: Clindamycin: a review of fifteen years of experience. Rev Infect Dis 4:1133–1153, 1982.

87. Rosenblatt JE, Edson RS: Metronidazole. Mayo Clin Proc 58:154–157, 1983.

88. Four B, Mandell GL: Rifampin. Med Clin North Am 66:157–173, 1982.

89. Kapusnik JE, Parenti F, Sande MA: The use of rifampin in staphylococcal infections: a review. J Antimicrob Chemother 13 (Supp C):61–66, 1984.

90. Finland M, Kass EH, Platt R, eds: Summary of the Symposium, Sessions 1, 2, and 3: Trimethoprim-sulfamethoxazole revisited. Rev Infect Dis 4:185–195, 1982.

91. Geraci JE, Hermans PE: Vancomycin. Mayo Clin Proc 58:88–91, 1983.

92. Matzke GR, Zhanel GG, Guay DRP: Clinical pharmacokinetics of vancomycin. Clin Pharmacokinet 11:257–282, 1986.

Robert L. Merkow, M.D.

CHAPTER

17

Hand Infections

INTRODUCTION

Hand infections are common and may lead to significant impairment, resulting in severe disabilities including stiffness, contracture, and amputation. In the early 1900s, Allen B. Kanavel published his classic book, entitled *Infections of the Hand*,[1] which described the detailed surgical anatomy and treatment of infections of the hand in the pre-antibiotic era. During the 1920s and 1930s, serious hand infections were difficult problems, frequently leading to devastating losses of hand function, and, in many instances, were even limb- or life-threatening. Since Kanavel's time, many authors have had an interest in the problems of recognition and treatment of hand infections. Koch,[2-4] Mason,[5] Bailey,[6] Sneddon,[7,8] Eaton and Busch,[9] McKay and associates,[10] Carter,[11] Carter and co-authors,[12,13] Linscheid and Dobyns,[14] Neviaser,[15] Kilgore,[16,17] and others have written numerous articles providing useful information with regard to the diagnosis and management of hand infections. The advent of antibiotics has significantly improved our ability to treat most infections of the hand; however, in some instances the sole reliance on antibiotic treatment without appropriate attention to the overall principles of treating hand infections has led to a compromised outcome. Although the frequency and morbidity of hand infections is generally much lower than in the past, the importance of proper diagnosis and early appropriate treatment must be recognized by emergency and primary care physicians and surgical specialists who are called upon to care for these frequent problems.

GENERAL PRINCIPLES OF CARE

Most hand infections respond favorably when general principles of care are followed. These principles include appropriate rest, elevation, immobilization (with early mobilization), bacterial identification, appropriate antibiotic coverage, surgical incision, and drainage and debridement, when indicated. A specific cause or causes for the increased severity or chronicity should be sought in cases that do not promptly respond favorably when these principles are followed. Predisposing systemic conditions include diabetes, hematologic malignancies, and circulatory disorders, such as Raynaud's disease or Buerger's disease. Predisposing local factors that may be responsible for poorly responding infections include retained foreign body, necrotic or sequestered tissue, or ineffective drainage.

An appropriate medical history is important in the evaluation of patients with hand infections in order to determine whether the patient is at additional risk because of associated systemic conditions such as diabetes, vascular disease, or immunosuppression. Patients with hematological malignances or immunocompromised status caused by medications should be recognized as a special group who are vulnerable to serious hand infections. Additionally, a specific history of the circumstances surrounding a particular hand infection may be helpful in determining the likely offending organisms.

The initial treatment of a significant hand infection should include rest and elevation of the hand above the level of the heart and immobilization in the "safe" position (Fig. 17–1). Certain infections, such as rapidly progressive gangrene, acute fulminant pyogenic flexor tenosynovitis, or acute suppurative arthritis, may necessitate immediate surgical drainage to avoid uncontrollable spread or

From the Department of Orthopaedic Surgery, Hennepin County Medical Center, Minneapolis, Minnesota.

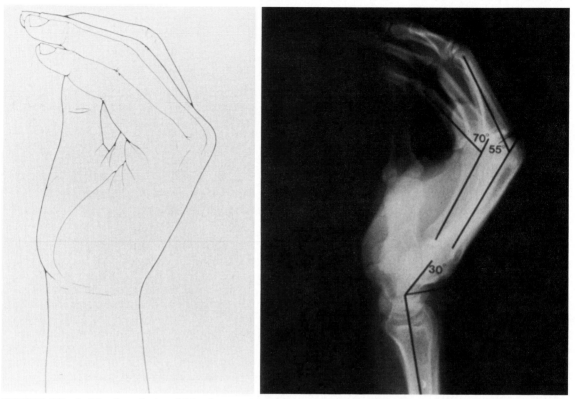

FIGURE 17–1. The hand should be immobilized in a balanced protective position with the wrist in approximately 20 to 30 degrees of extension. The metacarpophalangeal joints are flexed between 50 and 70 degrees and the interphalangeal joints are in relative extension or slight flexion.

damage to the flexor tendons or articular cartilage; however, most hand infections benefit from a brief period of immobilization, elevation and antibiotic saturation to better localize the process. Antibiotic coverage is begun based on Gram stain if available material is diagnostic. However, in most cases, antibiotics are begun on an empiric basis (Table 17–1),

chosen to cover the most likely organism in a specific situation.

Frequent re-evaluation over 12- to 48-hour intervals is important to determine whether the infection is responding favorably or not. Most infections are characterized by considerable associated cellulitis and swelling, which are diminished following this initial treatment,

TABLE 17–1. Empirical Choice of Antibiotics for Hand Infections

Suspected Organism	Antibiotic	
	PREFERRED	ALTERNATE
Staphylococcus	Penicillinase-resistant penicillin	Cephalosporin: vancomycin, clindamycin erythromycin
Beta-hemolytic *Streptococcus*	Penicillin	Chloramphenicol, erythromycin, cephalosporin
Gram-negative organisms	Aminoglycoside broad-spectrum penicillin or third-generation cephalosporin	Chloramphenicol, erythromycin
Mixed flora	Cephalosporin (first-, second-, or third-generation)	Chloramphenicol, tetracycline
Anaerobic organisms	Penicillin G; cefoxitin	Chloramphenicol(?)

thus making subsequent drainage and debridement, when required, easier, safer, and more effective.

Surgical treatment may be needed to effect adequate drainage of abscesses, removal of foreign body such as glass or wood, or debridement of sequestered bone or avascular necrotic soft tissues such as tendon, fascia, and collateral ligament.

A clear knowledge and understanding of the intricate anatomy of the hand, with recognition of anatomical spaces as described by Kanavel, are important before surgical intervention is undertaken. Proper timing, placement of incisions, and surgical equipment and technique as well as postoperative management are all important in order to effect a prompt resolution of the infective process and to prevent additional injury to the complex gliding structures of the hand.

ORGANISMS AND ANTIBIOTICS

The most common organism involved in hand infections still remains staphylococci, although other bacterial infections commonly encountered may involve streptococci or gram-negative bacteria such as *Proteus* or *Pseudomonas* (Table 17–2).[14, 18]

Infections following human or animal bites are frequently associated with anaerobes[19-21] such as *Bacteroides*. Certain animal bites are associated with an increased risk of specific bacterial infections, such as *Pasteurella multocida*, in association with cat bites,[21] and *Eikenella corrodens*, more recently being associated with a significant percentage of human bites.[19, 22] Mycobacterial infections, though uncommon, still represent the most common granulomatous infections[14] of the hand. These may involve *Mycobacterium tuberculosis* or the atypical *Mycobacterium* species. Anaerobic bacterial infections may be caused by several of the *Clostridium* species, *Bacteroides*, *Lactobacillus* and others. The most common viral infections include herpes simplex, herpes zoster, and common warts. Fungal infections may be caused by *Candida albicans* in chronically ill or immunosuppressed patients. Sporotrichosis may be contracted by gardeners following a puncture from a rose thorn. Coccidioidomycosis and histoplasmosis are other specific fungal infections with a regional association.

The correct use of a variety of antibiotic medications is important in the effective management of most hand infections. Antibiotics alone should not be relied upon to cure most

TABLE 17–2. Common Organisms and Infections

Bacterial	
Most common	
Aerobes	Staphylococcal
	Streptococcal
	Pseudomonas
	Proteus
Anaerobes	*Clostridium*
	Bacteroides
	Peptococcus
	Actinomyces
	Fusobacterium
	Lactobacillus
	Eubacterium
	Veillonella
	Bacteroides melaninogenicus
Others	*Mycobacterium tuberculosis*
	Atypical mycobacterium
	Anthrax
	Erysipeloid
	Gonorrhea
	Pasteurella multocida
	Eikenella corrodens
	Haemophilus influenzae
	Brucellosis
Viral	Herpes simplex
	Herpes zoster
	Vaccinia
	Warts
	Rabies
	Orf
Fungal	Sporotrichosis
	Blastomycosis
	Ringworm
	Coccidioidomycosis
	Onychomycosis
	Maduromycosis
	Nocardiosis
	Actinomycosis
	Candida albicans
	Geotrichum candidum

infections. Some infections, if recognized and treated within the first 12 to 48 hours, may be successfully treated with the use of antibiotics, splints, and elevation alone, thus avoiding the necessity for surgery.

Culture of drainage or aspiration when the patient is initially seen can give the most useful information to guide the antibiotic selection. However, if material for culture cannot be obtained, antibiotic selection is based on empirical considerations.

Antibiotics are generally required for only 5 to 10 days unless deep bone infection is present or complicating circumstances arise. Intravenous administration of antibiotics for the initial 3 to 5 days is the route of choice. Following this, with significant improvement of the infection, a course may be completed using oral antibiotics and monitoring the clinical progress.

SPECIFIC INFECTIONS

A spectrum of infections occur in the skin and subcutaneous tissues, ranging from infected abrasions or cellulitis, furuncles and paronychia, to deep subcutaneous abscess formation of the digital pulp or palmar spaces.

Cellulitis

Cellulitis commonly occurs secondary to a small puncture wound or an abrasion. Depending on the type and level of contamination, as well as the virulence of the organism, the severity of the infection may vary from mild to severe. Commonly, over a 12- to 24-hour period, the involved area of the hand may become swollen and painful (deep throbbing pain or night pain is a reliable symptom of deep abscess formation). The patient occasionally will be febrile, and examination will show an area of erythema with increased warmth and occasional forearm streaking. Forearm or lymphagetic spread may be indicative of a streptococcal infection, although staphylococci are the most common cause of cellulitis. Occasionally, if the epidermal insult was in a moist environment, *Pseudomonas* cellulitis can be recognized by the characteristic fruity odor and green discoloration of tissues. Cellulitis may also be caused by mixed bacteria or anaerobes.

The treatment for cellulitic infections without deep abscess consists of cleansing of the skin and tissues of the hand, unroofing of any epidermal blisters, and immobilization and elevation with antibiotic coverage dictated by Gram strain or empiric considerations. Once the acute cellulitis begins to reverse, a compression glove and early range of motion can be instituted to prevent swelling and stiffness.

Furuncles

Furuncles or carbuncles are infections seen in association with hair follicles. The usual organism is *Staphylococcus,* and treatment consists of appropriate antibiotics, rest, immobilization, elevation, and drainage of any superficial abscess once formed.

Pyogenic Granuloma

Pyogenic granuloma represents a hypertrophic growth of granulation tissue raised above the surface of the skin. This is usually caused by maceration owing to excessive moisture in the dressings. Frequently, exposure to the air, skin grafting, or removal of any foreign body material when present will allow resolution of the problem. In some cases, surgical excision is required, and in the chronic situation, one should excise the lesion for culture and pathologic examination to rule out the possibility of unusual infection or malignancy.

Subcutaneous Abscess

Subcutaneous abscess formation is seen on a continuum with the more superficial skin infections; however, in this situation, a frank subcutaneous collection of pus is present. An abscess may occur following a puncture wound with or without a retained deep foreign body. Another common etiology is injection of nonsterile chemicals or drugs with contaminated needles.[10] These patients commonly present with cellulitis and tenderness along the course of a major vein. The patient may have a history of drug abuse problems or evidence on physical examination of frequent contaminated needle use. Appropriate treatment for these infections includes immobilization, rest, elevation, and antibiotic saturation based on aspirated material or empiric coverage (Fig. 17–2). Following an initial observation period of 12 to 48 hours, the infection will either resolve, at which time functional rehabilitation and range of motion may be slowly begun, or will localize, at which time incision, drainage, and debridement should be carried out in the operating room. Marsupialization technique is used (excising an ellipse of tissue) to ensure adequate drainage (Fig. 17–3). Dressings are then changed postoperatively at 48 to 72 hours, and local care and functional treatment are continued as needed.

Paronychia

Paronychia is a common infection that occurs along the margin of the nail plate in the nail fold. An abscess may be present in the periungual soft tissues on the dorsum of the fingertip involving the area adjacent to the lateral nail fold and may extend superficially or deep into the germinal matrix. These infections are commonly caused by manipulation, manicure, puncture, or nail biting. In the chronic situation, infections may also be caused by fungus or yeast or they may be secondary to other lesions, including malignant

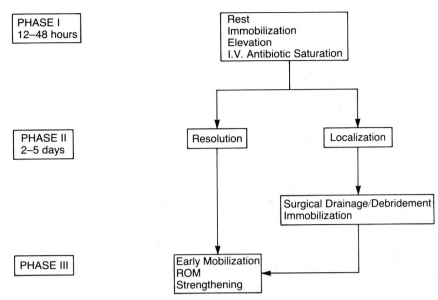

FIGURE 17–2. Treatment scheme for soft tissue hand infections. Rapidly progressive necrotizing infections, fulminant suppurative tenosynovitis, or pyogenic arthritis may necessitate immediate surgical decompression, irrigation, and debridement.

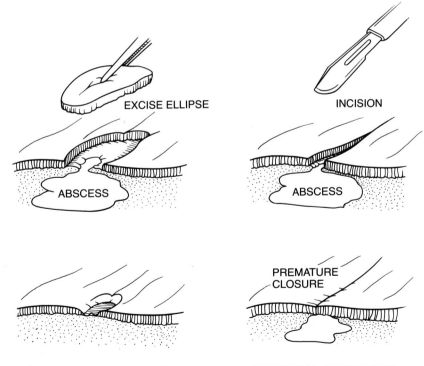

FIGURE 17–3. Marsupialization technique. Removal of an ellipse of tissue ensures that the wound will stay open, providing continued adequate drainage while the wound heals by secondary intention. Healing is usually cosmetically excellent, especially if the incisions have been made in proper orientation with the natural skin creases (see Fig. 17–7A–F).

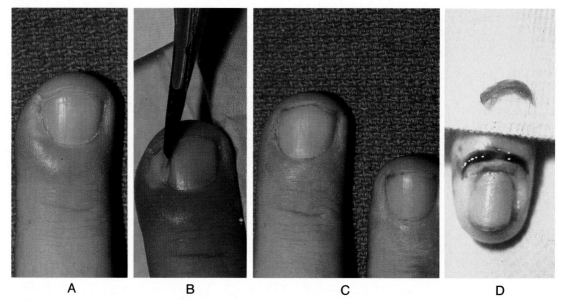

FIGURE 17–4. *A,* The paronychia as demonstrated here shows swelling along the eponychial margin with visible pus. *B,* Direct incision and drainage of the paronychia. *C,* Resolution of the infection. *D,* Marsupialization technique of Keyser for chronic paronychial infection. A crescent-shaped block of subcutaneous tissue is excised just proximal to the nail fold. Care must be taken not to injure the underlying germinal nail matrix, which is exposed by the eponychial marsupialization.

tumors. They present with swelling, erythema, and pus collection along the periphery of the nail. The bacterial infections are most commonly *Staphylococcus* but may also be mixed organisms. In the early stage of the lesions prior to abscess formation, antibiotics, a dry dressing, and observation are indicated.

Once an abscess has formed and pus is visible under the nail margin (Fig. 17–4A), decompression by eponychial incision, or partial or complete nail plate excision, is indicated to allow for drainage of the infection (Fig. 17–4B,C). In the chronic infection, the nail plate should be removed and a crescent-shaped wedge of tissue removed just proximal to the eponychial fold (Fig. 17–4D).[23] Cleansing is performed and a dry dressing is utilized at 24- to 48-hour intervals. Complications include involvement of the distal phalanx and tuft with osteitis or osteomyelitis and severe damage to the nail bed or eponychial folds.

Felon (Pulp Abscess)

Felon is a closed space abscess occurring in the septal compartments of the finger pulp. It is a fairly common infection that may occur several days following puncture to the finger pulp. The most frequent organism recovered,

again, is *Staphylococcus.* Pulp infections occur with a wide spectrum of severity, from cellulitis and induration of the finger pulp (which is not truly a felon or abscess) to a fulminant deep infection involving the digital pulp and bony distal phalanx.

Occasionally, in the milder situation, the treatment with antibiotics, immobilization, and elevation effects a resolution and conservative treatment can be continued. However, if a true abscess collection is present, surgical drainage is necessary for resolution of the infection. In the full-blown situation, the patient will present with severe throbbing pain in the digital pulp area. Significant swelling, warmth, erythema, and exquisite tenderness are present. Surgical drainage, when necessary, should be performed in the operating room under tourniquet control and careful planning. Lateral "hockey stick" or full "fish-mouth" type of approaches should be kept dorsal (Fig. 17–5A–E) running along the hyponychium just under the nail plate in order to avoid the complication of denervation and devascularization, leaving a depressed tender scar with an atrophied digital pad (Fig. 17–5G). If the incision is kept dorsally, the volar-based blood and nerve supply to the pulp will remain intact, allowing for healing without disruption of the tactile pad.

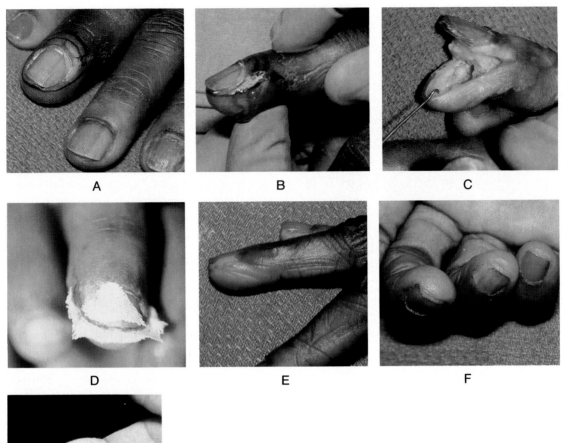

A   B   C

D   E   F

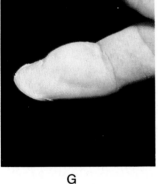

G

FIGURE 17–5. *A,B,* When a felon is drained through a "fish mouth" type incision, the line of incision must be kept dorsally at the level of the hyponychium. *C,* If the incision is kept well dorsal, the entire volar flap is protected from devascularization by maintenance of the incoming vascular and nervous supply. *D,* Zeroform may be interposed in the wound to insure adequate drainage until the first dressing change at 48 hours. *E,F,* Follow-up photographs demonstrating resolution of the felon infection and satisfactory healing without injury or atrophy of the pulp tissue. *G,* Postoperative result following "fish mouth" type incision of a felon which was made too volar. Atrophy of the soft tissues between the incision and the dorsal bone is evident.

An alternative approach, when the felon is pointing in a particular area of the pulp, is to drain the abscess over the area of maximum intensity with a direct incision into the pulp. A small ellipse of skin should be removed in order to ensure proper continued drainage. One should also be wary of the complications of osteomyelitis of the distal phalanx, septic arthritis of the distal interphalangeal (DIP) joint, tendon sheath infection, or retained necrotic tissue or foreign body, in which case chronic drainage following surgical decompression may persist.

Herpetic felons (Fig. 17–6) may mimic bacte-

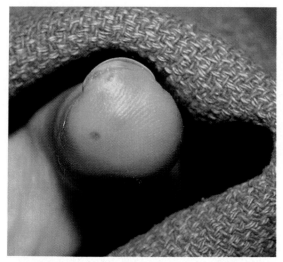

FIGURE 17–6. Herpetic felon with vesicles in varying stages of healing; this may simulate a pyogenic felon.

rial pulp abscess infections and should be differentiated because these infections are caused by a virus and should not be surgically drained.[24] In such cases, small herpetic vesicles or blisters will be noted on the fingertip. These are effectively treated with protection, rest, and immobilization with or without antiviral medication. Herpetic infections can be expected to resolve over a 10- to 21-day period.

Palmar Space Infection

Palmar space infections may occur in the thenar or hypothenar spaces.[1, 25] Similar type abscesses may occur in the web spaces of the palm. These types of infections most frequently occur following a puncture wound in the palmar and digital areas, with or without retention of a foreign body. Deep, painful infection may evolve over the ensuing 3 to 5 days. The most common organism is *Staphylococcus*, although other bacteria may be recovered. The patient may present with obvious findings of abscess formation with deep throbbing pain, redness, tenderness, and fluctuance; however, often the swelling may be subtle, with brawny induration, erythema, and tenderness in the palm. A small wound or perforation on the surface may lead to a large underlying deep abscess, as in the "collar button" situation. Treatment should include intravenous antibiotic saturation followed by incision, drainage, and debridement in a fully equipped

operating room. Continued drainage of the abscess is provided by leaving the wound open, with placement of either a small gauze or rubber drain, or, preferably, by the more effective method of marsupialization (wound enlargement) in order to ensure adequate, continued drainage (Fig. 17–7A–F). Postoperatively, intravenous antibiotics are continued along with immobilization and elevation, with a dressing change at 24 to 48 hours. Possible complications include injury to the deep vital structures in the hand, including nerve tendons or muscles, and one should remain alert to the possibility of acute suppurative tenosynovitis.

Tendon Sheath Infections

Tendon sheath infections involve the flexor tendon sheaths, which extend from the midpalm level to the distal phalanges. The thumb and little finger tendon sheaths may communicate with the radial, ulnar, or carpal bursa. Flexor tenosynovitis occurs with a spectrum of severity, and two types should be recognized. Acute, suppurative flexor tenosynovitis, as described by Kanavel, is rather rare, and may occur secondary to a puncture wound of the finger with purulent staphylococcal or streptococcal infection within the flexor tendon sheath. The cardinal signs of this type of infection, as originally described by Kanavel, are presented in Table 17–3. More frequently occurring infections mimicking a tendon sheath infection, such as subcutaneous abscess or septic proximal interphalangeal (PIP) arthritis, also present with a posture of partial flexion and pain with passive extension; however, the swelling is usually fusiform rather than uniform, and tenderness along the flexor sheath does not extend into the base of the finger in the palmar area.

A milder form of flexor tenosynovitis may be seen in which a subcutaneous or local infection causes a tenosynovitis with a sympathetic effusion. Bacteria may be present in the synovium without fulminant purulence in the tendon sheath. This milder type of flexor tenosynovitis may be treated effectively with intravenous antibiotics, immobilization, and elevation. Early surgical treatment, when needed, should consist of a limited incision and drainage of the tendon sheath proximally and distally, with irrigation and use of a small catheter. However, if a fulminant, purulent flexor tenosynovitis is present, more extensive surgi-

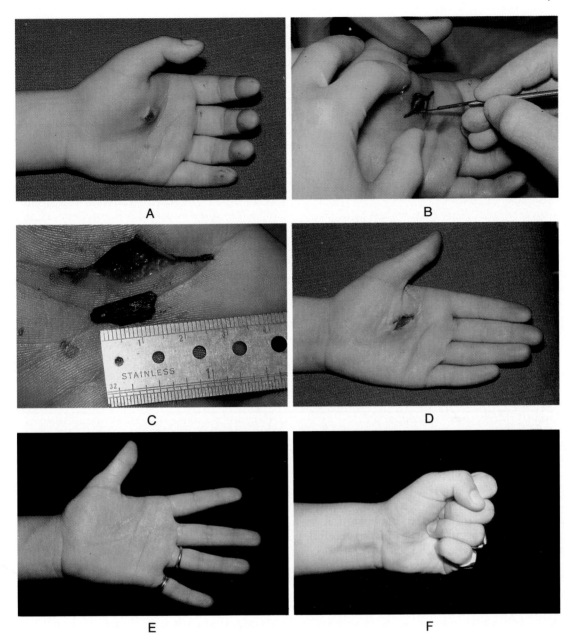

FIGURE 17 – 7. *A,* Palmar abscess with extension into the thenar bursa. *B,* Incision and drainage by use of excision of an elliptical block of tissue. Pus and granulation tissue were removed and the wound copiously irrigated. *C,* Removal of a foreign body, a piece of wood, which was found in the depths of the wound. *D,* Rapid healing and resolution of the infection, swelling and cellulitis 48 hours after incision and drainage. *E,F,* Complete healing of the elliptical defect at 3 weeks with good maintenance of hand function.

cal exposure with wide incision, drainage and debridement is indicated. The A2 and A4 pulleys should be preserved, if at all possible, in order to maintain effective finger flexion. Early mobilization must be carried out within the first 3 to 5 days in order to prevent tendon adherence and stiffness of the fingers.

If tendon necrosis is present, the degenerated tendon material will serve as a sequestered focus of infection. In this situation, excision of the tendon or tendons may be necessary before the infection can be controlled. Later, one- or two-stage tendon reconstruction is necessary to restore function.

TABLE 17–3. Kanavel's Cardinal Signs

1. Uniform swelling of the involved finger
2. Tenderness along the flexor tendon sheath extending into the palm*
3. Partial flexion posture of the finger
4. Severe pain with passive extension

* Most diagnostic sign.

Bites

Animal and human bites are a common cause of hand infections,[11, 19, 21, 22, 26, 27] which, if recognized and treated early, can minimize the morbidity and ultimate impairment of hand function. Unfortunately, many bite type infections are seen after a delay in medical care and treatment, leading to more serious infections. Specific organisms are associated with various animal bites and are discussed in this section. Human bites may be of different types, with a spectrum occurring from self-inflicted, inadvertent nail bites to violent partial amputations. One of the more common types of bites is the "clenched fist" or "fist in mouth" type injury, where following a blow to the tooth a "bite" in the "knuckle," or metacarpophalangeal (MCP) area, has occurred.

Streptococci and staphylococci remain the most frequent organisms; however, following human bites, up to 43 percent of patients may have a mixed infection with both gram-positive and gram-negative bacteria. Both aerobic and anaerobic bacteria may be present, and *Eikenella corrodens,* a gram-negative bacterium, has been reported to occur in up to 20 percent of cases. As a result of the high incidence of both penicillin-sensitive organisms, such as anaerobes and *Eikenella corrodens,* and the high incidence of *Staphylococcus aureus,* the recommended empiric coverage should include both penicillin and a penicillinase-resistant medication.

A bite wound should never be closed, but if seen early, it can be irrigated, debrided, left open, immobilized, and treated with antibiotic coverage. If seen later, when an established infection is present, formal debridement and surgical drainage in the operating room are usually necessary. X-rays should always be taken to check for intra-articular injury or foreign body. Bacterial infection and contamination are usually involved in the extensor tendons or in the MCP joint owing to the contamination along the gliding plane of the extensor tendon. Once the infection is brought under control, early mobilization of the hand can usually be effected by the fifth to tenth day.

Domestic cat or dog bites may become infected with *Pasteurella multocida* in a significant percentage of cases.[21] Staphylococci and streptococci and anaerobic species may also be recovered, and these bites should be treated similarly to human bites with penicillin coverage for the *Pasteurella* and anaerobes and penicillinase-resistant medication for the staphylococci.

Septic Arthritis

Septic arthritis in the hand may occur secondary to inoculation by direct penetration as the result of a puncture-type wound or from the spread of infection from an adjacent wound originating from subcutaneous abscess or tendon sheath infection. These infections can be severe and disabling, causing destruction of the joint or osteomyelitis of the phalanges or metacarpal, with significant loss of hand function. In Kanavel's text, septic arthritis was a devastating injury, especially when the PIP joint was involved, and frequently resulted in the necessity of a finger amputation.

As with other large joint infections, such as the knee, hip, or shoulder, septic arthritis must be recognized early and treated with arthrotomy, surgical debridement, and drainage. Early functional mobilization is used in order to preserve joint integrity and function.

Depending on the circumstances surrounding the joint infection, the organisms may be either gram-positive or gram-negative, with *Staphylococcus* and *Streptococcus* being the most frequent. Human or animal bites may be the cause of septic arthritis, and in these cases as recommended in the above section, antibiotic coverage for the appropriate organisms should be initiated.

The clinical presentation of a septic joint is that of severe pain with motion, marked swelling, erythema, and tenderness of the involved

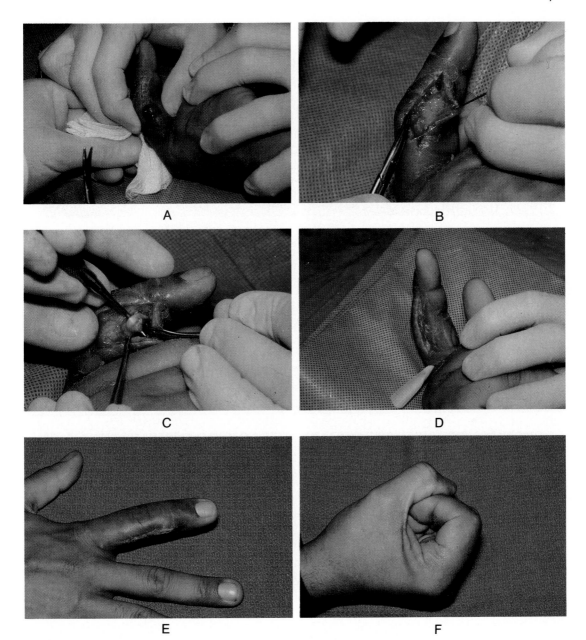

FIGURE 17–8. *A,B,* Interoperative photographs of a septic PIP joint being drained through midaxial incision. *C,* Identification of the collateral ligaments and partial excision to allow for adequate continued joint drainage. *D,* Proximal drain and the ulnar placement of the midaxial incision. *E,F,* Early mobilization, active range of motion, and satisfactory healing following septic PIP joint drainage.

joint. Needle aspiration may be of help in establishing the diagnosis with certainty and identifying the bacteria involved. In borderline cases, a period of immobilization, elevation, and antibiotic saturation can be instituted with close monitoring of the progress. If joint infection is present, surgical drainage with irrigation and debridement should be carefully performed in the operating room. PIP joint infections are most effectively drained through unilateral or bilateral mid-axial incisions,[28] taking care to keep the incision dorsal enough so as not to cause flexion contracture upon wound healing. The volar portion of the collateral ligament should be excised in order to ensure adequate and continued drainage of

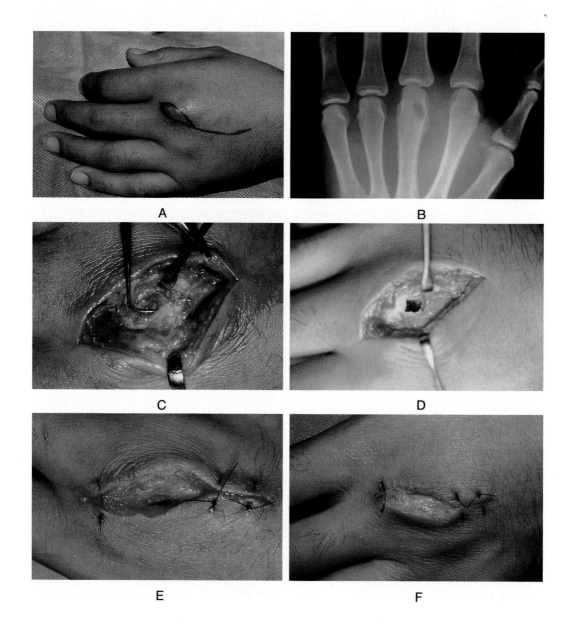

FIGURE 17–9. *A,B,* Preoperative photograph and x-rays of a patient with osteomyelitis involving the head and neck of the third metacarpal bone with dorsal swelling. *C,D,* Interoperative photograph showing a defect in the metacarpal bone with granulation tissue and interosseous abscess. This was windowed, irrigated, and debrided to provide adequate drainage. *E,F,* Partial closure of wound at surgery and at 48 hours showing satisfactory control of infection. *G,H,* Early radiographs of the interosseous abscess and later healing of the bone defect. *I,J,* Satisfactory clinical healing and range of motion at 6 weeks postoperatively.

the joint. If severe joint destruction is already present, primary arthrodesis in an appropriate degree of flexion is occasionally required. Early mobilization of the joint should be employed, particularly if the PIP joint is involved (Fig. 17–8*A–F*). This can be instituted with active flexion and extension on the second or third postoperative day. Local care and intravenous antibiotics are continued until the wound is clearly healing without evidence of retained infection. By the fifth to seventh day, usually pain, swelling and drainage have decreased, allowing for increased movement and function.

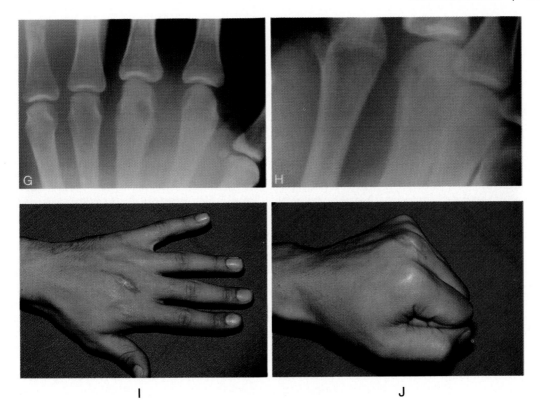

FIGURE 17–9 *Continued*

OSTEOMYELITIS

Osteomyelitis following the bones in the hand is relatively unusual.[4] In adults, osteomyelitis usually results from extension of contiguous soft tissue infection, such as a severe, neglected paronychia or felon, or from an adjacent wound infection or joint infection. Certain puncture injuries that penetrate directly into the bone may also cause osteomyelitis, such as the tooth in mouth injuries. In children, bone infection of the metacarpals or phalanges may be caused by hematogenous seeding secondary to bacteremia. The most common organism involved in both the adult and pediatric age group is *S. aureus.*

Treatment consists of incision, drainage, immobilization, and intravenous antibiotics. Access to the metacarpals is best through a dorsal incision (Fig. 17–9A–J) and the phalanges through a mid-axial incision. The infections should be cultured and a biopsy should be performed in all cases to obtain culture and sensitivity of the infecting organism and to rule out underlying pathological diagnosis. Drill holes should be made in the cortex with a window for decompression, irrigation, and debridement of the infection. Obvious necrosis or sequestrum should be excised and the wound should be left completely open or partially open to allow for adequate ongoing drainage. Early functional treatment of the hand should be allowed with range of motion, intermittent splinting, and local wound care performed. Intravenous antibiotics are continued for 2 to 6 weeks, depending on the clinical response.

CHRONIC INFECTIONS

Several types of chronic infections and tenosynovitis may be caused by atypical mycobacteria, tuberculosis, *Mycobacterium lepraemurium* or fungi.[14, 17, 18] The most common mycobacterial infection is caused by *M. marinum,* in which the patient may present with a history of a penetrating wound which occurred in an aquatic environment, such as a fresh water lake, the ocean, or from domestic fish tanks. Other mycobacteria, such as *M. kansasii* or *M. avium–intracellulare,* may also cause tenosynovial infections. The patient typically will have a chronic, minimally symptomatic swelling along the fingers and palm or in the volar aspect of the wrist. In these patients, tenosynovectomy is indicated and culture of the biopsy must be plated on Lowenstein-Jensen medium at a temperature of 30 to 32° C. Histologically, one may see noncaseating granulomas and acid-fast bacilli on staining. Surgical treatment is tenosynovectomy performed through oblique interaxial palmar incisions in the fingers or oblique incisions in the palm or through the carpal canal as indicated by the extent of the disease process. A brief period of postoperative splinting for 5 to 10 days with early active motion gives the best results. Antituberculous medication must be started on an empiric basis, unless the acid-fast stains are positive, because definitive cultures take 6 weeks for growth. The anti-tuberculous drugs of choice are rifampin, isoniazid, and ethambutol, which should be continued for 1 to 2 years.

Mycobacterium tuberculosis[15] may present in a similar fashion to the atypical mycobacterial infections and may involve not only synovium but the small joints of the hand as well. Tuberculous infections can also produce bony subperiosteal reaction and proliferation. Tenosynovectomy is indicated in chronically involved areas, and rarely surgical excision or curettage of the metacarpals or phalanges may be indicated when significantly involved with the infective process. Anti-tuberculous drugs are utilized for 1 to 2 years.

Leprosy is caused by *M. lepraemurium* and may commonly involve the hands, as it has a predilection for the cooler areas of the body. Ulnar neuropathy may cause intrinsic motor paralysis with typical interosseous atrophy, clawing, and weakness of pinch. Fingertip ulcerations can result secondary to the insensate tactile pads. A program of educating the patient to protect anesthetic fingers is important in the treatment program. The principal drug used in the treatment of leprosy is diaminodiphenylsulfone, and surgical reconstructive procedures may be indicated in some cases for substitution of losses due to specific neurologic deficits.

Fungal infections may be superficial or deep. Most common fungal infections are superficial and involve the nail and surrounding tissues. These may be treated with removal of the nail, scrapings for definitive diagnosis, and local topical antifungal agents.

When deep mycoses are present, they may be difficult to treat or eradicate. Ulceration and sinus formation may communicate with deep tendon or synovial tissues, or even involve the bones and joints. The most important modality of treatment is medical, with the appropriate antifungal agent. Occasionally surgical debridement of tenosynovium, bones, or joints may be necessary.

GANGRENOUS INFECTIONS

The gangrenous infections may be caused by clostridial species or other anaerobes, commonly microaerophilic *Streptococcus*, as in Meleney's infection[29] or a variety of mixed organisms in the diabetic setting.

Clostridial gangrene of the hand is rare, but may occur following severe mutilating or crushing-type injuries when a combination of contaminated traumatized ischemic tissue is present. A variety of different clostridial species may be involved. Gram-positive rods on Gram stain are diagnostic. The clinical presentation is that of fulminant, rapidly progressing infection with gas and crepitation in the subcutaneous tissues. Typically, brawny edema and rapidly advancing cellulitis with purplish skin discoloration and intracuticular bullae formation are present. Other gas-forming organisms, such as coliforms, streptococci, or *Bacteroides* may also cause a similar infection.

The principles of treatment include prompt resuscitation of the patient; massive doses of intravenous antibiotics, including penicillin; and adequate surgical debridement. Hyperbaric oxygen has also been shown to be beneficial in improving the mortality and limb salvage caused by these devastating infections.

Meleney's infection may present with a similar picture and is caused by microaerophilic *Streptococcus*. Patients are treated most effectively, in a fashion similar to that for clostridial gangrene, with massive intravenous penicillin, early surgical debridement, and hyperbaric oxygen.

Diabetic gangrene of the hand is a different disease.[30] The patient often presents in poor health with a history of frequent hospital admissions and previous lower extremity amputations. Nutrition and wound healing capacity are poor, and following debridement or amputation of gangrenous digits, the wound may be unable to be healed. Mortality is high, at least 50 percent within 2 years of infection.

The principles of treatment in such cases include aggressive medical support, with early adequate amputation and loose tension-free primary or delayed primary closure of wounds.

References

Cited References

1. Kanavel AB: Infections of the Hand: A Guide to the Surgical Treatment of Acute and Chronic Suppurative Processes in the Fingers, Hand, and Forearm, 7th ed. Philadelphia, Lea & Febiger, 1943.
2. Koch SL: Felons, acute lymphangitis and tendon sheath infections: differential diagnosis and treatment. JAMA 92:1171, 1929.
3. Koch SL: Acute rapidly spreading infections following trivial injuries of the hand. Surg Gynecol Obstet 59:277, 1934.
4. Koch SL: Osteomyelitis of the bones of the hand. Surg Gynecol Obstet 64:1, 1937.
5. Mason ML: Infections of the hand. Surg Clin North Am 22:455, 1942.
6. Bailey D: The Infected Hand. London, HK Lewis & Co, Ltd, 1963.
7. Sneddon J: The Care of Hand Infections. Baltimore, Williams & Wilkins Co, 1970.
8. Sneddon J: Dressings in hand sepsis. Br Med J 1:372–373, 1969.
9. Eaton RG, Butsch DP: Antibiotic guidelines for hand infections. Surg Gynecol Obstet 130:119–122, 1970.
10. McKay D, Pascarelli EF, Eaton RG: Infections and sloughs in the hands in drug addicts. J Bone Joint Surg 55A:741–746, 1973.
11. Carter PR: Common hand injuries and infections: A practical approach to early treatment. XIV. Philadelphia, WB Saunders Co, 1983.
12. Carter SJ, Burman SO, Mersheimer WL: Treatment of digital tenosynovitis by irrigation with peroxide and oxytetracycline. Ann Surg 163:645–650, 1966.
13. Carter SJ, Mersheimer WL: Infections of the hand. Orthop Clin North Am 1:455–466, 1970.
14. Linscheid RL, Dobyns JH: Common and uncommon infections of the hand. Orthop Clin North Am 6:1063–1104, 1975.
15. Neviaser RJ: Closed tendon sheath irrigation for pyogenic flexor tenosynovitis. J Hand Surg 3:462–466, 1978.
16. Kilgore ES Jr, Brown LG, Newmeyer WL, Graham WP, Davis TS: Treatment of felons. Am J Surg 130:194–197, 1975.
17. Kilgore ES: Hand infections. J Hand Surg 8:723–726, 1983.
18. Strickland JW: Infections of the hand. In Cowan NJ, ed: Practical Hand Surgery. Miami, Symposia Specialist, 1980, pp 493–510.
19. Goldstein EJC, Miller TA, Citron DM: Infections following clenched-fist injury: a new perspective. J Hand Surg 3:455–457, 1978.
20. Mann RJ, Hoffeld TA, Baring-Farmer C: Human bites of the hand: twenty years of experience. J Hand Surg 2:97–104, 1977.
21. Peeples E, Boswick JA Jr, Scott FA: Wounds of the hand contaminated by human or animal saliva. J Trauma 20:383–388, 1980.
22. McDonald I: *Eikenella corrodens* infection of the hand. Hand 11:224–227, 1979.
23. Keyser JJ, Eaton RG: Surgical cure of chronic paronychia and eponychial marsupialization. Plast Reconstr Surg 58:66–70, 1976.
24. Louis DS, Silva J Jr: Herpetic whitlow: herpetic infections of the digits. J Hand Surg 4:90–94, 1979.
25. Boyes J: Bunnell's Surgery of the Hand, 4th ed. Philadelphia, JB Lippincott Co, 1964.
26. Chuinard RG, D'Ambrosia RD: Human bite infections of the hand. J Bone Joint Surg 59A:416–418, 1977.
27. Guba AM Jr, Mulliken JB, Hoopes JE: The selection of antibiotics for human bites of the hand. Plast Reconstr Surg 56:538–541, 1975.
28. Wittels NP, Donley JM, Burkhalter WE: A functional treatment method for interphalangeal pyogenic arthritis. J Hand Surg 9A:894–898, 1984.
29. Meleney F: Clinical Aspects and Treatment of Surgical Infections. Philadelphia, WB Saunders Co, 1949.
30. Lagaard SW, McElfresh EC, Premer RF: Diabetic Gangrene of the Upper Extremity. Transactions of the 41st Meeting, American Society for Surgery of the Hand, New Orleans, Vol 10, No. 2, 1986.

Uncited References

Glass KD: Factors related to the resolution of treated hand infections. J Hand Surg 7:388–394, 1982.
Robins RHC: Tuberculosis of the wrist and hand. Br J Surg 54:211–218, 1967.
Stern PJ, Staneck JL, McDonough JJ, Neale HW, Tyler G: Established hand infections: a controlled, prospective study. J Hand Surg 8:553–559, 1983.

Claude R. Hitchcock, M.D., Ph.D.

CHAPTER

18

Gas Gangrene

INTRODUCTION

Gas gangrene caused by the anaerobic bacterium *Clostridium* usually occurs in soft tissue. Only rarely does bone become involved with *Clostridium* in the form of osteomyelitis. This type of infection is acute and frequently follows skeletal trauma, in which soft tissues are damaged during the fracturing of bones. This chapter presents the problem of gas gangrene as it exists without antecedent trauma and occurs as a "primary" infection following customarily "clean" surgery.

Among organisms in the scale of life, the anaerobic bacteria may be one of the earliest life forms. All living matter in the world contains anaerobic bacteria. The classic description of "gas gangrene" implies infection with *Clostridium,* which produces powerful exotoxins. Other bacteria are commonly present; Chapter 19 discusses gas-forming infections with organisms other than *Clostridium.*

Clostridia are found as spore forms or vegetative forms in soil and intestinal tracts of animals and man. Wherever animal life exists on our earth, clostridia are found in abundance.[1] The earliest anaerobic organism studied by Louis Pasteur in France (1861) was a bacterium that forms butyric acid anaerobically and that he named *Clostridium butyricum.* Pasteur subsequently identified another pathogenic form of *Clostridium,* which he named "septicum" in 1877. The most virulent form of *Clostridium* that we know, *"Clostridium perfringens,"* was discovered independently in three countries: in the United States in 1892 Welch and Nuttall called it *Bacillus aerogenes capsulatus;* in Germany in 1893 Frankel named it *Bacillus phlegmonis emphysematosae;* and in France in 1897 Veillon and Zuber called it *Bacillus perfringens.* Following an extensive experience with gas gangrene in World War I, the name "perfringens" gained popularity and is most commonly used today for this species. However, in Germany the organism is frequently still known as "Frankel's bacillus" and in some English-speaking countries the *perfringens* species is still referred to as *Clostridium welchii.*[1]

For more than two decades, the author has had an extensive experience with gas infections; of a total of 303 such infections, 247 were caused by clostridial organisms. Chapter 19 deals with a group of 56 patients, who were managed by the author, with gas infection from nonclostridial bacteria.

In these 22 years, our clinic has treated 107 patients with clostridial gas gangrene following trauma, 71 patients with this infection following a clean surgical procedure (postoperative infection), and 69 patients with clostridial gas gangrene appearing as a "primary" infection without antecedent trauma or surgery. Current literature still perpetuates some misconceptions about clostridial infections, which are often described as a threat only, following trauma or when significant devitalized tissue is present. Some authors speak of this infection as "gas gangrene" only if necrosis of muscle is present. Some physicians still consider *C. perfringens* to be the only *Clostridium* species of significance as a pathogen for humans. Our experience indicates the need for change in many of these concepts, which are emphasized at various places in this chapter.

We have used a simple classification for these clostridial infections, dividing them into patients with myositis and those with serious "cellulitis" only.[2] The myositis cases were further divided into a "diffuse spreading" type as contrasted with a "localized" form. Also, we recognized a "diffuse spreading cellulitis" as contrasted with a "localized" form. Cellulitis, in our description, is a serious infection involving cells of several types of tissues and frequently leading to death.

From the Hennepin County Medical Center, Minneapolis, Minnesota.

BACTERIOLOGY OF THE CLOSTRIDIA

The clostridia are true saprophytes and can be found in the intestinal tract of animals and man. Less commonly, they may colonize the external ear canal and perineal skin. They are gram-positive rods with a large and well-formed central or subterminal spore (particularly in *C. perfringens*). They are anaerobic and occasionally are difficult to recover in the laboratory. Care must be taken in securing appropriate culture material from the patient, and the infected material should go to the laboratory in anaerobic containers (see Chapter 5).[1, 3]

Clostridia, with rare exception, lack the enzymes cytochrome oxidase, catalase, superoxide dismutase, and peroxidase. Most bacteria produce hydrogen peroxide (H_2O_2) when grown in the presence of oxygen. If catalase or peroxidase, which acts upon H_2O_2, are not present, presumably the accumulation of H_2O_2 can reach a concentration sufficient to kill the organisms. Also, free oxygen or, more specifically, the free radical form of O_2 — superoxide (O_2) — is harmful to anaerobes.[4] If effective reducing agents (such as sodium thioglycolate or amino triazole) are not present in cultures, these oxidative enzyme processes may raise the redox potential to levels inhibitory to *Clostridium*.[3, 4]

Necrotic tissue and blood are rich in catalase and provide an optimal environment for the growth of *Clostridium*. However, there can be a lowering of redox potential of localized areas of tissue (hypoxia) without necrosis, and there can still be catalase or peroxidase present, allowing conversion of clostridial spore forms to rapidly growing vegetative forms capable of producing exotoxins.

The redox potential requirements of *Clostridium* vary from one species to another. There is a variation in the tolerance to oxygen and peroxide. For instance, *C. perfringens* is more tolerant of peroxide than are some other species.[5, 6]

Clostridia are found on all mucous membranes of the human body, from the mouth through the anus. They can inhabit the meatus of the urethra in both the male and female and can produce every type of infection known in humans, such as cellulitis, fasciitis, myositis, abscess, and empyema. The organisms are present in the tartar of teeth and under the subgingival margins, in cerumen, and transiently on skin.

Primary isolation of *Clostridium* from infective material may be difficult, and meticulous culture techniques may be required. Some species of *Clostridium* may take several days and then grow only poorly or "die out" in the laboratory. Thus, species identification may not always be possible. Still others may be speciated only through reference laboratories, further complicating precise associations with disease. Most forms of *Clostridium* characteristically produce any of several well-known exotoxins. *C. perfringens*, for example, produces nine that are responsible for many of the pathophysiological characteristics of the infection (Fig. 18–1).

Alpha toxin (lecithinase) is a hemolytic toxin causing necrosis. It hydrolyzes lecithin to phosphorocholine and diglycerides. This toxin also hydrolyzes cephalin and syringomyelin. Because lecithin is found in membranes of many different cells, the opportunities for attack by this toxin are numerous. In its action, lecithinase inactivates enzyme systems that are dependent on lecithin.

Theta toxin is a hemolytic and lethal toxin that causes hemolysis and necrosis and is cardiotoxic. It is oxygen- and heat-labile. Kappa toxin is a collagenase that lyses proteins, hydrolyzes hyaluronic acid, and acts as a spreading factor; it is lethal.

Mu toxin is a hyaluronidase that hydrolyzes hyaluronic acid and acts as a spreading factor. Nu toxin is a deoxyribonuclease that affects the DNA of cells. Fibrinolysin is a protease that lyses fibrin. Neuraminidase destroys the immunologic receptors on erythrocytes and cleaves tertiary sialic acid. Hemagglutinin is a toxin that inactivates blood group factor A on erythrocytes. The circulating factor of *Clostridium* is a toxin that inhibits phagocytosis.

These and other toxins are produced in varying amounts by different organisms under varying conditions. The author believes that differing clinical manifestations of gas gangrene are perhaps due to varying amounts and patterns of the known toxins and in turn the species of *Clostridium* recovered from a patient's wound.

Invasiveness of the species involved in an infection is influenced by the effect of normal serum on the proteinases produced by that organism. The kappa exotoxin of *C. perfringens* (collagenase) is not inhibited by normal serum, and this bacterium is the most clinically invasive of all the clostridia. *C. histolyticum* and *C. septicum* are similar but clinically are less invasive. Normal serum, however, does inhibit the proteinases of *C. tetani*, *C. botulinum*, *C. sporo-*

EXOTOXINS OF CL. PERFRINGENS TYPE A

Alpha	(Lecithinase C.)	Lethal	hydrolyses lecithin to phosphoro choline + diglycerides. hemolysis - necrosis
Theta	(Hemolysin)	Lethal	cardiotoxic - necrosis hemolysis - O + heat labile
Kappa	(Collagenase)	Lethal	lyses proteins
Mu	(Hyaluronidase)		hydrolyses hyaluronic acid. spreading factor
Nu	(Deoxyribonuclease)		affects DNA of cells
Fibrinolysin	(Protease)		lyses fibrin
Neuraminidase			Destroys immunologic receptors on erythrocytes – cleaves tertiery sialic acid
Hemagglutinin			Inactivates blood group factor A on erythrocytes
Circulating factor		Inhibits phagocytosis	

FIGURE 18 – 1. Exotoxins of *Clostridium perfringens* Type A. (From Hitchcock CR: Gas gangrene in the injured extremity. In Gustilo RB, ed: Management of Open Fractures and Their Complications, Vol IV. Philadelphia, WB Saunders Co, 1982, p 186.)

genes, and *C. novyi.* These organisms are not invasive to a similar degree.

The spore forms are resistant to heat, drying, and disinfectants. They can survive for untold periods of time in a dry state of preservation. Some spores can survive boiling in water or alkaline fluids for more than 1 hour. Some can resist dry heat to 150° C for more than 1 hour, and most are relatively impenetrable to dyes.

The ability of these bacteria to survive in all climates and under vastly varying conditions is noteworthy. All soil must be considered contaminated with the spores of *Clostridium* and, to a higher degree, particularly soils exposed to animal droppings, as in a barnyard. Also, decaying vegetable matter is a universal milieu for propagation of these bacteria.

An oxygen-rich environment induces sporogenesis to occur, whereas an oxygen-poor environment stimulates proliferation of the bacteria as the actively dividing toxin producing vegetative form. A normal redox potential in human tissue suppresses growth of *Clostridium.* Anything causing a reduction in the redox potential induces the appearance of the vegetative form. The author has found the following to be predisposing factors to *Clostridium*

infection: trauma, surgery, foreign bodies, malignancy, aerobic infections, suppressed immune reaction, vascular disease, epinephrine injection, cold, shock, and edema. Analysis of the author's 207 cases has indicated one or more of the previous factors to have been involved in the etiology of gas gangrene.

PATHOGENESIS OF CLOSTRIDIAL INFECTION

Contamination of tissue with spores or vegetative forms of *Clostridium* is a prerequisite for the development of the infection. Transient hypoxia of localized areas of tissue at the site of contamination causes spores to germinate; lowered redox potential of the tissue favors growth of the vegetative form of the anaerobe. Proliferating vegetative forms produce exotoxins, which cause severe local edema and tissue destruction. Normal plasma does not inhibit the proteinases of *C. perfringens* and *C. septicum,* and these bacteria invade surrounding tissues avidly.[7]

Edema appears within 2 to 4 hours after active bacterial growth begins. Necrosis of local muscle, fat, and fascia by proteinases takes place. Thrombosis of local blood vessels leads to increased hypoxia in the region of the infection (Fig. 18–2).

Hydrogen sulfide and carbon dioxide gases are produced and begin to dissect outward into surrounding tissues. Edema follows the dissecting gases and exotoxins. Further thrombosis of vessels takes place. The infection becomes self-perpetuating. Within 12 to 20 hours, the patient can be overwhelmed by the infection, particularly with *C. perfringens*. Some patients have arrived at the author's hospital in a moribund state only 24 to 30 hours after trauma (or clean surgery or establishment of a primary infection). They died before resuscitative and therapeutic measures could be instituted.

In some patients with disseminating "cellulitis," there is no grossly obvious necrosis of muscle or other tissues but there may be small abscesses diffusely spread throughout the fat, muscle, and fascia. This is the type of clostridial infection that physicians generally fail to recognize as "gas gangrene." The author continues to receive calls from physicians who describe a patient of this type, declaring: "It

seems to be a bad infection, but, of course, it is not gas gangrene since there is no necrosis of muscle." This *is* gas gangrene. Cells of all layers of tissues are affected to produce a true generalized "cellulitis."

X-rays of the tissue demonstrate foci of gas, as noticed in Figures 18–3 and 18–4. The exotoxins are present, and the patient frequently is irrational or in a state of coma. Figure 18–5 demonstrates such an infection in a young woman who suffered an open fracture of the right radius and ulna when she fell from her horse in a farmyard. The picture was taken 30 hours after injury, and the patient was under therapy in the author's hospital. The patient was toxic, irrational, and in mild shock upon arrival. She required major therapy with extensive fasciotomies; massive antibiotic administration, including intravenous penicillin (to be described later); and hyperbaric oxygen. Noteworthy here is the degree of intense edema and subfascial pressure as evidenced by the wide-spreading wound edges following fasciotomy. This patient survived, and the arm was saved for normal, useful function. Figure 18–6 shows the patient upon discharge from

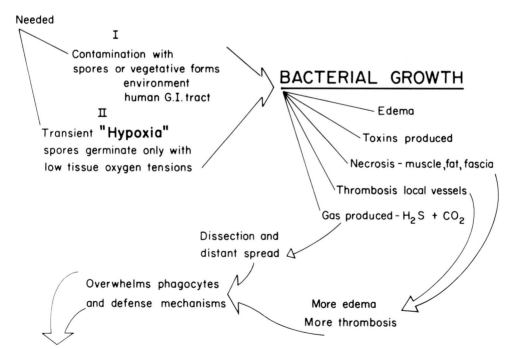

FIGURE 18–2. Pathogenesis of clostridial infections. (From Hitchcock CR: Gas gangrene in the injured extremity. In Gustilo RB, ed: Management of Open Fractures and Their Complications, Vol IV. Philadelphia, WB Saunders Co, 1982, p 188.)

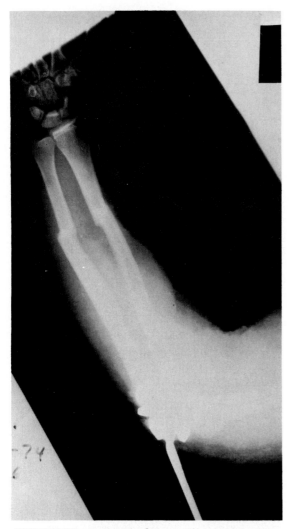

FIGURE 18–3. X-ray of the patient's right arm. Note the fuzzy appearance of soft tissue due to small bubbles of gas. (From Hitchcock CR: Gas gangrene in the injured extremity. In Gustilo RB, ed: Management of Open Fractures and Their Complications, Vol IV. Philadelphia, WB Saunders Co, 1982, p 190.)

the hospital with wounds closed and her arm in a cast.[8]

The skin overlying a clostridial infection develops a peculiar "bronze" color. This often progresses to formation of blebs and bullae and a black discoloration. The bronze color indicates the advancing margin of the infection. Some authors still ascribe serious gas gangrene only to infection with *C. perfringens, C. septicum,* or *C. tertium.* In the author's series, other species of *Clostridium* have been responsible for life-threatening infection (Table 18–1).

CLINICAL PICTURE OF GAS GANGRENE

Early Evidence of Disease

The majority of gas gangrene infections occur following trauma or an elective surgical procedure. In the author's series, there were 107 patients with gas gangrene secondary to trauma, 71 with infection secondary to elective surgery, and 69 patients in whom the infection was "primary" in nature.

In trauma patients, particularly those with extremity injuries such as an open fracture or soft tissue injury, the principal factor leading to successful therapy is "awareness" on the part of all concerned (physicians and nurses). In treating these patients, physicians should think *infection,* they should think *anaerobic infection,* and they should think *clostridial infection.*[8]

A wound that is developing a clostridial infection is unusually tender over and above that which would be anticipated. Pain is present in excess of that which is normally expected, and the patient commonly complains bitterly of the rapidly worsening pain. Edema appears early and can progress to frightening proportions within 2 to 6 hours. The edema often is present in areas quite distant from the site of the trauma. It is not uncommon for an entire lower extremity to be markedly edematous 6 to 12 hours following a relatively innocuous open tissue injury of the foot.

Within the first few hours, there is a serosanguineous drainage from these wounds. This early drainage is relatively innocuous in appearance and frequently is mistaken for "normal" or "expected" drainage. After approximately 12 to 18 hours, the drainage becomes offensive in odor and looks like pus. Clinicians with proper awareness, observing the serosanguineous drainage, will be alerted to the need for a Gram stain smear of the drainage to de-

TABLE 18–1. Species of *Clostridium* in 247 Infected Patients*

C. perfringens	194	C. bifermentans	5
C. speticum	21	C. sartagoformum	1
C. tertium	3	C. sporogenes	2
C. paraputrificum	2	C. sordelli	1
C. butyricum	3	C. capitovale	1
C. sardiensis	1	C. ramosum	1
C. fallox	1	C. clostridiforme	1
		Unknown species	14

* In some patients, more than one species was isolated.

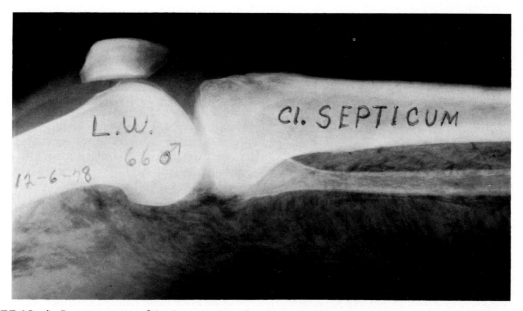

FIGURE 18–4. Gas gangrene of the lower extremity. Note streaks of gas throughout the muscle mass. (From Hitchcock CR: Gas gangrene in the injured extremity. In Gustilo RB, ed: Management of Open Fractures and Their Complications, Vol IV. Philadelphia, WB Saunders Co, 1982, p 192.)

termine the possible presence of gram-positive rods, often with a relative paucity of white blood cells (WBCs) indicating the likelihood of clostridial infection. Early detection is important, since the disease can be significantly reduced in intensity and virulence with massive

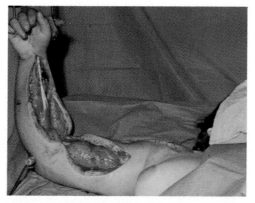

FIGURE 18–5. Gas gangrene of the right arm of a 15-year-old girl following open fracture of the distal radius and ulna. No necrotic muscle is present; this is typical "cellulitis." Early fasciotomy prevented necrosis by relieving subfascial pressure secondary to edema. (From Hitchcock CR: Gas gangrene in the injured extremity. In Gustilo RB, ed: Management of Open Fractures and Their Complications, Vol IV. Philadelphia, WB Saunders Co, 1985, p 188.)

antibiotic therapy and appropriate wide and thorough debridement early in the course of events.

Fever is commonly of low grade during the first 8 to 29 hours. The presence of secondary organisms, such as *Staphylococcus aureus*, *Streptococci*, *Enterobacter* species, *Escherichia coli*, and *Klebsiella*, will induce a more febrile reaction. Clinicians should be aware of the possibility of clostridial infection progressing rapidly, even though a febrile reaction is minimal.

Bronzing of the skin will take place as early as 6 to 8 hours following the trauma. This color change can spread rapidly to include an entire hemicorpus of the patient within 12 hours. It indicates the extent of spread of gas and toxins.

The emotional aspect of the patient is of great importance and should be watched carefully by physicians and nurses. Patients in whom gas gangrene infection is developing become unduly anxious and apprehensive. They are fearful of their surroundings and circumstances and are often concerned about dying. They may become frantic in their anxiety.

In the author's experience, it is not uncommon for nurses' notes to provide a classic picture of developing gas gangrene as they describe the patient's emotional changes. The need for physicians to read nurses' notes frequently during the course of each day is obvious. Patients with open fractures or severe lac-

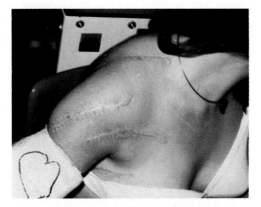

FIGURE 18–6. Upon discharge from hospital, fasciotomy wounds have healed nicely and the arm is in a plaster cast for final healing of the radius and ulna. (From Hitchcock CR: Gas gangrene in the injured extremity. In Gustilo RB, ed: Management of Open Fractures and Their Complications, Vol IV. Philadelphia, WB Saunders Co, 1982, p 185.)

erations of the extremity should be observed at 1- to 2-hour intervals by qualified surgeons or physicians. They should be considered at high risk no matter how well they have responded clinically to resuscitation and early surgery.

Late Evidences of the Infection

Hydrogen sulfide and carbon dioxide gas are produced within the tissues immediately upon multiplication of the bacteria. Crepitation can be detected by palpation. X-rays of the body tissues (specified for maximum differentiation of soft tissue densities) frequently demonstrate gas in the tissues. By x-ray the gas can appear as blebs along fascial planes or as a mottled configuration caused by myriads of tiny gas bubbles interspersed in tissue mass (Figs. 18–3 and 18–4). Failure to demonstrate gas in tissues by palpation or x-ray should not rule out the possibility of gas gangrene. Gram-positive rods in wound drainage is the principal presumptive criterion upon which early therapy should be based.

The skin of an infected extremity can become edematous and dark brown to black within 4 to 6 hours, and blebs and bullae appear shortly thereafter. Hemolysis of blood takes place to varying degrees and in the most severe cases can be suspected by examination of the peripheral blood smear. Most patients with well-established gas gangrene will experience a significant drop in hemoglobin within the first 12 to 24 hours. Severe hemolysis causes urine to darken to a black color and the patient's hemoglobin to drop to a level of 4 to 6 gm. Breakdown products of hemoglobin are injurious to the kidneys. The tubular damage can lead to acute tubular necrosis and renal shutdown. The author has instituted acute hemodialysis for several weeks in such patients before achieving recovery of renal function.

Patients with rapidly progressing clostridial infection can go into shock within 8 to 10 hours with a systolic blood pressure as low as 50 to 60 mm Hg. These patients are usually irrational. The author has received referral patients in a moribund state as early as 24 hours after the onset of a gas gangrene infection; they frequently died within minutes of the onset of resuscitative measures.

The astute and careful clinician who has the support of well-trained and observant nurses can detect the early signs of developing gas gangrene and make a "presumptive" diagnosis. This is the "golden opportunity" for start of therapy. Appropriate resuscitative measures and supportive intravenous fluid therapy, coupled with adequate antibiotic therapy with emphasis on lavage intravenous doses of penicillin G, as well as early opening and debridement of infected areas can lessen the disease and increase salvage of lives and limbs.

FRACTURE

All open fractures are contaminated. Patients with an open fracture must be considered at risk for serious infection.[9] The degree of contamination influences the risk of clostridial infection. Agricultural accidents involving farmyards, animal pens, or farm equipment have the greatest potential for clostridal contamination. However, in the author's group of 79 patients with gas gangrene following an extremity injury, 47 patients had "non-farm" outdoor accidents involving automobiles (16), motorcycles (nine), ladders (eight), mowers (one), and so on. Of 31 accidents on farms, nine involved animals and 22 involved farm equipment such as combines (harvesting machines) and tractors.

All patients with open fractures should receive intravenous broad-spectrum antibiotics started upon admission to the emergency room. Formerly, it was common practice for such patients to begin antibiotic therapy following completion of surgery. Wound infection has been reduced with antibiotic therapy started immediately upon the patient's arrival at the emergency room.

Even in major trauma hospitals, a delay of 2 to 4 hours is common before surgical correction of an open fracture can be achieved. Postponement of antibiotic therapy during these hours is no longer acceptable practice. The best antibiotic pattern to use is aqueous penicillin G in a dosage of 12 to 16 million units per 24 hours coupled with a cephalosporin and an aminoglycoside (e.g., cefazolin and gentamicin).

Crushed or badly contused soft tissue is more likely to have a lower redox reduction potential and to favor growth of anaerobes than is vital and non-injured soft tissue. However, debridement at this time should remove only tissue that is obviously devitalized. Immediate mechanical stabilization of the bony skeleton is desirable wherever possible.

The most common error in the management of open fractures is closure of the wound at the time of initial surgery. Leaving the extremity wound open reduces risk of infection from anaerobes by improving oxygenation of tissues through improved capillary blood flow. Fasciotomy can also help by reducing subfascial tissue pressure as edema develops.

The individual surgeon's ingenuity and preferences will determine how the tissues are to be managed when the wounds are left open. To prevent clostridial infections, the cardinal principle should be as follows: *Leave the wound open following debridement and skeletal fixation.*

SURGICAL PROCEDURES

General anesthesia should be used for the surgical procedures. All dead tissue must be excised. However, if hyperbaric therapy is available, only devitalized and obviously dead tissue should be excised. Borderline tissues frequently will survive following therapy with hyperbaric oxygen (HBO).

Judgment is necessary in the debridement of extremities with respect to projected function of the limb following removal of the mass of muscle. If resection of large muscle mass is necessary and residual limb function would be seriously impaired, the limb should be amputated. Amputation should be performed at the lowest possible site. Hyperbaric oxygen therapy has been shown to permit a lower level of amputation and increased salvage of the residual limb. Amputation stumps should be of the guillotine type and left open. Saline-moistened dressings are useful on the open stumps. If HBO therapy is available, borderline viable tissues can be left at the time of initial debridement. The patient can be returned to the operating room for subsequent additional debridement if necessary. In the author's experience, the use of HBO has reduced the level of amputation required in 26 of 31 patients (84 percent).

The patient with established gas gangrene infection should receive an antibiotic regimen, including aqueous penicillin G intravenously (IV) at a dosage of 24 to 30 million units per 24 hours (for a normal adult). Patients sensitive to penicillin can be treated with clindamycin phosphate (Cleocin) in an IV dosage of 1200 to 2400 mg daily. The patient should receive parenteral aminoglycoside, such as gentamicin, in a dosage of 3 to 5 mg/kg every 6 to 8 hours daily. Also, a cephalosporin such as cephalothin (Keflin), 1 gm every 4 to 6 hours, or cefazolin (Ancef), 1 gm every 8 hours, can be added for supplementary coverage of other organisms.[10]

The management of patients with established gas gangrene poses serious problems for a local community hospital. The author's hospital served as a referral center for such patients for 22 years (1964–1986), and the survival of such patients has been noteworthy (92 percent for all patients with extremity trauma). When comparison of patients was made relative to distance traveled, it was obvious that patients coming from "out of state" experienced as good survival with equally serious infections as patients who were transported short distances within the immediate local area. Modern transport facilities, including ambulances for surface movement and ambulance airplanes or helicopters for longer distances, have proved highly successful.

Surgeons have been concerned about the presence of a "foreign body," such as metal plates and other fixation devices in wounds. In the author's experience, these fixation devices have not hindered healing. They have been successfully left in septic wounds of the gas gangrene type with good wound healing, providing maximal therapy was given as outlined.

ANTITOXIN FOR GAS GANGRENE

Gas gangrene antitoxins produced from plasma of hyperimmunized horses formerly were available for treatment of established infections and prophylaxis if gas gangrene was suspected. Sensitivity to horse serum limited its usefulness. The globulin-modified polyvalent antitoxin produced by the Lederle Pharmaceutical Co. contained 10,000 units of antitoxin for *C. perfringens*, 10,000 units for *C. septicum*, 3000 units for *C. histolyticum*, 1500 units for *C. novyi*, and 1500 units for *C. sordellii*.

Clinical evaluation in the author's cases failed to support any benefit from antitoxin administration. This polyvalent antitoxin is no longer produced by Lederle.

SOFT TISSUE INJURIES OF THE EXTREMITIES

Soft tissue injuries of the extremities are equally at risk for development of gas gangrene when they occur in an agricultural setting. Life-threatening gas gangrene has developed following a puncture wound of the sole of the foot with a rusty nail. It is important, here also, to follow a plan of "open treatment of the wound."

A patient with a soft tissue wound of the lower extremity is best served by a short term of hospitalization, with the wound left open following irrigation and with appropriate therapy on the fifth to sixth post-injury day; the wound can be safely sutured at that time. If a surgeon elects to close such a wound (and it is frequently done), the patient should receive adequate antibiotic therapy following treatment and should be instructed to return for observation by the surgeon no later than 8 hours following the surgical closure. *Such follow-up is mandatory.*

The dressing must be removed and the wound inspected. Undue pain at the wound site, drainage, and increased tenderness should be indications for removal of the sutures and hospitalization of the patient. The rapidity with which gas gangrene develops once the bacteria begin to propagate is alarming to the patient and confusing to the physician. A delay of 12 to 18 hours, in the author's experience, has meant the difference between salvage of the limb and amputation.

As with open fractures, soft tissues should be adequately debrided to remove devitalized tissue at the initial surgical treatment of the wound. All bleeding points must be adequately tied off or cauterized. Larger wounds should be left open and the patient hospitalized at bed rest with mild elevation of the extremity. Fasciotomy is frequently needed to prevent an increase of subfascial pressure, which can result in capillary obstruction. The treatment of such patients with established gas gangrene is similar to those with open fractures.

THERAPY FOR GAS GANGRENE

The use of oxygen under hyperbaric conditions for treatment of anaerobic infections was popularized by Brummelkamp and colleagues in 1961.[11] They showed the benefit of HBO in the treatment of patients with clostridial infection (classic gas gangrene). Subsequent studies in animals and clinical experience have shown the usefulness of HBO in arresting clostridial infections.

A major hyperbaric chamber facility was installed at Hennepin County Medical Center and began operation during March 1964.[2, 12-16] Since that time to March 1986, 247 patients with clostridial infection were treated at the hospital. Following the plan of Brummelkamp, we have treated patients under 3 atmospheres absolute pressure (3 ATA), which is 2 atmospheres over pressure (2 atmospheres above ambient atmospheric pressure).[11] One treatment cycle is 2 hours at 3 ATA with the patient breathing 100 percent oxygen by demand type of mask.

Since 1 atmosphere of pressure (14.7 pounds/square inch or 760 mm Hg pressure) is equal to a depth of 33 feet in sea water, the treatment is described at a depth of "66 feet" for a 2-hour "bottom time." The patient, in essence, is surrounded by air at a pressure of sea water pressing inward on the sides of a submarine at 66 feet of depth in the ocean. Under these conditions, a significant increase in physically dissolved oxygen in the blood and plasma of the body is achieved when the patient breathes 100 percent oxygen.

Under these circumstances, the body acts as a reservoir of liquid and three basic physical gas laws relating gases to liquids apply:[17]

Henry's law (1803) states: "A quantity of a gas dissolved into a liquid increased directly as the pressure exerted on the liquid by the gas."

Dalton's law of partial pressures (1807) states: "With a mixture of gases, the quantity of a specific gas dissolved by a liquid depends upon the partial pressure of that gas in the ambient mixture."

The *law of Boyle* states: "When temperature

is constant the gas volume is inversely proportional to pressure exerted on the gas."

Those making use of hyperbaric facilities also should remember that gases are compressible and liquids are not.[17] Thus, every gas-containing viscus in the body is influenced by the increased pressure surrounding the patient's body.

For patients who are unconscious or whose condition cannot accomplish adequate equilibration of the pressure within the inner ear and the nasopharynx through the eustachian tube, myringotomy must be performed prior to pressurization within the chamber. Patients with pulmonary blebs or vesicles are in danger of rupture when they are brought from "depth" to ambient pressure at the end of the treatment cycle.

Cerebral oxygen toxicity in the form of mild tremors or convulsions does occur but is not serious. Removal of the oxygen mask for 3 to 5 minutes, permitting the patient to breathe the ambient air of the chamber, suffices to control these cerebral toxicity manifestations. Of greater importance is the risk of pulmonary damage with progressive pulmonary fibrosis (the *Lorrain Smith* effect). This occurred once in our series following the fifth treatment cycle

in a 19-year-old patient suffering gas gangrene secondary to an elective abdominal operation. This was the only death attributable to complications from chamber treatment (0.01 percent). The hyperbaric chamber facility in use at Hennepin County Medical Center is shown in Figure 18 – 7.

The partial pressure of oxygen in femoral arterial blood can be raised under HBO of 3 ATA and 100 percent oxygen from a normal level of 90 mm Hg partial pressure to a determined level of 1600 to 2000 mm Hg partial pressure. The theoretical level of 2233 mm Hg pressure (2280 minus 47 mm Hg partial pressure of water vapor in the lungs) is never achieved because of arterial-venous shunting in the lungs. However, experiments with dogs have shown that with 3 ATA and the animal breathing 100 percent oxygen through an endotracheal tube, the pulmonary alveolar gas will contain a P_{O_2} of 1975 mm Hg (normal 63 mm Hg), major venous blood will contain a P_{O_2} of 89 mm Hg (normal 25 mm Hg), lymph of the thoracic duct will contain a P_{O_2} of 588 mm Hg (45 mm Hg in the normal dog), and the superior mesenteric vein blood will contain a P_{O_2} of 580 mm Hg.

Adequate circulation of blood through tis-

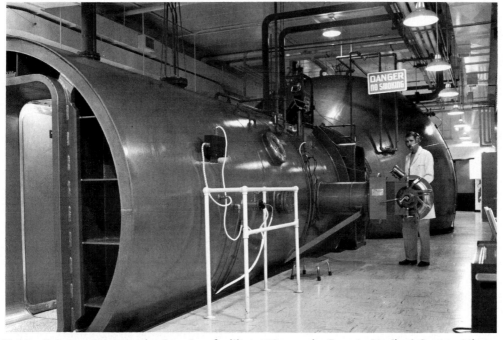

FIGURE 18 – 7. Large hyperbaric chamber facility at Hennepin County Medical Center, Minneapolis. Chambers can be pressurized to 7 atmospheres absolute. (From Hitchcock CR: Gas gangrene in the injured extremity. In Gustilo RB, ed: Management of Open Fractures and Their Complications, Vol IV. Philadelphia, WB Saunders Co, 1982, p 198.)

sues must be maintained to achieve benefits from increased levels of physically dissolved oxygen. The diffusion of oxygen through tissue at 37° C is measured in micra (100 to 200 micra). Providing increased oxygen to the surface of a wound fails to increase the oxygenation of deeper lying tissues. Fasciotomy of extremities prevents impairment of circulation through deep-lying capillary beds compromised by high interstitial pressures and facilitates the increase in redox potential of tissue that can be achieved with HBO.

Experiments in animals have shown that hyperbaric oxygen treatment of actively growing cultures of *C. perfringens* stops spore germination, reduces the gas production from sugars, and inhibits the bacterial growth in younger cultures.[5] Blood, when added to cultures, protects the organisms from the effect of HBO. Catalase, when added to cultures, also has a protective effect for the bacteria. Thus, adequate debridement is needed to remove nonviable tissue (rich in catalase) and blood from wounds.[6]

Experiments in dogs in the author's laboratories simulated clinical experience. Infection was established in the hamstring muscle group with injection of a standard slurry containing a measured number of *Clostridium* spores and epinephrine; no additional trauma was applied. Hypoxia in the area of the inoculum resulted from the epinephrine effect on vessels. All animals showed a progressing infection in the extremity and died within 24 hours if no effective remedial therapy was applied. In experimental groups (20 dogs each), therapy was initiated at 12 to 14 hours following inoculation:

1. If HBO alone was used, there were no survivors.

2. Surgical debridement alone resulted in no survivors.

3. HBO plus surgical debridement resulted in no survivors.

4. Antibiotics, including penicillin and cephalothin sodium (Keflin) (when started at 12 to 14 hours), permitted a survival rate of 50 percent.

5. The addition of surgical debridement plus penicillin and Keflin plus HBO yielded a survival rate of 95 percent.

The HBO therapy was similar to that used in our human cases and consisted of treatment of each animal in the hyperbaric chamber at 3 ATA with 100 percent oxygen administered through an indwelling endotracheal tube. The treatment cycles were given every 6 hours during the first 24 hours, every 12 hours during the second 24 hours, and once during the third 24 hours following initiation of therapy.[18]

In an attempt to assess the value of hyperbaric oxygen in the clinical cases, the overall group of patients was divided into those receiving antibiotics plus HBO (125), and a group of patients (30) who received surgical debridement and antibiotics only. These 155 patients all had either myositis or cellulitis with necrosis of tissue, which are considered serious and far advanced infections. There was a 78 percent survival in the 125 patients receiving surgery, antibiotics, and HBO versus a 56 percent survival in the 30 patients who received surgery and antibiotics only.

In some institutions, small portable hyperbaric chambers made of transparent plastic have been used. The author considers these cumbersome for such critically ill patients. Supportive measures, such as intravenous fluid administration, respirator support, and suction drainage of cavities, must continue during the HBO therapy treatments. This can be done best in a chamber of a size that enables accessory equipment and attendant personnel to be in the chamber with the patient.

The obvious goal of everyone involved in the care of patients with open fractures and severe soft tissue injuries of the extremities should be primary healing of the injured parts and prevention of a serious infection such as gas gangrene. If a clostridial infection does occur, however, the author encourages transport of the patient to a major treatment center with adequate hyperbaric facilities and availability of all supportive services required in the management of such critically ill patients.

References

1. Smith DT, Conant NF: Zinsser's Textbook of Bacteriology, 10th ed. New York, Appleton-Century-Crofts, Inc, 1952, pp 536–568.
2. Hitchcock CR, Baker RC, Foss DL, Haglin JJ: Selection of patients with gas gangrene for hyperbaric oxygen therapy. In Wada J, Iwa T, eds: Proceedings of the Fourth International Congress on Hyperbaric Medicine. Tokyo, Igaku Shoin, Ltd, 1970, pp 269–275.
3. Finegold SM, Baron EJ: Anaerobic gram-positive bacilli. In Baily and Scott's Diagnostic Microbiology, 7th ed. St Louis, CV Mosby Co, 1986, pp 519–532.
4. Davis BD: Energy production. In Davis DB, Dulbecco R, Eisen HN, Ginsburg HS, eds: Microbiology, 3rd ed. Hagerstown. Harper & Row Publishers, 1980, pp 33–44.
5. Demello FJ, Hashimoto T, Hitchcock CR, Haglin JJ:

The effect of hyperbaric oxygen on the germination and toxin production of *Clostridium perfringens* spores. In Wada J, Iwa T, eds: Proceedings of the Fourth International Congress on Hyperbaric Medicine. Tokyo, Igaku Shoin, Ltd, 1970, pp 276–281.

6. Hill GB, Osterhout SS: In vitro and in vivo effects of hyperbaric oxygen on *Clostridium perfringens.* In Brown IW Jr, Cox BG, eds: Washington DC, Hyperbaric Medicine, National Academy of Science–National Research Council Publication, 1966, Vol 1404, p 538.

7. Demello FJ, Anderson WR, Hitchcock CR, Haglin JJ: Ultrastructural study of experimental clostridial myositis. Arch Pathol 97:118–125, 1974.

8. Hitchcock CR: Gas gangrene in the injured extremity. In Gustilo RB, ed: Management of Open Fractures and Their Complications. Philadelphia, WB Saunders Co, 1982, pp 183–208.

9. Nelson GD, Gustilo RB, Hitchcock CR: Gas gangrene infections related to compound fractures. Minn Med 54:249–251, 1971.

10. Hitchcock CR, Bubrick MP: Anaerobic and necrotizing infections including gas gangrene. In Rakel RE, ed: Conn's Current Therapy. Philadelphia, WB Saunders Co, 1985, pp 29–32.

11. Brummelkamp WH, Hogendijk J, Beorema I: Treatment of anaerobic infections (clostridial myositis) by drenching the tissues with oxygen under high atmospheric pressure. Surgery 49:299, 1961.

12. Bubrick MP, Hitchcock CR: Necrotizing anorectal and perineal infection. Surgery 86(4):655–662, 1979.

13. Hitchcock CR: Anaerobic infections. In Najarian JS, Delaney JP, eds: Critical Surgical Care. New York, Stratton Intercontinental Medical Book Corporation, 1977, pp 507–514.

14. Hitchcock CR, Bubrick MP: Gas gangrene infections of the small intestine, colon and rectum. Dis Colon Rectum 19(2):112–119, 1976.

15. Hitchcock CR, Demello FJ, Haglin JJ: Gangrene infection: new approaches to an old disease. Surg Clin North Am 55(6):1403–1410, 1975.

16. Hitchcock CR, Haglin JJ, Arnar O: Treatment of clostridial infections with hyperbaric oxygen. Surgery 62:759–769, 1967.

17. Bert P: Barometric Pressure (translated by Hitchcock and Hitchcock). Columbus, Ohio, College Book Company, 1943.

18. Demello FJ, Haglin JJ, Hitchcock CR: Comparative study of experimental *Clostridium perfringens* infection in dogs treated with antibiotics, surgery and hyperbaric oxygen. Surgery 73:936–941, 1973.

Claude R. Hitchcock, M.D., Ph.D.

CHAPTER

19

Non-clostridial Necrotizing Skin and Soft Tissue Infections

INTRODUCTION

Gas infections secondary to bacteria other than species of *Clostridium* do occur and are equally lethal for the infected patient. In Chapter 18 we considered gas infections secondary to clostridia; in this chapter we are concerned with gas-forming bacilli that are in the nature of cocci and gram-negative bacilli.

Table 19–1 presents the bacteria categorized as to anaerobic versus aerobic. Predominant in the anaerobic group are the various forms of cocci, such as peptostreptococcus, that cause gas gangrene with classic characteristics. Also, in the anaerobic group are the gram-negative bacilli such as *Bacteroides fragilis.* Among the aerobes that cause gas gangrene are *Streptococcus pyogenes* and *Staphylococcus aureus* among the cocci, and *Escherichia coli, Klebsiella pneumoniae, Enterobacter,* and *Proteus* as the various aerobic forms of gram-negative bacilli.

The author has had experience with 56 such infections in a study from 1964 to 1986 that ran concurrently with the study of the 247 clostridial infections. Survival was almost identical to that of the clostridial group—78 percent for the non-clostridial gas infections and 75 percent for the clostridial gas infections. As in the group of infections with *Clostridium,* the author divided the cases into those secondary to trauma, those that were secondary to clean surgery as postoperative infections, and those that appeared as a primary infection without antecedent trauma or surgery.

There were 19 non-clostridial gas infections secondary to trauma, and survival was 84 percent; there were three non-clostridial gas in-

fections that occurred postoperatively from clean surgery, and survival was 100 percent; and there were 34 patients with a non-clostridial gas infection that appeared as a primary disease, and survival was 70 percent.

With the exception of the infections occurring in the postoperative group, survivals were close to those for the clostridial gas infection.

Table 19–2 lists the types of infection occurring in the trauma, postoperative, and primary infection groups. Most were soft tissue infections that commonly followed involvement of the gastrointestinal tract or one of its appendages.

PATHOGENESIS

In contrast to clostridial bacteria, this group of non-clostridial organisms does not produce exotoxins. The rapidity of the infection is a major problem, and the disease can spread almost as rapidly, as is frequently noted with clostridial infections. Local damage to tissue is frequently more superficial involving fascia and subcutaneous fat and skin. In our experience with this type of infection, we have had to denude extensive areas of the body, including the fascia. Fasciitis and gas deep to the fascia occur with these bacteria.

In contrast to the clostridia, this group of organisms does not produce the characteristic "bronzing" of the skin. More likely, an erythematous and mottled appearance of the skin is seen. At times, the erythema is strikingly intense. Edema can also be extensive with infections with this group of organisms. The gas formed by the non-clostridial bacteria does dissect widely from the point of origin, and it is not uncommon to see evidence of crepitation far distant from the focus of the infection. As

From the Hennepin County Medical Center, Minneapolis, Minnesota.

TABLE 19 – 1. Gas-Producing Microorganisms

	Anaerobes	Aerobes
Gram-negative bacilli	*Bacteroides fragilis*	*Escherichia coli* *Klebsiella pneumoniae* *Enterobacter* *Proteus*
Gram-positive bacilli	*Clostridium perfringens* *Clostridium septicum* *Clostridium tertium* *Clostridium paraputrificum* *Clostridium butyricum* *Clostridium sardiensis* *Clostridium bifermentans* *Clostridium sartagoformum* *Clostridium sporogenes* *Clostridium sordellii* *Clostridium capitovale* *Clostridium ramosum* *Clostridium beiferinckii* *Clostridium fallox*	
Cocci	Peptostreptococcus	*Streptococcus pyogenes* *Staphylococcus aureus*

in the clostridial group, x-rays of soft tissue are important in the diagnosis. The author considers the appearance of gas in the tissues to be late evidence of the infection.

The Gram stain is important in the initial assessment of the problem. In this condition, gram-negative bacilli or gram-positive cocci, rather than gram-positive or gram-variable bacilli, are typically seen. Subsequent cultures should be performed to delineate the specific

TABLE 19 – 2. Types of Gas Infections

Trauma
  Extremities
    Soft tissue only
    Fractures plus soft tissue
  Abdomen
    Blunt
    Penetrating

Postoperative
  Gastrointestinal tract surgery (stomach, small bowel, colon)
  Cholecystectomy
  Appendectomy
  Anal and perianal surgery
  Extremities (clean surgery)
  Vascular reconstruction—ischemia

Primary
  Diabetes (extremities, abdominal)
  Rectum, anus, perineum
  Fournier's disease (scrotum)
  Lymphadenitis and abscess

organism involved. Commonly, several organisms can be cultured from any patient with such an infection. Knowledge of the type of organisms is important in establishing the antibiotic therapy for the patient.

Surgical debridement is mandatory immediately upon recognition of the infection. All devitalized tissue must be excised. Whenever there is doubt about the presence of infection in the abdomen, a laparotomy must be performed and all organs inspected carefully and any areas of devitalized tissue removed. Infections that appear to be primary in the thigh of diabetics or immunosuppressed patients often are extensions of peritoneal cavity infections that burrow through muscle groups and down fascial planes. The appendix and colonic diverticula are frequently the source of the infection.

In injuries to the extremities, the same factors relative to the need for amputation apply as in clostridial infections. We must achieve adequate debridement of all devitalized tissue and fractures must be stabilized—preferably with fixators and external splints. The soft tissue injuries should be left open and dressings changed at 4-hour intervals during the early post-trauma period. Usually, moist dressings utilizing antibiotic solutions, diluted betadine, 25 percent acetic acid, or saline are best.

There is no evidence that the addition of hyperbaric oxygen to the therapy program benefits these patients. The organisms respond to appropriate antibiotics, and supportive care must be maximized. Proper fluid by intravenous route to maintain adequate blood volume and adequate urine output is important. Blood transfusions and plasma should be used to maintain an adequate post-trauma hemoglobin (10 to 14 gm/dl). Respiratory support is frequently needed, and patients often require indwelling endotracheal tubes with positive pressure respiration support for prolonged periods of time. Frequently, several debridement procedures may be needed in order to adequately remove all devitalized tissue.

ANTIBIOTIC THERAPY FOR NON-CLOSTRIDIAL GAS INFECTIONS

Table 19–3 portrays the antibiotics that are most effective in the treatment of the gram-positive cocci, gram-negative bacilli, and coliform organisms. Here it can be seen that so-dium penicillin G is excellent for the gram-positive cocci and that clindamycin, cephalosporins, and tetracycline are also well suited.

In the group of the gram-negative bacilli, including *Bacteroides fragilis,* we can use clindamycin, metronidazole, cefoxitin, chloramphenicol, and carbenicillin. The coliforms are best treated with aminoglycosides, cephalosporins, extended-spectrum penicillins, and chloramphenicol. Antibiotic therapy should be continued until the patient is well beyond the acute phases of the infection. Frequently, a change in antibiotic therapy is indicated during the reconstructive phases of surgery. Continual assessment of the type of organisms present and the antibiotic sensitivities is helpful in determining the appropriate antibiotics during this aspect of the therapeutic program.

The loss of extensive areas of fascia in these patients—particularly in the circumstance of abdominal infections—frequently leads to the need for Marlex mesh closure of the abdominal wall. The principles here are the same as for such a closure in the patients suffering from a clostridial gas infection. Here, also, early recognition of the infection and early institution of appropriate therapy with properly selected antibiotics are important to the outcome for the patient. In my experience, transport of these patients over long distances in appropriate aircraft or major surface vehicles, such as ambulances, is not detrimental to the outcome. On the contrary, the therapy that can be provided at a major treatment center often overbalances the possible deleterious effects of travel.

TABLE 19–3. Antibiotic Therapy for Gas Infections

Gram-positive bacilli	
Clostridium	Sodium penicillin G
	Clindamycin
	Metronidazole
	Chloramphenicol
	Cephalosporins
Gram-positive cocci	
Peptostreptococcus (anaerobic streptococcus)	Sodium penicillin G
	Clindamycin
	Cephalosporins
	Tetracycline
Gram-negative bacilli	
Bacteroides fragilis	Clindamycin
	Metronidazole
	Cefoxitin
	Chloramphenicol
Coliforms	Aminoglycosides
	Cephalosporins
	Extended-spectrum penicillins
	Chloramphenicol

References

Bubrick MP, Hitchcock CR: Necrotizing anorectal and perineal infections. Surgery 86(4):655–662, 1979.

Hitchcock CR, Bubrick MP: Anaerobic and necrotizing infections including gas gangrene. In Rakel RE, ed: Conn's Current Therapy. Philadelphia, WB Saunders Co, 1985, pp 29–32.

Hitchcock CR, Demello FJ, Haglin JJ: Gangrene infection: new approaches to an old disease. Surg Clin North Am 55(6):1403–1410, 1975.

Smith DT, Conant NF: Zinsser's Textbook of Bacteriology, 10th ed. New York, Appleton-Century-Crofts, Inc, 1952, pp 536–568.

Margaret L. Simpson, M.D.
Rafael S. Recto, M.D.
Antonio M. Montalban, M.D.

CHAPTER

20

Mycobacterial Infections of Bones and Joints

INTRODUCTION

Mycobacterial infection of the musculoskeletal system develops from lymphohematogenous dissemination or direct extension from a primary pulmonary or gastrointestinal focus of infection.[1] Tuberculosis of bones and joints ranks third as sites of extrapulmonary tuberculosis, after lymphatic and pleural involvement. Although the number of cases of pulmonary tuberculosis in the United States has been decreasing, the number of cases of extrapulmonary tuberculosis has remained constant.[2] In the Philippines, tuberculosis is a major health problem, with skeletal tuberculosis being the most problematic form of extrapulmonary tuberculosis. Skeletal tuberculosis occurs in 1 percent of patients with tuberculosis.[3] In the United States, patients with skeletal tuberculosis will have a predisposing problem such as joint trauma, intravenous drug abuse, intra-articular steroid injection, chronic systemic illness, or the systemic use of immunosuppressants.[4,5]

With the introduction of effective chemotherapy against *Mycobacterium* species, medical therapy has provided a useful adjunct to the previously utilized surgical procedures. In some instances surgery is primarily used as a diagnostic procedure.

Almost all infections of the spine are caused by *Mycobacterium tuberculosis.* Mycobacterial arthritis is usually due to *M. tuberculosis,* but

atypical mycobacteria may also cause this type of infection.

PATHOPHYSIOLOGY

The primary lesion of musculoskeletal tuberculous disease is usually a combination of osteomyelitis and arthritis. Invasion of the joint space may occur via the bloodstream or from lesions in epiphyseal bone eroding into the joint space. Initially, an inflammatory reaction develops, followed by the formation of a granulomatous reaction in the synovium or bone. The pannus of granulation tissue will erode and destroy cartilage and later cancellous bone. This leads to progressive demineralization and caseous necrosis with loss of support below the articular surface.[1] This process may take months or years to develop. Early disease affects peripheral cartilage first, initially preserving the joint space. Since *Mycobacterium* does not produce collagenase, the cartilage of joint spaces or intervertebral discs is not destroyed. In the spine the sequestered but intact intervertebral disc remains a barrier to spontaneous fusion.

In later disease paraosseous "cold" abscesses may develop in tissue surrounding the joint. Erosion and sinus tract formation may eventually develop. During the healing process, fibrous tissue, which may result in ankylosis of the joint, is formed.[1]

TUBERCULOSIS OF THE SPINE

Half of skeletal tuberculosis cases occur in the spine.[6] Because of the serious morbidity that may result from involvement of the spine,

Dr. Simpson is at the Department of Internal Medicine, Division of Infectious Disease, Hennepin County Medical Center, University of Minnesota, Minneapolis. Drs. Recto and Montalban are from the Department of Orthopedics, University of the Philippines – Philippine General Hospital, Manila.

this is the most important form of skeletal tuberculosis. Tuberculous infection of the spine is frequently called Pott's disease.

Persons with spinal tuberculosis present with pain in a segmental distribution corresponding to the site of involvement. As the infection progresses, severe muscle spasm worsens the initial back discomfort. Occasionally, other systemic symptoms such as fever, weight loss, or those of active pulmonary tuberculosis may be present. The thoracic spine is involved most frequently followed by the lumbar region, with cervical and sacral involvement the least common.

The process begins in the anterior portion of a vertebral body. The disc space between two involved vertebrae is usually destroyed, producing the characteristic finding of anterior wedging of two adjacent vertebrae with loss of the intervening disc space (Fig. 20–1).

Pus from a vertebral focus characteristically ruptures anteriorly, causing the development of an abscess. Because of confinement by tight ligament connections, these abscesses may dissect along tissue planes for long distances. Sinuses may rupture through fascial planes in the triangle of Petit, Pouport's ligament, the iliac crest, or other contiguous sites, including other vertebrae.[2]

Motor and sensory abnormalities from cord problems may occur as a result of multiple etiologies. Pressure from a paraspinal abscess may produce ischemic changes in the subjacent cord. Caseous or granulating tissue may extrude from the posterior aspect of the vertebral body, resulting in anterior cord compression. An inflammatory thrombosis of the anterior spinal artery or a sudden cord transection from loss of structural integrity may occur rarely.

Because skeletal tuberculosis is a form of reactivation tuberculosis, in almost all cases a tuberculosis skin test will be positive.[6] The white blood cell count is usually normal, and anemia may or may not be present. The erythrocyte sedimentation rate (ESR) is elevated in 80 percent of cases, an average of 37 mm/hour. The chest x-ray is abnormal in two thirds of patients with spinal tuberculosis, many demonstrating active pulmonary disease.[7, 8]

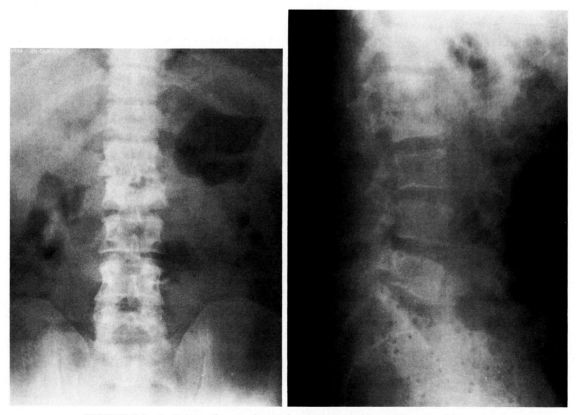

FIGURE 20–1. Pott's disease involving L1 and L2 in a 46-year-old man.

Spinal x-rays will demonstrate destruction of the anterior margins of one or more vertebral bodies. Progressive disease will result in vertebral body wedging frequently involving two or three vertebrae.[1] Calcification of a paravertebral abscess is almost pathognomonic for tuberculosis. Narrowed disc spaces will be present on x-ray in 64 percent, collapsed or compressed vertebrae in 61 percent, and lytic lesions in 46 percent. Sclerosis of vertebral edges is less common (28 percent), and paravertebral abscesses are found by x-ray in only 26 percent.[9] Kyphotic and scoliotic angulations were less than 40 and 30 degrees, respectively, at presentation.[7] Routine spinal x-rays probably underestimate the extent of vertebral involvement. Computerized axial tomography is very useful in assessing exact location of involvement in addition to delineating extent of involvement.

Confirmation by obtaining tissue for pathology, acid-fast stain, and mycobacterial culture is necessary in any worrisome spinal lesion. Earlier studies revealed that relying on radiological and clinical data might cause a diagnostic error in as many as 30 percent of lesions.[1] Bacterial and fungal infections as well as malignancies may appear similar to the spine lesions associated with tuberculosis. Computerized axial tomography guided by biopsy has allowed acquisition of an appropriate specimen leading to the diagnosis of tuberculosis in up to 82 percent of cases.[10] A pathology report of granulation tissue with typical Langhans' cells is classic for tuberculosis.[6] Because the culture may take 6 to 8 weeks before growth develops, pathology typical for tuberculosis allows for the beginning of appropriate anti-tuberculosis therapy.

The chemotherapy of skeletal tuberculosis is discussed later in this chapter. Before an operation is performed, if one is necessary, anti-tuberculosis therapy should be administered for 2 weeks to prevent miliary seeding. Patients without neurological involvement will show a satisfactory result in up to 90 percent with adequate chemotherapy and early ambulation.[11] Casting and surgery add little in the nonadvanced case. A more prominent gibbus may form without the use of surgery, and areas of normal kyphosis will be aggravated by the presence of disease.[12, 13] The use of bone graft/fusion versus debridement only in somewhat more advanced cases remains controversial. One comparative study of the two procedures demonstrated slightly earlier healing with bone graft/fusion, but later results were similar to those with debridement only.[11] The use of bone graft and fusion requires a more prolonged course of bed rest and recovery.[11-13] In persons with paraplegia, decompression and usually stabilization with bone grafting and fusion need to be performed.[12, 14]

For children with three or more vertebral bodies collapsed, a two-stage procedure may be performed — debridement and anterior fusion followed by posterior fusion 2 weeks after the first surgery. Paraspinal abscesses will disappear more rapidly with drainage and debridement. Stabilization is needed in some cases when there is extensive involvement.

In the thoracic region, a standard thoracotomy is done. The incision is made two rib levels higher than the apex of the kyphosis. The left side is preferred because the pulsating aorta can be utilized as a landmark and can be better protected from iatrogenic injuries. The right side is occasionally used, however, when there is associated lung extension from a thoracic focus. In the presence of lung penetrations, the abscess should be opened and its contents drained. With bone grafting, kyphotic angulation can be corrected as well as its progression minimized.[12-14] Routinely, bone struts from the ribs or iliac or fibular shaft are used in all surgical cases.

In the thoracolumbar region, a retropleural–retroperitoneal approach is used. This enables one to do away with tube thoracostomy. The diaphragm can be detached from its peripheral and psoas muscle attachment and incised for better exposure. Lesions of L3 to L5 are approached via the standard lumbotomy incision. The abscess is drained.[14-16] Necrotic bone and cartilage are debrided, and the vertebrae are fused. Specimens are sent for histopathologic examination, and culture and isolation studies as well as acid-fast bacilli stains are done. Two or three grafts are needed when the kyphotic angulation is 40 degrees and above. The choice of grafts depends on the number of vertebrae involved, weight of the patient, and the angle of kyphosis.[12] As a general rule, fibular grafts are utilized if longer segments are involved and in young children with three or more levels involved.

X-rays are taken postoperatively to confirm acceptance of the graft. A bony fusion rate of over 90 percent is usually achieved in 2 years.[12] Postoperative immobilization consists of a Minerva jacket or four posterior braces for cervical lesions and body jacket or braces for thoracolumbar lesions for at least 4 months.

TUBERCULOUS ARTHRITIS

Tuberculous arthritis usually presents as an insidious monoarticular arthritis. Weight-bearing joints are frequently affected, with the knee, hip, or ankle being involved in over 50 percent of cases. The joint symptoms may be present for months or years. Over 50 percent of patients will also show evidence of active or previous tubercular disease, either in the lungs or at another site.[9] Other systemic symptoms may be present at the same time as the monoarticular arthritis in up to 80 percent. In the 10 percent of cases with polyarticular tuberculous arthritis, other sites of active tuberculosis are almost always present.

Tuberculous involvement of peripheral joints is a combination of osteomyelitis and arthritis. Because of the nature of hematogenous seeding and the lack of effective phagocytosis in the metaphyseal region, tuberculosis involves the subchondral bone and synovial reflection (Fig. 20–2) early in the infectious process.[4] As the disease progresses, soft tissue abscesses and draining sinuses may also develop.

In almost all persons with tuberculous arthritis, a skin test for tuberculosis will be positive. If a person is taking immunosuppressants, the skin test may be negative.[6] Early x-ray changes reveal soft tissue swelling and subchondral osteoporosis. Later, varying amounts of cortical and cartilage destruction occur.[6] One important test that needs to be performed

consists of analysis and culture of synovial fluid. Early infections are characterized by a fluid consistent with a chronic effusion; later in the course, the fluid develops a gelatinous appearance. The range of synovial fluid white blood cell count ranges from 1000 to greater than 10,000 cells/mm.[3] Polymorphonuclear leukocyte counts are also quite variable, 10 to 90 percent being the range.[17] The most specific tests are synovial biopsy for histology and tuberculous culture and synovial fluid for tuberculous culture. Staining of synovial fluid for acid-fast bacilli will yield a positive result in 20 percent of cases of tuberculous arthritis.[17] Culture of synovial fluid will yield tuberculous organisms in 80 percent of cases. Synovial biopsy histology and culture will delineate the appropriate diagnosis in over 90 percent of cases.[17] In a person with a persisting monoarticular arthritis and sterile bacterial cultures, cultures for tuberculosis and fungus need to be performed and a synovial biopsy for histology and tuberculous/fungal cultures should be considered.

During the early synovial stage of the disease, chemotherapy alone will result in a very good outcome.[1, 18] Chemotherapy may be started with the finding of histologic evidence of tuberculosis pending culture results. When extensive synovial involvement is present, the use of synovectomy in addition to chemotherapy has been shown to decrease the duration of hospitalization, but this procedure remains controversial.[18] When the loss of joint space

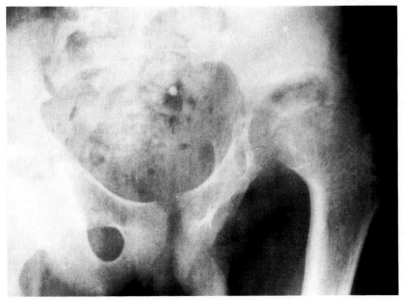

FIGURE 20–2. Tuberculosis in the left hip of a 14-year-old boy.

has occurred or disease of surrounding bone is present or persistent joint swelling and stiffness is present, synovectomy with debridement and possible fusion should be considered.[18, 19] Primary fusion may be preferable to the Girdlestone procedure for the hip in young people. Joint replacements are contraindicated during active tuberculosis. If possible, extensive therapeutic surgical procedures should be done after 2 weeks of anti-tuberculous chemotherapy.

CHEMOTHERAPY OF SKELETAL TUBERCULOSIS

In the past, three- or four-drug anti-tuberculosis therapy for 18 to 24 months has been the standard method of treatment of pulmonary and extrapulmonary tuberculosis. However, two-drug therapy with isoniazid and rifampin is now the recommended therapy for pulmonary tuberculosis with sensitive organisms.[20] One study has demonstrated a success rate of 95 percent in the treatment of extrapulmonary tuberculosis with isoniazid and rifampin therapy for 9 months.[21]

Presently, the principal mycobacterial medications utilized include isoniazid, rifampin, streptomycin, and pyrazinamide. Ethambutol is a bacteriostatic agent that is still utilized as a third drug with some of the previously listed agents. Combining rifampin and isoniazid has enabled shortened regimens to be utilized in the therapy of tuberculosis.

Isoniazid is used in a dose of 300 mg/day in adults and 10 to 20 mg/day in children.[20] The most common adverse effect is hepatotoxicity, occurring in 1 to 2 percent of persons. Liver function tests and gastrointestinal symptoms need to be closely monitored initially. Peripheral neuropathy is another side effect that may be prevented by using pyrodoxine with isoniazid.[20]

Rifampin is administered at a dose of 600 mg/day in adults and 10 mg/kg/day in children.[20] Hepatotoxicity is a side effect with this medication. In addition, intermittent administration may result in thrombocytopenia, myalgias, hemolytic anemia, and acute renal failure.

Streptomycin is administered intramuscularly at a dose of 15 mg/kg/day in adults and 20 to 40 mg/kg/day in children. Its major side effect is ototoxicity. Pyrazinamide is given at a dose of 15 to 30 mg/kg/day and also may cause hepatotoxicity. Ethambutol is given at a dose of 15 to 25 mg/kg/day, with retrobulbar neuritis being the most common adverse effect.[20]

In the United States, where the rate of drug resistance is very low, treatment may be initiated with only two drugs, primarily isoniazid and rifampin. While sensitivities are pending, some will utilize a third drug (streptomycin, pyrazinamide, or ethambutol) to provide extra bactericidal activity as well as cover for the possibility of resistant organisms. Persons from areas (Asia) that are associated with higher rates of drug resistance by *M. tuberculosis* may need up to four drugs initially. Isoniazid and rifampin may be given in regimens utilizing twice-weekly administration.[20]

In a study by Dutt and colleagues, 21 persons with Pott's disease were treated for 9 months.[21] Treatment failure occurred in one patient, and a repeat debridement and bone graft were necessary in another patient. Two further failures may have occurred as a result of isoniazid drug resistance. In this same study, new bone lesions developed in two of 26 patients with other bone and joint tuberculosis who were receiving therapy; however, no other complications occurred.

At this time it is hard to assess the 9-month regimen of two drugs for skeletal tuberculosis, particularly with spinal involvement. In early skeletal disease, 9-month therapy with isoniazid and rifampin is probably adequate if the organism is sensitive and the clinical course uncomplicated. Longer therapy (12 to 18 months) is probably needed for persons with significant bony involvement requiring surgical debridement and drainage. Response is improved when abscesses and sequestrum are debrided and drained. For resistant organisms or areas in which resistant organisms occur more frequently, up to 18 months of therapy with three to four medications will need to be used.

SUMMARY

Primarily *M. tuberculosis* disease has been discussed. Bone and joint infections with nontuberculous mycobacteria may also occur. Both surgery and anti-tuberculosis chemotherapy are probably needed for treatment for nontuberculous mycobacterial infections.[22] Atypical presentation may also occur with *M. tuberculosis*, including sacroiliitis and tuberculous arthritis and meningitis.[23, 24]

Tuberculous infection of bones and joints needs to be considered when no easily identified bacteria or malignancy can be found as an etiology of an invasive process. Because of the absence of systemic symptoms, the diagnosis of tuberculosis may be delayed. This will cause further local damage, which may be preventable with this treatable disease.

References

1. Hoover NW: Extrapulmonary tuberculosis: diagnosis and treatment—skeletal tuberculosis. In Pfuetze KH, Radner DB, eds: Clinical Tuberculosis. Springfield, Ill, Charles C Thomas, 1966, p 299.
2. Des Prez RM, Goodwin RA: Mycobacterium tuberculosis. In Madell GL, Douglas RG, Bennett JE, eds: Principles and Practice of Infectious Diseases. New York, John Wiley and Sons, 1985, p 1383.
3. American Thoracic Society: The present status of skeletal tuberculosis. Am Rev Respir Dis 88:272, 1963.
4. Berney S, Goldstein M, Bishko F: Clinical and diagnostic features of tuberculous arthritis. Am J Med 53:36, 1972.
5. Forlenza SW, Axelrod JL, Grieco MH: Pott's disease in heroin addicts. JAMA 241:379, 1979.
6. Davidson PT, Horowitz I: Skeletal tuberculosis: a review with patient presentations and discussion. Am J Med 48:77, 1970.
7. Silao JV, Montalban AN, Nitollama R, Frando VJ: Profile of Pott's disease in PGH. Acta Medica Philippina 15A:4, 1980.
8. Friedman B: Chemotherapy of tuberculosis of the spine. J Bone Joint Surg 48A:451, 1966.
9. LaFond E: An analysis of adult skeletal tuberculosis. J Bone Joint Surg 40A:346, 1958.
10. Adapon BD, Legada BD, Lini EV, Silao JV, Cruz AD: CT-guided closed biopsy of the spine. J Comput Assist Tomogr 5:73, 1981.
11. Medical Research Council Working Party on Tuberculosis of the Spine, Seventh Report: A controlled trial of anterior spinal fusion and debridement in the surgical management of tuberculosis of the spine in patients on standard chemotherapy: a study in two centers in Africa. Tubercle 59:79, 1978.
12. Hodgson AR, Stock FE, Fang SY, Ong GBB: Anterior spinal fusion: the operative approach and pathological findings in 412 patients with Pott's disease of the spine. Br J Surg 48:172, 1960.
13. Fourth Report of the Medical Research Council Working Party on Tuberculosis of the Spine: A controlled trial of anterior spinal fusion and debridement of the surgical management of tuberculosis of the spine in patients on standard chemotherapy: a study in Hong Kong. Br J Surg 61:853, 1974.
14. Yaw AC, Hodgson AR: Penetration of the lung by the paravertebral abscess in tuberculosis of the spine. J Bone Joint Surg 50A:243, 1968.
15. Hsu LCS, Yaw AC, Hodgson AR: Tuberculosis of the spine. In Evarts CM, ed: Surgery of the Musculoskeletal System. New York, Churchill Livingstone, 1983.
16. Vander Brink KD, Edmonson AS: The spine. In Edmonson AS, Crenshaw AH, eds: Campbell's Operative Orthopedics. St. Louis, CV Mosby, 1980, p 2088.
17. Wallace R, Cohen AS: Tuberculous arthritis: a report of two cases with review of biopsy and synovial fluid findings. Am J Med 61:277, 1976.
18. Marks KE: Nonspinal tuberculosis. In Evarts CM, ed: Surgery of the Musculoskeletal System. New York, Churchill Livingstone, 1983.
19. Anderson LD: Infection. In Edmonson AS, Crenshaw AH, eds: Campbell's Operative Orthopedics. St. Louis, CV Mosby, 1980, p 1079.
20. American Thoracic Society: Treatment of tuberculosis and tuberculosis infection in adults and children. Am Rev Respir Dis 134:355, 1986.
21. Dutt AK, Moers D, Stead WW: Short-course chemotherapy for extrapulmonary tuberculosis. Ann Intern Med 104:7, 1986.
22. Marchevsky AM, Damsker B, Green S, Tepper S: The clincopathological spectrum of non-tuberculous osteoarticular infections. J Bone Joint Surg 67A:925, 1985.
23. Ludmerer KM, Kissane JM: Severe right hip pain in a 73-year-old woman. Am J Med 81:117, 1986.
24. Maier WP, Wilmer CI, Wilson CH. Meningitis associated with tuberculous arthritis of the knee. Am J Med 80:151, 1986.

Robert P. Gruninger, M.D.

CHAPTER

21

Fungal Infections in Bones and Joints

It is quite possible to spend a lifetime in active orthopedic practice and never encounter some of the following forms of osteomyelitis.

P. H. CURTISS[1]

Orthopedic infections caused by fungi are uncommon. Most of these infections have occurred as part of disseminated deep mycotic infection, as superinfection in immunocompromised host, as secondary infection in trauma or surgical wounds, or by extension to contiguous joint or bone from a cutaneous infection. Uncommonly, these bone infections present as the initial clinical problem and then usually in the normal host. Although more than 275 fungi have been reported to cause disease in humans,[2] only a few cause most of the musculoskeletal infections.[3, 4] There are numerous case reports of uncommon fungi causing bone or joint infections. Unfortunately, insufficient documentation to distinguish acceptable from questionable etiology[2, 5] in some reported cases precludes knowing the actual number of fungi that have caused these infections. According to their pathogenicity in humans, fungi can be divided into *true pathogens* (TPs) and *opportunistic pathogens* (OPs) (Table 21–1).[3] TP fungi, which include the deep or systemic mycoses such as *Histoplasma capsulatum*, *Blastomyces dermatitidis*, *Coccidioides immitis* and others, infect the normal host as well as the compromised host and come from the environment. In contrast, OPs either indigenous to humans (e.g., the *Candida* species) or derived from the environment (e.g., *Aspergillus* species) rarely infect the normal

host.[3] Opportunistic fungi are commonly isolated in the laboratory, and therefore the clinical significance of these opportunistic fungi must be carefully documented.[2, 5]

Certain factors are important in diagnosis of all fungal infections of the skeletal system (Table 21–2).[4] Attention to epidemiology is critical. Exposure to most TPs occurs in predictable geographic areas, whereas the OPs are ubiquitous. In infection with TP, there is often a predilection for specific joint/bone sites, particularly in the normal host (Table 21–3). These true fungal infections usually have a predictable extraskeletal clinical presentation (e.g., pulmonary, skin). Clinical presentation and the site of skeletal opportunistic infections more likely are determined by the nature of the underlying disease. Radiologic findings in both are helpful and occasionally may be diagnostic, particularly if there is definitive evidence of fungal infection elsewhere (e.g., lung, skin). However, the most definitive diagnosis of skeletal fungal infection necessitates positive culture and histopathology (see Chapter 5).[4, 6, 8] Fungal serologic studies may be helpful, but it is unlikely to be definitive and at times could be misleading. Laboratory detection of fungal antigen, except in cryptococcosis and histoplasmosis[9] and possibly candidiasis, is not readily possible.[6, 7] The therapy for fungal infections is most challenging, as there are only a limited number of acceptable antifungal agents.[10–12] They are not universally effective and may be associated with serious side effects; surgery has been used, but there is often insufficient evidence to know when it is necessary; and the outcome of the infection is more dependent upon host factors and extent of extraskeletal disease. Each of these factors is developed in this chapter according to specific fungi with the exception of therapy, which is reviewed collectively, with

From the Department of Pathology and the Section of Infectious Diseases, the Department of Medicine, Hennepin County Medical Center and the Musculoskeletal Sepsis Unit, Metropolitan Medical Center, Minneapolis, Minnesota.

TABLE 21–1. Fungi Associated with Bone and Joint Infections

True Pathogens
  Blastomyces dermatitidis
  Coccidioides immitis
  Paracoccidioides brasiliensis
  Histoplasma duboisii
  Sporothrix schenckii
  Cryptococcus neoformans

Opportunistic Fungi
  Candida sp.
  Aspergillus sp.

Miscellaneous Fungi
  Pseudallescheria boydii
  Drechslera rostrata and *spiciferum*
  Saccharomyces sp.
  Fusarium solani
  Phialophora parasitica and *richardsiae*
  Rhizopus sp.
  Chrysosporium sp.

emphasis on principles rather than precise treatment regimens, as few exist.

TRUE PATHOGENS

Blastomycosis

Bone and joint infection with *Blastomyces dermatitidis* (BD) is the third most frequent clinical form of primary blastomycosis. Pulmonary infection, which is the most common, and cutaneous infection occur more frequently.[3, 4] It is estimated skeletal infections occur in 8 to 59 percent of the patients with BD.[4] Fewer patients present with asymptomatic monarticular arthritis or rarely an occult osteolytic bone lesion.[3]

BD most commonly causes illness in middle-aged men. Although the exact geographic distribution and natural habitat of this dimorphic fungus remains unsettled,[3] infection occurs in North America extending throughout the Appalachian states and the watersheds of the Ohio, Mississippi, Missouri, and St. Lawrence rivers.[3, 13, 14] To a lesser extent, blastomycosis has been found in Africa, Asia, and Europe.[3, 4] BD has been isolated from microfoci composed of moist acid soil, which is high in organic matter;[15] pigeon manure;[16] and decaying material. Infection has been described in dogs,[17] and, oddly, spread from dog to human has been reported,[18] although not from human to human. Skeletal infection occurs in the normal host primarily by hematogenous spread from the lungs and to a lesser extent by direct extension from a cutaneous BD infection.[19, 20, 20a] Endogenous reactivation from a previous infection with BD also occurs.[21]

Bone is more commonly involved than joints, although both may be involved at the same time. Skeletal lesions have occurred in all bones and usually occur in association with x-ray evidence of pulmonary disease.[19] The ribs, vertebrae, and tibia are the most common sites. Skull involvement was a common site in one reported series of patients[22] but absent in another review of 45 patients.[19] BD bone lesions are suppurative or granulomatous. Contiguous soft tissue involvement may or may not occur.

BD arthritis is uncommon. It usually appears in association with pulmonary and, less commonly, cutaneous blastomycosis.[20, 23] Most often, it is monarticular and involves the knee, ankle, or elbow joint in that order. Primary or secondary contiguous osteomyelitis occurs in less than one third of the patients with arthritis.[23] In distinction to arthritis resulting from other fungi and tuberculosis (TB), the patients tend to present with an *acute* synovitis and joint fluid is usually purulent.

Osseous blastomycosis may be diagnosed by x-ray when associated with pulmonary or cutaneous blastomycosis, although no pathognomonic roentgen pattern has been described. Gehweiler and associates carefully described the various x-ray findings in 45 patients with 89 bone lesions.[19] One third of their patients had two or more bone lesions, and 73 percent had concurrent pulmonary disease. They observed focal and diffuse osteomyelitis in short bones, long bones, and sesamoid bones. The diffuse osteomyelitis in all three groups of

TABLE 21–2. Important Factors in Diagnosis of All Fungal Infections of Bones and Joints

Epidemiology
  Exogenous or endogenous source
  Geographic exposure

Site Predilection
  Bone, joint, both

Host Factors
  Immune status
  Underlying disease
  Primary or principal site of infection

Definitive Criteria
  Radiologic
  Direct examination of specimen
  Culture and precise fungus identification
  Immunologic: detection of antibody/antigen

TABLE 21–3. Site of Skeletal Infection of Common Fungi

Disease	Bone	Joint	Both (Simultaneously)
Blastomycosis	Common (ribs, vertebrae, tibia)	Uncommon (acute monarticular: knee, ankle, elbow)	Occasional
Coccidioidomycosis	Common (vertebrae, ribs, tendon and ligament insertions, bony prominences)	Common (allergic) Uncommon (infectious and chronic monarticular)	Uncommon
Paracoccidiomycosis	Uncommon (except in acute juvenile disease: disseminated)	?	?
Histoplasmosis			
H. capsulatum	Rare	Rare (allergic or infectious)	?
H. duboisii	Common (metaphysis of long bones, though any may be involved)	?	?
Sporotrichosis	Not uncommon (metacarpals and phalanges)	Not uncommon (knee)	Unusual
Cryptococcosis	In 5–10% of all patients (bony prominences in extremity, skull, and vertebra)	Usually spared	?
Candidiasis	Uncommon (usually secondary to arthritis)	Common (site varies, although large joints and vertebra more common)	Uncommon
Aspergillosis	Uncommon (orbital, vertebra with disc)	Rare	?

bones showed rapid destruction with a remarkable propensity to penetrate into adjacent joints or soft tissue and produce fistulas. The lesions usually originate in the subchondral or epiphyseal-metaphyseal region of the long bones. An exception to this occurs when a soft tissue BD abscess erodes into compact cortical bone along the shaft of a long bone. Then a slowly enlarging, circumscribed, saucer-shaped defect occurs. It characteristically excludes the medullary cavity. Lesions of the vertebrae are similar to those of TB with destruction of disc spaces. However, in contrast to TB it erodes vertebrae anteriorly and may show skip segments of vertebral involvement. Extension into an adjacent rib at the articulation with the transverse process of the vertebrae in particular occurs with BD. These observations may help differentiate focal blastomycosis from tuberculosis, as this rarely occurs in TB. Paraspinal masses and dissecting lesions under the anterior longitudinal ligament also occur. Lesions in flat bones occur primarily by erosion from paraspinal abscesses or pleural collections. Less commonly, an expansile lesion in rib will extend to the pleural

space. The list of differential diagnostic possibilities in osseous blastomycosis is extensive. It includes other granulomatous disease, namely TB, sarcoid, bone infarcts, gout, rheumatoid arthritis, and both primary and secondary tumors. A bone survey may help in the differential diagnosis.

The x-ray findings in BD arthritis may be negative, may show osteolytic lesions or effusion, or, least likely, may reveal juxta-articular osteomyelitis.[20, 23]

Definitive diagnosis may be made early by demonstrating the characteristic broad-based budding yeast (tissue phase) of BD by direct microscopic examination of a joint or bone lesion aspirate.[8, 24] Confirmation of the diagnosis can be made by culture of BD yeast (37° C) and mold form (30° C), although it may take 1 to 5 weeks for growth to occur. Detection of the BD specific exoantigen of the mycelial form will aid in identifying nonsporulating isolates or mold forms that do not convert to yeast at 37° C.[25, 26] If the yeast form is recovered in the laboratory, specific identification may be made by fluorescent antibody (FA) detection of the BD–specific antigen A.[26]

If characteristic yeasts are not seen, differentiation from *Coccidioides immitis, Cryptococcus neoformans, Histoplasma capsulatum* (including var. *duboisii*), or *Paracoccidioides brasiliensis* yeast forms may be difficult. Misidentification of these yeast forms may be avoided with the use of BD–specific FA reagents.[25, 27]

The serodiagnosis of BD using the complement fixation (CF) and double immunodiffusion (DID) antibody test remains controversial[24] because of low sensitivity and cross-reacting antibodies with other systemic fungi. However, some suggest that it is possible using the enzyme immunoassay (EIA) and immunodiffusion (ID) tests using the BD–specific A antigen.[25] An EIA titer of 1:32 or greater alone, or a titer of 1:8 or 1:16 with a positive ID, is considered diagnostic in 85 percent of the cases and falsely positive in only 2 percent of patients.[25]

Coccidioidomycosis

The clinical forms of bone and joint infection due to *Coccidioides immitis* (CI) are the most encompassing of all the true pathogenic fungi. The spectrum extends from a self-limited hypersensitivity arthralgia and arthritis (desert rheumatism) associated with a primary pulmonary infection to multiple bone and joint disease in disseminated coccidioidomycosis.[3, 28, 29]

CI is a dimorphic fungus[30] found in the soil in semi-arid and arid regions of the Western hemisphere 40° N and 45° S of the equator. Most infections occur in California, Arizona, Texas, and contiguous areas of Mexico.[31] Primary infection through inhalation of CI spores occurs commonly in late summer and in the vicinity of soil excavation. Rarely, direct cutaneous infection occurs, albeit extension to bone or joints does not follow this type of primary CI infection.[32, 33]

HYPERSENSITIVITY ARTHRITIS (PRIMARY PULMONARY COCCIDIOIDOMYCOSIS)

Approximately 60 percent of persons with primary CI infection remain asymptomatic. Of the symptomatic patients, most will have a self-limited flu-like syndrome with cough, chest pain, and fever. In this group, a diffuse evanescent macular rash will develop in 10 percent. The "valley fever" constellation of erythema nodosum or erythema multiforme with arthralgias will develop in fewer; an even lower

number will be affected by arthritis. The arthritis rarely occurs without the skin manifestation.[34] This joint involvement is more often multiple and migratory.[35] There is little, if any, effusion and no x-ray abnormalities. An eosinophilia is common. This hypersensitivity arthritis is self-limited, resolving in 2 to 4 weeks,[35] and no specific diagnostic or antifungal therapeutic intervention is required.[3, 28, 29, 34]

INFECTION

Disseminated Coccidioidomycosis. CI bone and joint infections occur in approximately 20 percent of the acute disseminated cases of coccidioidomycosis.[28] Skin is the only extrapulmonary site that is more commonly involved in disseminated coccidioidomycosis.[29] Dissemination tends to occur early in the CI infection. It is more common in males, particularly of dark-skinned races.[33] Any bone may be involved, although there is predilection for areas of tendon and ligament insertions or bony prominences.[28, 29] Vertebrae are the most common infected site, and multiple vertebral involvement is common.[28, 36] In contrast to tuberculosis, intervertebral disc involvement with gibbus formation is uncommon; if it occurs, it is a late manifestation.[28] Paraspinous abscess and contiguous rib destruction often occur in these patients.

Nondisseminated Coccidioidomycosis. The most common form of CI skeletal infection occurs in the less acutely ill patient with nondisseminated coccidioidomycosis. Often there is single bone involvement, although as many as four to eight bones have been involved in 10 percent of the cases.[29] The bones involved, in descending order of frequency, include the vertebrae, tibia, skull, metatarsals, femur, and ribs.[28, 37] Typically, osteolytic lesions in the diaphysis and metaphysis of long bones occur early. Older lesions of subacute or chronic infection and those that are resolving become sclerotic. Skull lesions may be circumscribed and irregular and may involve both bony tables or only the outer table.[28, 37] The lesions of long bones and outer table of the skull are similar to those of blastomycosis.[28, 37]

Asymptomatic Coccidioidomycosis. Occult bone lesions, with a distribution similar to the clinical forms of bone infection described above, occur in patients who have been in the endemic areas of CI. These lesions should appear sclerotic rather than purely osteolytic.[28]

The definitive diagnosis of CI bone infection requires a positive culture of tissue or purulent material. A presumptive diagnosis may be made by observing characteristic CI spherules with endospores in direct examination of pus or with special stains on tissue sections. Because yeast may be confused with immature CI spherules, the culture is most important.

Serologic studies have been helpful in diagnosis of coccidioidomycosis. In spite of newer immunodiffusion serologic tests, the traditional CF test is the most useful.[38-40] The CF titer directly parallels the disease activity, and titers of 1 : 32 to 1 : 64 are hallmarks of disseminated disease. In contrast, the skin test is negative in this situation and therefore is more valuable as an epidemiological tool. It is not useful in diagnosis or in evaluation of active CI bone infections.

Arthritis. CI joint infection, although long recognized,[41] is less common than bone infection. It usually occurs as an extension from a contiguous osteomyelitis or directly by hematogenous seeding.[35, 36] Interestingly, each of these routes of joint infection provides a different roentgenographic corollary. The former route shows parasynovial bone lesions antedating the synovitis; the latter route, with an indolent onset and much delayed changes in joint space integrity, reveals no evidence of osteomyelitis.[35] Thus, CI arthritis may present as a chronic synovitis.[33] If unrecognized or ineffectively treated, CI arthritis progresses to villonodular arthritis, pannus formation, erosive articular chondritis, and, finally, extension into surrounding structures. Involvement occurs predominantly in weight-bearing joints, particularly the knee (70 percent of cases).[35] Effusion occurs in a majority of patients. Diagnosis is often delayed because of minimal extra-articular symptomatology, the x-ray may show thickened synovial membrane and intact articular surfaces only,[33] and there may be a low yield on synovial fluid cultures (<5 percent of reported cases).[35] Diagnosis is best made by obtaining synovial tissue for histopathologic study and culture. Arthroscopy with macroscopic observation alone may be misleading, as the lesions appear similar to those of rheumatoid arthritis. Serologic evidence may be helpful in this situation, but a skin test is not.

Tenosynovitis without joint or bone infection is another rare manifestation of disseminated coccidioidomycosis.[28]

PARACOCCIDIOIDOMYCOSIS

Paracoccidioidomycosis is caused by the dimorphic fungus *Paracoccidioides brasiliensis* (Pb). Its ecologic characteristics are notable because the disease occurs in restricted geographic areas in Central and South America, although it has been reported in the United States[3, 42, 43] and for this reason is included here. The presumed source of Pb is limited to soil, dust, and plants that occur in an acid environment that maintains a year-round constant humidity.

Paracoccidioidomycosis is a disease of adult males. It most often is seen with mucosal ulcerations of the mouth and nose. The disease may be self-limited, although usually there is a progressive course extending over weeks to decades. Other sites of infection include lungs; skin; lymph nodes; liver; spleen; adrenals; and, less frequently, bone. The bone lesions are usually present in areas of good blood supply and consist of osteolytic foci.[3, 43] Rarely, diffuse osteomyelitis occurs. Bone involvement may be more common than previously appreciated.[3]

An exception to the common form of this disease is *acute juvenile paracoccidioidomycosis*. This usually is a fulminant disease of pubescence with positive blood and bone marrow cultures, widespread organ involvement, and often osteolytic lesions of several skeletal areas.[3, 43] In younger and older children, Pb infection is more benign and protracted. Diagnosis of Pb is established by direct potassium hydroxide (KOH) examination of pus or exudate, histopathological examination, and/or culture of tissue. The KOH preparation usually reveals the characteristic budding yeast. They must be distinguished from *B. dermatitidis*, which may occur in the same endemic region. Biopsy specimens can confirm the diagnosis in 90 to 95 percent of cases, provided that the multiple budding cell is observed. Culture should be obtained. If the culture is positive, it indicates active disease.[44] Serologic diagnosis is possible using an immunodiffusion test and is frequently decisive.[43] These precipitin antibodies usually appear within 30 days of onset of the infection and are the first antibodies to disappear.[42] This test may be used as a measure of therapeutic response, although the CF antibodies that appear later correlate better with response to treatment.[44]

Histoplasmosis

Histoplasmosis is caused by *Histoplasma capsulatum* (HC) in the United States or *Histoplasma duboisii* (HD) in Africa. HD is included here because of its predilection for bone[3, 4, 45] in contrast to HC.[3, 4, 46] It has been estimated that osteoarticular lesions occur in less than 0.01 percent of HC infections and in 40 to 59 percent of HD infections.[4] Bone infection with HC rarely occurs in spite of the near-universal infection of residents living in highly endemic areas.[4, 47] Both fungi are dimorphic and exist in soil and animal excreta. Each may infect various animal species. HC is found in the central United States, primarily along major rivers (the Ohio and Mississippi) and corresponding valleys, whereas HD is limited to the humid and high rainfall areas of central and western Africa.[3, 14, 45]

Although it is clear that the portal entry for HC is pulmonary, it is unclear whether the skin or possibly a pulmonary route is the primary portal of entry for HD. HC infection results in a benign pulmonary disease in a majority of cases. Occasionally, a disseminated primary or reactivation illness occurs in which bone marrow involvement is common, although concomitant bone or joint lesions usually are lacking.[3, 47a] Patients with HD characteristically present with skin and lymph node and/or bony lesions and rarely with concomitant pulmonary disease. Only a few cases of focal infectious arthritis,[48–50] bone or tenosynovitis in disseminated disease,[51, 52] and migratory polyarthritis[53] have been described with HC. The last was considered to be a protean manifestation of a primary pulmonary infection not unlike that occurring with coccidioidomycosis.[47]

Features of the infectious form of HC included insidious onset, progressive focal disease often with a delay in diagnosis of several months,[48–50] and lack of characteristic x-ray changes. Definitive diagnosis was made by tissue histopathology/culture or a culture of purulent joint fluid.[3] Since blastomycosis exists in the endemic areas of HC and may show similar clinical and histopathological findings, care must be taken to observe distinguishing features of the budding yeast. HC lacks the broad-based bud as seen in BD.[2, 3] In contrast, HD usually presents as a local chronic papulomatous skin lesion or local osteolytic lesion. It occurs primarily in the metaphysis of long bones, although small bones of the hands, flat bones, ribs, vertebrae, and skull have been infected.[45, 53a] Disseminated HD involves multiple lesions in bone, skin, lymph nodes, liver, and spleen. Bone, unlike in HC, and especially the bone marrow are most commonly involved.[4] Differences in the histopathology of bone lesions exist. Giant cells are infrequent in HC, whereas they compose most of the lesion in HD.

The serologic response in HC differs considerably, depending upon the clinical form of HC; thus, it is not a reliable diagnostic test. However, antibody titers to yeast-phase antigens of 1 : 32 or greater are highly suggestive of active HC, whereas titers of 1 : 8 or 1 : 16 are only presumptive evidence of active disease. Some studies suggest that antibodies to the H antigen correlate with acute disease, whereas antibodies to the M antigen suggest either acute or chronic disease. Antibodies to both H and M antigens appearing simultaneously, although uncommon, are diagnostic of HC.[54] Complement fixation antibodies to mycelial antigen of 1 : 8 or greater and immunodiffusion antibody band to M or H antigens are as diagnostic as a CF titer of 1 : 32 or greater. The presence of both antibodies (regardless of titer) is suggestive of active HC.[54, 55] In contrast, diagnostic HD serologic studies are not available.

Sporotrichosis

Sporotrichosis, which is caused by the dimorphic fungus *Sporothrix schenckii* (SS), is primarily a nodular and ulcerative cutaneous and subcutaneous infection.[3, 14] It occurs on the extremities and characteristically follows the lymphatics. Secondary spread to articular surfaces, bone, and muscle is *not* infrequent.[56] SS is a ubiquitous fungus and is commonly found in a saprophytic relation with a variety of plant life.[57] Infection most commonly occurs following skin trauma and inoculation of conidia (spores), resulting in the characteristic lymphocutaneous form of disease.[3, 58] A distinct syndrome of chronic ulceronodular skin lesion with chronic arthritis or osteomyelitis has been described.[58] Less common is a fixed, cutaneous form with only a single skin lesion. Rarely, a mucocutaneous form may appear as an aphthous ulcer on a mucous membrane. Alternatively, a primary infection may occur in the lungs, resulting in chronic cavitary disease or a primary lymph node infection.[59] Often, the latter rapidly progresses with parenchymal spread in lung and adjacent tissues. Although historically seen as a skin infection, SS is now recognized as an important source of pulmonary infection.[56] Spread from the lung to joint without a skin lesion has been reported.[59] Disseminated disease is rare. Skeletal involvement is the third most common site of infection, and most often there is a cutaneous lesion prior to bony involvement. An exception occurs in knee infections when the primary infection occurs by direct injection of SS.[3] In contrast, the metacarpals and phalanges are the most commonly involved bones when associated with a primary skin lesion. Less commonly, the tibia, other extremity bones, and ribs have been involved with skin lesions. Arthritis, in addition to direct injection, may occur secondary to a skin lesion or following dissemination from pulmonary infection.[60] The x-ray findings include osteolytic bone lesions, periostitis, and destructive synovitis. These findings may be confused with rheumatoid disease or a tenosynovitis.[61] In the absence of a skin infection or a diagnosed pulmonary disease, a delay in diagnosis from the onset of symptoms averages 2 years.[3, 60] Joint fluid is serosanguineous with an increased white blood cell (WBC) count and protein. The culture is usually positive. A synovial biopsy is preferred. It will show a typical granulomatous inflammatory lesion, and SS may be seen with special stains. Both should be done, as the diagnostic yield will be higher.[62] In addition to culture, a serodiagnosis may be made with immunodiffusion or latex slide and tube agglutination tests, particularly with arthritis.[3, 62]

Cryptococcosis

Cryptococcosis is a systemic infection caused by one of the four serotypes of the yeastlike fungus, *Cryptococcus neoformans* (CN). Bone is involved in 5 to 10 percent of patients, and joints are usually spared.[3, 4, 63] CN is a ubiquitous saprophyte with worldwide distribution. It has been isolated in nature from pigeon excreta and the soil. Primary infection occurs by inhalation of spores sexually produced by the "perfect state" of CN (*Filobasidiella* var. *neoformans/bacillispora*).[64, 65] Exposure to CN is common, and asymptomatic infection occurs according to skin test surveys. Apparently, a high natural resistance occurs. In contrast to other aerosol-borne mycoses, symptomatic CN illness rarely occurs in clusters, in occupational surroundings, or in other high-exposure circumstances. Clearly, the patients in whom clinical illness with CN develops are characteristically males, more often caucasian and immunocompromised,[66, 67] although not invariably.[3, 67] Clearly, transient pulmonary colonization and asymptomatic infection occur in many normal persons.[68]

Cryptococcosis is an acute, subacute, or chronic infection,[3, 67] usually affecting the pulmonary parenchyma in its primary clinical form.[68] Hematogenous dissemination results in metastatic foci, most commonly in the meninges, where natural resistance is poor; the kidney; skin; subcutaneous tissue; and bone.[66, 67]

The most common osseous sites of infection are the bony prominences in extremity bones, cranial bones, and vertebrae.[69, 70] The lesions are usually multiple, widely disseminated, discrete, and chronic. They are destructive and characteristically slow to change. Thus, they tend to have a constant appearance. In contrast to conditions caused by other mycoses, periosteal proliferation is usually lacking.[70, 71] The lesions resemble the cold abscesses seen in tuberculosis.[63, 72] Occasionally, a solitary osseous lesion is the only evidence of cryptococcal disease.[71, 73] Definitive diagnosis is made by histopathologic study and a positive culture of bone tissue or cold abscess pus. Both are important in order to avoid a misdiagnosis of osteogenic sarcoma or of Hodgkin's disease because of similar histologic findings[3, 63, 74] on the one hand and distinction in culture from nonpathogenic cryptococci on the other.[2, 3, 63]

In contrast to osteomyelitis, CN monarticular synovitis has been reported rarely.[46] The most common site is the knee, and in half of the patients with symptoms and signs of subacute synovitis, there was x-ray evidence of pre-existing adjacent osteomyelitis.[46] Diagnosis is established by histopathological study and culture.

OPPORTUNISTIC FUNGI

Candidiasis

The incidence of candidal bone and joint infection, once considered extremely rare, has increased in recent years.[75] There are over 100 species of *Candida*, but only a few (Table 21–4) are regularly recovered from humans; *Candida albicans* (CA) is the prototype.[76] CA is a normal human and animal commensal.[77] Other species may live in the environment.[76] Most candidal infections are of endogenous origin. A normal immune system usually protects humans from clinical disease.[78] If a person's status is immunocompromised by naturally occurring events, such as diabetes mellitus, pregnancy, or therapeutic or self-inflicted invasive interventions, *Candida* may become pathogenic. Then, depending upon the anatomic site colonized, the type of the intervention[79] (e.g., central hyperalimentation line)[80] or disease any one or more of the well-known myriad of clinical manifestations of candidal infection

TABLE 21–4. *Candida* and *Aspergillus* Species in Bone and Joint Infections

Candida*

C. albicans (most common)	C. parapsilosis
C. glabrata (Torulopsis glabrata)	C. stellatoidea
C. guilliermondii	C. tropicalis
C. holmii (Torulopsis holmii)	C. sp. (unknown)

***Aspergillus*†**

A. fumigatus	A. nidulans
A. flavipes	A. niger
A. flavus	A. terreus

* Arthritis more common than osteomyelitis and occasionally more than one species in same site of infection.

† Common contaminant in the laboratory that rarely causes osteomyelitis.

may occur, including arthritis and osteomyelitis.

ARTHRITIS

Candidal arthritis is more common than osteomyelitis.[81] The predisposing factors have included candidemia,[82] intra-articular corticosteroids,[83] leukemia and antibiotics,[84] immunocompromised status in infancy,[85, 86] prosthetic joints,[87] and, more recently, intravenous (IV) drug use.[88–90] Clinical presentation includes joint pain, swelling, and effusion. The course is indolent in one third and acute in two thirds of the patients. The x-ray findings are often negative.[81, 89] Larger joints are more commonly involved.[81, 88] Polyarticular presentation occurs in about one third of the patients.[81]

OSTEOMYELITIS

Candidal osteomyelitis in association with candidal arthritis is usually secondary rather than primary in contrast to most other fungal infections.[80, 81] Seeding of the joint occurs via the hematogenous route from a primary infection in the urine, gastrointestinal tract, skin, or other pathway.[81] A positive joint fluid culture is sufficient for diagnosis because *Candida* is an unlikely contaminant in the laboratory.[91]

Candidal osteomyelitis without joint involvement is rare, and prior to 1973 it was not well documented.[75] In that year, the first cases of a postoperative costochondral osteomyelitis following thoracotomy were reported.[92, 93] More recently, costochondral candidal osteomyelitis has been reported in heroin addicts.[88] Other sites of osteomyelitis include the intervertebral disc space and contiguous vertebrae[88, 90, 94–96] and, less commonly, the ribs, humerus, and ileum.[75] In addition to *C. albicans*, *C. glabrata*[97, 98] and *C. holmii*[99] have been implicated in osteomyelitis of the vertebrae,[97] hip,[98] and hand.[99] Although there are no characteristic x-ray findings,[99a] x-ray evidence of osteomyelitis is important for diagnosis. For a definitive diagnosis of candidal osteomyelitis, direct microscopic demonstration of the yeast (KOH or histopathologic) and a positive bone culture are required. In contrast to candidal arthritis, the histological evidence of fungal infection is important.[5, 75, 77] Serodiagnosis by detection of antibodies or *Candida* antigen, although promising, awaits further development.[100, 101]

Aspergillosis

Osseous infections caused by *Aspergillus*, although uncommon, are becoming more frequent.[75, 102, 103] *Aspergillus* is a ubiquitous environmental saprophytic mold found throughout the world.[3, 104, 104a] Of the approximately 200 *Aspergillus* species,[3] only six (Table 21–4) have been reported in osteomyelitis.[75, 103, 105–109] Commonly, *Aspergillus* is a culture contaminant in the clinical laboratory. For this reason, the diagnosis of an *Aspergillus* osseous infection necessitates, in addition to a positive culture, the demonstration of the fungi by microscopic examination of the initial specimen. Direct KOH demonstration or characteristic branching septate hyphae is necessary.[2, 5, 75, 104a] Unfortunately, this documentation is lacking in some reported cases.[110, 111]

The major clinical forms of *Aspergillus* are allergic, noninvasive colonization (including aspergilloma), and invasive disease. Invasive aspergillosis of the bone is rare. With few exceptions, it occurs in a patient compromised by disease, chemotherapy, trauma, surgery, or drug addiction.[103, 107, 112] Orbital osteomyelitis is the most common form and characteristically is related to extension from a paranasal sinus infection.[113] Vertebral osteomyelitis involving the adjacent intervertebral disc is the second most common osseous form. It has occurred after laminectomy in patients who have received glucocorticoids and antibiotics[103] and secondary to mycotic pseudoaneurysm following aortic bypass graft.[114] Contiguous spread from a pulmonary infection[106, 115] or hematogenous dissemination in the immunocompromised host may occur.[103] Children with chronic granulomatous disease seem uniquely susceptible to aspergillosis osteomyelitis.[103] Other sites of infection include ribs,[106, 110, 115] tibia and knee,[75] hip,[103] sternum, wrist, and metacarpals.[111]

Pseudallescheriasis and Miscellaneous Fungi

The spectrum of bone and joint infections associated with *Pseudallescheria boydii*[116-119] and a variety of other soil fungi[120-129] (see Table 21–1) is largely limited to *mycetomas*, although isolated cases of infectious arthritis or osteomyelitis have been described.[3] It is beyond the scope of this chapter to sort out the particularly confusing taxonomy of these fungi and, correspondingly, whether an infectious arthritis or osteomyelitis occurs de novo or in conjunction with a *mycetoma*.[3] However, it is important to understand that mycetoma is a distinct clinical syndrome. It presents as localized indolent, swollen lesions and sinuses involving cutaneous and subcutaneous tissue initially.[3, 129a] Ultimately, fascia and bone become involved if lesions are not recognized and treated properly. In contrast to a draining sinus associated with a septic arthritis or osteomyelitis, the term mycetoma should be restricted to the triad of tumefaction, draining sinuses, and *grains*.[3] In this context, the etiologic agents of mycetoma in humans include several actinomyces (*Actinomyces, Nocardia, Actinomandura,* and *Streptomyces*), true fungi (*Pseudallescheria, Aspergillus, Curvularia*), and bacteria (called botryomycosis rather than mycetoma).[3]

Although a diagnosis of mycetoma can be made clinically and by the detection of grains in wound discharge, culture and laboratory identification of the etiologic agent are always indicated. This is imperative for the institution of appropriate drug therapy, which most often is accompanied by extensive local surgery. The other skeletal infections caused by these soil fungi are similar to those of *Aspergillus*. The differences are basically related to the species of fungus (see Table 21–1) and its sensitivity to available antifungal drugs. As with mycetoma, it is virtually impossible to be entirely sure how many reported cases represent actual infection versus a wound or an occasional laboratory contaminant. Thus, the rules for definitive diagnosis require visualization of fungal elements on direct specimen examination, culture with precise identification, and histopathological evidence of tissue invasion.

THERAPY OF FUNGAL BONE AND JOINT INFECTIONS

The treatment of fungal infections of bones and joints, like that of the most common bacterial forms of osteomyelitis and septic arthritis, revolves around the basic principles of surgical intervention and chemotherapy. Therapy has varied considerably, and thus it would be presumptuous to suggest that optimal therapy is known for fungal bone and joint infections.[130-133] Rather, it is important to recognize each case unto itself. It is axiomatic that surgical debridement of diseased bone and removal of significant accumulations of pus, exudate, or infected synovium resistant to treatment are indicated. Equally important is treatment of the underlying disease or control of immunosuppressive therapy.[10, 11] Judicious use of one or more of the few antifungal agents[11, 12, 134] is indicated in most of these patients (Table 21–5). However, this therapy must not be undertaken lightly, as use of these agents is associated with major side effects.[11] It is, therefore, probably as important to document the fungal infection as it is to initiate chemotherapy.[3] Once that is reached and antifungal therapy is planned, monitoring of efficacy and side effects is imperative.[11, 134]

The two major classes of antifungal agents (see Table 21–4) are polyenes[135, 136] and imidazoles.[137] Amphotericin B is the prototype polyene; it has been used both systemically (intravenously) and locally in focal infections with reports of success and failure.[138] The dose and duration, other than that recommended for disseminated systemic fungal diseases, is largely conjectural. Newer, less toxic forms of amphotericin B, such as a mixture with liposome, may permit more liberal use of this toxic drug in the future.[136] Two imidazoles, miconazole (intravenous) and the preferred ketoconazole (oral), have been used in osseous fungal infections with reported successes and failures.[128, 130, 131, 133, 139, 140] It appears that it is ineffective in candidal osteomyelitis. A third agent, 5-fluorocytosine (oral), has been used in combination with amphotericin B with reported success in some.[141] It should not be used alone. Combinations of the above drugs have been tried, but once again a firm consensus as to what is best in any patient, regardless of the particular fungal infection, is lacking.[69] Combinations of amphotericin B with agents such as rifampin and tetracycline show promise in laboratory and animal studies but await clinical studies to determine their role.[11, 142] More

TABLE 21–5. Guidelines for Antifungal Drug Therapy in Bone and Joint Infections

| | Amphotericin B (Intravenous and Intra-articular) | Imizoles | | | |
		Miconazole (IV)	Ketoconazole (p.o.)	5-FC (p.o.)	Other
Blastomycosis	Preferable	+* (PO alone if active and limited disease)	+	No	None
Coccidioidomycosis	Agent of choice (intra-articular 5–15 mg used)	+ (Suppressive)	+	No	None
Paracoccidioido- mycosis	Preferable	+ (PO effective)	+	No	Sulfonamides (3–5 years)
Histoplasmosis					
H. capsulatum	Preferable	+ (PO low dose effective)	+	No	?Sulfadiazine
H. duboisii	Preferable	?	?	No	?Trimethoprim-sulfa
Sporotrichosis	In relapse (intra-articular 5–15 mg effective)		No	No	Potassium iodide (preferable)
Cryptococcosis	Preferable	No	?	+†	None
Candidiasis	Preferable	+	+	+†	Yes, but not in orthopedic infections
Aspergillosis	Preferable	No	No	?†	?Rifampin with amphotericin B
Pseudallescheriasis	Preferable	+	?	No	None

* A plus sign (+) indicates effective, even though resistance may occur.
† Use in combination with amphotericin B, but not alone.
Abbreviations: 5-FC = 5-fluorocytosine; IV = intravenous; PO = by mouth.

than likely, no truly fungicidal agents for use in the host exist.[142]

In selected cases of SS, treatment with potassium iodide (KI), heat, or other remedies has been tried; however, convincing evidence of effectiveness, except for KI, is lacking.[3] Unique among fungal infections is the therapeutic effectiveness of sulfa drugs in paracoccidioidomycosis.[3] Either short-acting agents or analogues with a greater half-life have been effective.[3]

In summary then, aside from timely surgical intervention and correction of the predisposing host factors, therapy for osseous fungal infections must be individualized and development of more efficacious and less toxic drugs is awaited.

References

1. Curtiss PH: Some uncommon forms of osteomyelitis. Clin Orthop 96:84–87, 1973.
2. McGinnis MR: Laboratory Handbook of Medical Mycology. New York, Academic Press, 1980.
3. Rippon JW: Medical Mycology, 2nd ed. Philadelphia, WB Saunders Co, 1982.
4. Schwarz J: What's new in mycotic bone and joint diseases? Pathol Res Pract 178:617–634, 1984.
5. Ajello L: Comments on the laboratory diagnosis of opportunistic fungus diseases. Lab Invest 11:1033, 1962.
6. Drutz DJ: Antigen detection in fungal infections. N Engl J Med 314:115–117, 1986.
7. Klotz SA, Penn RL, George RB: Antigen dection in the diagnosis of fungal respiratory infections. Semin Respir Infect 1:16–21, 1986.
8. O'Hara M: Histopathologic diagnosis of fungal disease. Infect Control 7:78–84, 1986.
9. Wheat LJ, Kohler RB, Tewari RP: Diagnosis of disseminated histoplasmosis by detection of *Histoplasma capsulatum* antigen in serum and urine specimens. N Engl J Med 314:83–88, 1986.
10. Cartwright RY: Opportunistic mycoses of various body sites. In Speller DCE, ed: Antifungal Chemotherapy. New York, John Wiley & Sons, 1980, pp 365–404.
11. Pratt WB, Fekety R: The Antimicrobial Drugs. New York, Oxford University Press, 1986, pp 317–352.
12. Hermans PE, Keys TF: Antifungal agents used for deep-seated mycotic infections. Mayo Clin Proc 58:223–231, 1983.
13. Witorsch P, Utz JP: North American blastomycosis: a study of 40 patients. Medicine (Baltimore) 47:169–200, 1968.
14. Conant NF, Smith DT, Baker RD, Callaway JL: Manual of Clinical Mycology. Philadelphia, WB Saunders Co, 1971.
15. Schoenwetter WF, Williams DNB: Diagnosis of blastomycosis (Lt). N Engl J Med 315:762–763, 1986.
16. Sarosi GA, Serstock D: Isolation of *Blastomyces dermatitidis* from pigeon manure. Am Rev Respir Dis 114:1179–1183, 1976.
17. Sarosi GA, Eckman MR, Davies SF, Laskey WK: Ca-

nine blastomycosis as a harbinger of human disease. Ann Intern Med 91:733–735, 1979.

18. Gnann JW Jr, Bressler GS, Bodet CA, Avent CK: Human blastomycosis after a dog bite. Ann Intern Med 98:48–49, 1983.

19. Gehweiler JA, Capp MP, Chick EW: Observations on the roentgen patterns in blastomycosis of bone. Am J Roentgenol 108:497–510, 1962.

20. Sanders LL: Blastomycosis arthritis. Arthritis Rheum 10:91–98, 1967.

20a. Moore RM, Green NE: Blastomycosis of bone: a report of six cases. J Bone Joint Surg 64(A):1097–1101, 1982.

21. Lasley WL, Sarosi GA: Endogenous activation in blastomycosis. Ann Intern Med 88:50–52, 1978.

22. Colonna PC, Gucker T: Blastomycosis of skeletal system: summary of 67 recorded cases and case report. J Bone Joint Surg 26:322–328, 1944.

23. Bayer AS, Scott VJ, Guze LB: Fungal arthritis. IV. Blastomycotic arthritis. Semin Arthritis Rheum 9:145–151, 1979.

24. Moser SA: Laboratory diagnosis of blastomycosis. Clinical Microbiology Newsletter 7:53–57, 1985.

25. Turner S, Kaufman L: Immunodiagnosis of blastomycosis. Semin Respir Infect 1:22–28, 1986.

26. Sekhon AS, DiSalvo AF, Standard PG, Kaufman L, Terreni AA, Garg AK: Evaluation of commercial reagents to identify the exoantigens of *Blastomyces dermatitidis, Coccidioides immitis,* and *Histoplasma* species cultures. Am J Clin Pathol 82:206–209, 1984.

27. Green JH, Harrell WK, Johnson J, Benson R: Preparation of reference antisera for laboratory diagnosis of blastomycosis. J Clin Microbiol 10:1–7, 1979.

28. Deresinski SC: Coccidioidomycosis of bone and joint. In Stevens DA, ed: Coccidioidomycosis: A Text. New York, Plenum Medical Book Company, 1980, pp 195–211.

29. Drutz DJ, Catanzaro A: Coccidioidomycosis. Am Rev Respir Dis 117:559–585; 727–771, 1978.

30. Smith CE, Saito MT: Serologic reactions in coccidioidomycosis. J Chron Dis 5:571–579, 1957.

31. Pappagianis D: Epidemiology of coccidioidomycosis. In Stevens DA, ed: Coccicioidomycosis: A Text. New York, Plenum Medical Book Company, 1980, pp 63–85.

32. Wilson JW, Smith CE, Plunkett DA: Primary cutaneous coccidioidomycosis: criteria for diagnosis and report of a case. Calif Med 79:233–239, 1953.

33. Pollack SF, Morris JM, Murray WR: Coccidioidal synovitis of the knee. J Bone Joint Surg 49:1397–1407, 1967.

34. Catanzaro A, Drutz DJ: Primary coccidioidomycosis. In Stevens DA, ed: Coccidioidomycosis: A Text. New York, Plenum Medical Book Company, 1980, pp 139–145.

35. Bayer AS, Guze LB: Fungal arthritis II. Coccidioidal synovitis. Semin Arthritis Rheum 8:200–211, 1979.

36. Winter WG, Pappagianis D, Huntington RA, Larson RK: Coccidioidal arthritis and spondylitis, 1976. In Ajello L, ed: Coccidioidomycosis: Current Clinical and Diagnostic Status. Miami, Symposia Specialists, 1976, pp 169–175.

37. Iger M: Coccidioidial osteomyelitis. In Ajello L, ed: Coccidioidomycosis: Current Clinical and Diagnostic Status. Miami, Symposia Specialists, 1976, pp 177–190.

38. Calhoun DL, Osir EO, Dugger KO, Galgiani JN, Law JH: Humoral antibody response to specific antigens of *Coccidioides immitis.* J Infect Dis 154:265–272, 1986.

39. Pappagianis D: Serology and serodiagnosis of coccidioidomycosis. In Stevens DA, ed: Coccidioidomycosis: A Text. New York, Plenum Medical Book Company, 1980, p 97.

40. Wieden MA, Galgiani JN, Pappagianis D: Comparison of immunodiffusion techniques with standard complement fixation assay for quantitation of coccidioidal antibodies. J Clin Microbiol 18:529–534, 1983.

41. Rosenberg EF, Dockerty MB, Meyerding HW: Coccidioidal arthritis. Arch Intern Med 49:238–250, 1942.

42. Bouza E, Einston DJ, Rhodes J: Paracoccidioidomycosis (South American blastomycosis) in the United States. Chest 72:100–102, 1977.

43. Restrepo A, Robledo M, Giraldo R, Hernandez H, Sierra F, Gutierrez F, Londono F, Calle G: The gamut of paracoccidioidomycosis. Am J Med 61:33–42, 1976.

44. Restrepo MA, Gomez I, Cano LE, Arango MD, Gutierrez F, Sanin A, Robledo MA: Treatment of paracoccidioidomycosis with ketoconazole: a three year experience. Am J Med 74(1B):48–52, 1983.

45. Johnson AC: In Reeder MM, Palmer PES, eds: The Radiology of Tropical Diseases with Epidemiological, Pathological and Clinical Correlations. Baltimore, Williams & Wilkins, 1981, pp 347–419.

46. Bayer AS, Choi C, Tillman DB, Guze LB: Fungal arthritis. V. Cryptococcal and histoplasmal arthritis. Semin Arthritis Rheum 9:218–227, 1979.

47. Sellers TF, Price WN, Newberry WM: An epidemic of erythema multiforme and erythema nodosum caused by histoplasmosis. Ann Intern Med 62:1244–1262, 1965.

47a. Allen J: Bone involvement with disseminated histoplasmosis. Am J Roentgenol 82:250–254, 1959.

48. Gass M, Kobayashi GS: Histoplasmosis: an illustrative case with unusual vaginal and joint involvement. Arch Dermatol 100:724–727, 1969.

49. Key JA, Large AM: Histoplasmosis of the knee. J Bone Joint Surg 24:281–290, 1942.

50. Omer GE, Lockwood RS, Travis LO: Histoplasmosis involving the carpal joint. J Bone Joint Surg 45A:1699–1703, 1963.

51. Klingberg WG: Generalized histoplasmosis in infants and children. J Pediatr 36:728–741, 1950.

52. Pfaller MA, Kyriakos M, Weeks PM, Kobayashi GS: Disseminated histoplasmosis presenting as an acute tenosynovitis. Diagn Microbiol Infect Dis 3:241–255, 1985.

53. Class RV, Cascio FS: Histoplasmosis presenting as an acute polyarthritis. N Engl J Med 287:1133–1134, 1972.

53a. Cockshott WP, Lucas AO: Radiologic findings in *Histoplasma duboisii* infections. Br J Radiol 37:653–660, 1964.

54. Davies SF: Serodiagnosis of histoplasmosis. Semin Respir Infect 1:9–15, 1986.

55. Wheat J, French MLV, Kohler RB, Zimmerman SE, Smith WR, Norton JA, Eitzen HE, Smith CD, Slama TG: The diagnostic laboratory tests for histoplasmosis. Ann Intern Med 97:680–685, 1982.

56. Lynch PJ, Voorhees JJ, Harrell R: Systemic sporotrichosis. Ann Intern Med 73:23–30, 1970.

57. Travassos LR, Lloyd KO: *Sporothrix schenckii* and related species of *Ceratocystis.* Microbiol Rev 44:683–721, 1980.

58. Wilson DE, Mann JJ, Bennett JE, Utz JP: Clinical features of extracutaneous sporotrichosis. Medicine (Baltimore) 46:265–279, 1967.

59. Brook CJ, Ravikrishnan KP, Weg JG: Primary pul-

monary and articular sporotrichosis. Am Rev Respir Dis 116:141–143, 1977.

60. Bayer AS, Scott VJ, Guze LB: Fungal arthritis. III. Sporotrichial arthritis. Semin Arthritis Rheum 9:66–74, 1979.

61. Molstad B, Strom R: Multiarticular sporotrichosis. JAMA 240:556–557, 1978.

62. Morgan MA, Cockerill FR, Cortese DA, Roberts GD: Disseminated sporotrichosis with *Sporothrix schenckii* fungemia. Diagn Microbiol Infect Dis 2:151–155, 1984.

63. Chleboun J, Nade S: Skeletal cryptococcosis. J Bone Joint Surg 59A:509–514, 1977.

64. Miller GPG: The immunology of cryptococcal disease. Semin Respir Infect 1:45–52, 1986.

65. Diamond RD: *Cryptococcus neoformans*. In Mandell GL, Douglas RG, Bennett JE, eds: Principles and Practices of Infectious Diseases, 2nd ed. New York, John Wiley & Sons, 1985, pp 1460–1468.

66. Lewis JL, Rabinovich S: The wide spectrum of cryptococcal infections. Am J Med 53:315–322, 1972.

67. Littn ML, Walter JE: *Cryptococcus:* current status. Am J Med 45:922–932, 1968.

68. Kirkering TM, Duma RJ, Shadomy S: The evolution of pulmonary cryptococcosis. Ann Intern Med 94:611–616, 1981.

69. Bryan CS: Vertebral osteomyelitis due to *Cryptococcus neoformans*: case report. J Bone Joint Surg 59A:275–276, 1977.

70. Collins VP: Bone involvement in cryptococcosis (torulosis). Am J Roentgenol 63:102–112, 1950.

71. Burch KH, Fine G, Quinn EL, Eisses JF: *Cryptococcus neoformans* as a cause of lytic bone lesions. JAMA 231:1057–1059, 1975.

72. Chelboun J, Nade S: Skeletal cryptococcosis. J Bone Joint Surg 59:509–514, 1977.

73. Poliner JR: Localized osseous cryptococcosis. J Pediatr 94:597–599, 1979.

74. Zach TL, Penn RG: Localized cryptococcal osteomyelitis in an immunocompetent host. Pediatr Infect Dis 5:601–603, 1986.

75. Simpson MB Jr, Merz WG, Kurlinski JP, Soloman MH: Opportunistic mycotic osteomyelitis: bone infections due to *Aspergillus* and *Candida* species. Medicine (Baltimore) 56:475–482, 1977.

76. Hopfer RL: Mycology of *Candida* infections. In Bodey GP, Fainstein V, eds: Candidiasis. New York, Raven Press, 1985, pp 1–12.

77. Kozinn PJ, Taschdjian CL: Laboratory diagnosis of candidiasis. In Bodey GP, Fainstein V, eds: Candidiasis. New York, Raven Press, 1985, pp 85–110.

78. Rogers TJ, Balish E: Immunity to *Candida albicans*. Microbiol Rev 44:660–682, 1980.

79. Bodey GP, Fainstein V: Systemic candidiasis. In Bodey GP, Fainstein V, eds: Candidiasis. New York, Raven Press, 1985, pp 135–168.

80. Noble HB, Lyne ED: *Candida* osteomyelitis and arthritis from hyperalimentation therapy. J Bone Joint Surg 56A:825–829, 1974.

81. Bayer AS, Guze LB: Fungal arthritis. I. *Candida* arthritis. Semin Arthritis Rheum 8:142–150, 1978.

82. Edwards JE, Turkel SB, Elder HA, Rand RW, Guze LB: Hematogenous *Candida* osteomyelitis. Am J Med 59:89–94, 1975.

83. Ginzler E, Meisel AD, Munters M, Kaplan D: *Candida* arthritis secondary to repeated intra-articular corticosteroids. NY State J Med 79:392–394, 1979.

84. Poplack DG, Jacobs SA: *Candida* arthritis treated with amphotericin B. J Pediatr 87:898–990, 1975.

85. Adlers, Randall J, Plotkin SA: Candidal osteomye-

litis and arthritis in a neonate. Am J Dis Child 123:595–596, 1972.

86. Klein JD, Yamauchi T, Horlick SP: Neonatal candidiasis, meningitis, and arthritis: observations and a review of the literature. J Pediatr 81:31–34, 1972.

87. Goodman JS, Seibert DG, Reahl GE, Geckler RW: Fungal infection of prosthetic joints: report of two cases. J Rheumatol 10:494–495, 1983.

88. Dupont B, Drouhet E: Cutaneous, ocular, and osteoarticular candidiasis in heroin addicts: new clinical and therapeutic aspects in 38 patients. J Infect Dis 152:577–591, 1985.

89. Yarchoan R, Davies SF, Freid J, Mahowald ML: Isolated *Candida parapsilosis* arthritis in a heroin addict. J Rheumatol 6:447–450, 1979.

90. Holzman RS, Bishko F: Osteomyelitis in heroin addicts. Ann Intern Med 75:693–696, 1971.

91. Hurley R: Pathogenicity of the genus *Candida*. In Winner HI, Hurley R, eds: Symposium on *Candida* Infections. Edinburgh, Livingstone, 1966, p 13.

92. Williams CD, Cunningham JN, Falk EA, Isom OW, Chase RN, Spencer FC: Chronic infection of the costal cartilages after thoracic surgical procedures. J Thorac Cardiovasc Surg 66:592–598, 1973.

93. Chmel H, Grieco MH, Zickel R: *Candida* osteomyelitis: report of a case. Am J Med Sci 266:299–304, 1973.

94. Edwards JE, Turkel SB, Elder HA, Rand RW, Guze LB: Hematogenous *Candida* osteomyelitis: report of three cases and review of the literature. Am J Med 59:89–94, 1975.

95. Hirschmann JV, Everett ED: *Candida* vertebral osteomyelitis: case report and review of the literature. J Bone Joint Surg 58A:573–575, 1976.

96. O'Connell CJ, Cherry AV, Zoll JG: Osteomyelitis of cervical spine: *Candida guilliermondii*. Ann Intern Med 79:748, 1973.

97. Thurston AJ, Gillespie WJ: *Torulopsis glabrata* osteomyelitis of the spine: a case report and review of the literature. Aust NZ J Surg 51:374–376, 1981.

98. Gustke KA, Wu KK: *Torulopsis glabrata* osteomyelitis: report of a case. Clin Orthop 154:197–200, 1981.

99. Murdock CB, Fischer JF, Loebel D, Chew WH: Osteomyelitis of the hand due to *Torulopsis holmii*. South Med J 76:1460–1461, 1983.

99a. Reiser M, Rupp N, Färber D: Röntgenologische befunde bei der septischen Candida–Arthritis. ROEFO, 129:335–339, 1978.

100. Kahn FW: Jones JM. Latex agglutination tests for detection of *Candida* antigens in sera of patients with invasive candidiasis. J Infect Dis 153:579–585, 1986.

101. Gentry LO, Wilkinson ID, Lea AS, Price MF: Latex agglutination test for detection of *Candida* antigen in patients with disseminated disease. Eur J Clin Microbiol 2:122–128, 1983.

102. Barnwell PA, Jelsma LF, Raff MJ: *Aspergillus* osteomyelitis: report of a case and review of the literature. Diagn Microbiol Infect Dis 3:515–519, 1985.

103. Tack KJ, Rhame FS, Brown B, Thompson RC: *Aspergillus* osteomyelitis: report of four cases and a review of the literature. Am J Med 73:295–300, 1982.

104. Young RC, Bennett JE, Vogel CI, Carbone PP, DeVita VT: Aspergillosis: the spectrum of disease in 98 patients. Medicine (Baltimore) 49:147–173, 1970.

104a. Swatek F, Halde C, Rinaldi MJ, Shadomy HJ: *Aspergillus* species and other opportunistic saprophyteic hyaline hyphomyces. In Lennete EH, Balows

A, Hausler WJ, Shadomy HJ, eds: Manual of Clinical Microbiology, 4th ed. Washington, DC, American Society of Microbiology 584–594, 1985.

105. Grossman M: Aspergillosis of bone. Br J Radiol 48:57–59, 1975.

106. Redmond A, Carre IJ, Biggart JD, Mackenzie DWR: Aspergillosis (Aspergillus nidulans) involving bone. J Pathol Bacteriol 89:391–395, 1965.

107. Seligsohn R, Rippon JW, Lerner SA: Aspergillus terreus osteomyelitis. Arch Intern Med 137:918–920, 1977.

108. Glotzbach RE: Aspergillus terreus infection of pseudoaneurysm of aortofemoral graft with contiguous vertebral osteomylitis. Am J Clin Pathol 77:224–227, 1982.

109. Roselle GA, Baird IM: Aspergillus flavipes group osteomyelitis. Arch Intern Med 139:590–592, 1979.

110. Altman AR: Thoracic wall invasion secondary to pulmonary aspergillosis. Am J Roentgenol 129:140–142, 1977.

111. Shaw FW, Warthen HJ: Aspergillosis of the bone. South Med J 29:1070–1071, 1936.

112. Gustafson TL, Schaffner W, Lavely GB, Stratton CW, Johnson HK, Hutchinson RH: Invasive aspergillosis in renal transplant recipients: correlation with corticosteroid therapy. J Infect Dis 148:230–238, 1983.

113. Bennet JE: Aspergillus species. In Mandell GL, Douglas RG, Bennett JE, eds: Principles and Practice of Infectious Diseases, 2nd ed. New York, John Wiley & Sons, 1985, pp 1447–1451.

114. Brandt SJ, Thompson RL, Wenzel RP: Mycotic pseudoaneurysm of an aortic bypass graft and contiguous vertebral osteomyelitis due to Aspergillus fumigatus. Am J Med 79:259–262, 1985.

115. Caligiuri P, MacMahon H, Courtney J, Weiss L: Opportunistic pulmonary aspergillosis with chest wall invasion. Arch Intern Med 143:2323–2324, 1983.

116. Haapasaari J, Essen RV, Kahanapaa A, et al: Fungal arthritis simulating juvenile rheumatoid arthritis. Br Med J 2:285–286, 1982.

117. Kemp HBS, Bedford AF, Finchman WJ: Petreillidium boydii infection of the knee: a case report. Skeletal Radiol 9:114–117, 1982.

118. Ludwick LI, Rytel MW, Yanez JP, et al: Deep infections from Petreillidium boydii treated with miconazole. JAMA 241:272–273, 1979.

119. Travis LB, Roberts GD, Wilson WR: Clinical significance of Pseudallescheria boydii: a review of 10 years' experience. Mayo Clin Proc 60:531–537, 1985.

120. Rolston KVI, Hopfer RL, Larson DL: Infections caused by Dreschlera species: case report and review of the literature. Rev Infect Dis 7:525–529, 1985.

121. Ajello L, Iger M, Wybel R, Vigil FJ: Dreschlera rostrata as an agent of phaeohyphomycosis. Mycologia 73:1094–1102, 1980.

122. Stillwell WT, Rubin BD, Axelrod JI. Chrysosporium, a new agent in osteomyelitis. Clin Orthop 184:190–192, 1984.

123. Jakel C, Leek JC, Olsen DA, Robbins DL: Septic arthritis due to Fusarium solani. J Rheumatol 10:151–153, 1983.

124. Feld R, Fronasier VL, Brombardier C, Hastings DE: Septic arthritis due to Saccharomyces species in a patient with chronic rheumatoid arthritis. J Rheumatol 9:637–640, 1982.

125. Torstrick RF, Harrison K, Heckman JD, Johnson JE: Chronic bursitis caused by Phialophora richardsiae: case report (part 2). J Bone Joint Surg 61A:772–774, 1979.

126. Echols RM, Selinger DS, Hallowell C, et al: Rhizopus osteomyelitis: a case report and review. Am J Med 66:141–145, 1979.

127. Gardella S, Nomedeu B, Bombi JA, Munoz J, Puis de la Bellacasa J, Pumarola A, Rozam C: Fatal fungemia with arthritic involvement caused by Trichosporon beiselii in a bone marrow transplant recipient (letter). J Infect Dis 151:566, 1985.

128. Brabender W, Ketcherside J, Hodes GR, Rensachary S, Barnes WG: Acremonium kiliense osteomyelitis of the calvarium. Neurosurgery 16:554–556, 1985.

129. Kaell AT, Weitzman I: Acute monarticular arthritis due to Phialophora parasitica. Am J Med 74:519–522, 1983.

129a. Osyton JK: Mandura foot: a study of twenty cases. J Bone Joint Surg 43B:259–267, 1961.

130. Clafin K, Milbauer J, Sullivan B: Ketoconazole and blastomycotic osteomyelitis. Ann Intern Med 98:260–261, 1983.

131. Dismukes WE, Stamm AM, Graybill JR: Treatment of systemic mycoses with ketoconazole: emphasis on toxicity and clinical response in 52 patients. Ann Intern Med 98:13–20, 1983.

132. Drouhet E, Dupont B: Laboratory and clinical assessment of ketoconazole in deep-seated mycoses. Am J Med 74:30–47, 1983.

133. Clafin K, Milbauer J, Sullivan B: Ketoconazole and blastomycotic osteomyelitis (letter). Ann Intern Med 98:260–261, 1983.

134. Medoff G, Kobayashi GS: Strategies in the treatment of systemic fungal infections. N Engl J Med 302:145–155, 1980.

135. Medoff G, Kobayashi GA: The polyenes. In Speller DCE, ed: Antifungal Chemotherapy. New York, John Wiley & Sons, 1980, pp 3–33.

136. Sugar AM: The polyene macrolide antifungal drugs. In Peterson PK, Verhoef J, eds: The Antimicrobial Agents Annual 1. Amsterdam, Elsevier, 1986, pp 229–244.

137. Calhoun DL, Galgiani JN: The imidazoles: miconazole, ketoconazole. In Peterson PK, Verhoef J, eds: The Antimicrobial Agents Annual 1. Amsterdam, Elsevier, 1986, pp 218–228.

138. Stein SR: Coccidioides immitis infection of bone treated with local infusion of amphotericin B. In Ajello L, ed: Coccidioidomycosis: Current Clinical and Diagnostic Status. Miami, Symposia Specialists, 1976, pp 253–258.

139. Dismukes WE: National Institute of Allergy and Infectious Diseases Mycosis Study Group: treatment of blastomycosis and histoplasmosis with ketoconazole. Ann Intern Med 103:861–872, 1985.

140. Dijkmans BAC, Koolen MI, Mouton RP, Falke THM, Van Broek PJ, Van der Meer JWH: Hematogenous Candida vertebral osteomyelitis treated with ketoconazole. Infection 102:290–292, 1982.

141. Kauffman CA: Flucytosine. In Peterson PK, Verhoef J, eds: The Antimicrobial Agents Annual 1. Amsterdam, Elsevier, 1986, pp 213–217.

142. Speller DCE, ed: Antifungal Chemotherapy. New York, John Wiley & Sons, 1980, pp 213–224.

Ramon B. Gustilo, M.D.
Liberato A.C. Leagogo, M.D.

CHAPTER

22

Management of Infected Total Hip Replacement

INTRODUCTION

About 250,000 hips in the world are replaced annually, and 40 percent of these surgical procedures are performed in the United States.[1-5] The incidence of deep infection after total hip replacement has been reported to be as high as 10 percent,[6-9] and several reports indicate zero to 2.0 percent.[2, 10-15b] The increased morbidity of repeated surgical procedures, prolonged antibiotic therapy, hospitalization, and costs of $50,000 to $100,000 have characterized this dreaded complication of total hip replacement. Moreover, the ultimate results are less than ideal, with lifetime disability, sometimes a loss of a limb, or even death. The management of infected total hip replacement varies from early surgical debridement with prosthesis retained, prosthetic removal, prolonged antibiotic therapy, antibiotic beads, reimplantations, suppressive antibiotic therapy for life, arthrodesis, and amputation.

PATHOGENESIS, ETIOLOGY, AND CLASSIFICATION OF SEPSIS

Altered host resistance, diabetes mellitus, poor nutrition, and obesity have been mentioned by authors as contributing factors in total joint infections.[12, 16, 17] Patients with rheumatoid arthritis are more prone to infection because of the decreased chemotactic activity of the polymorphonuclear leukocytes.[6, 10, 18, 19] A high percentage of patients in whom sepsis develops had previous operations on the affected joint prior to the index arthroplasty.[6, 9, 20] The incidence is doubled in those who had undergone a hip nailing or osteotomy for fracture.[6] Concurrent sepsis from a remote site has been implicated in total hip and total knee arthroplasties,[8, 17, 18, 21, 22] and account for 10 percent of joint replacement patients having a distant site of infection preoperatively. Postoperatively, this can serve as a focus for hematogenous spread to the joint.

The etiology is either intraoperative contamination from the air in the operating room (airborne infection) or a direct inoculation from the normal skin flora or from the surgeon's hands, nostrils, or other source.

Infections that develop long after total joint arthroplasty are due to hematogenous seeding, such as urinary tract infection, catheterization, dental caries, ear infection, or to delayed growth or manifestations of indolent organisms present at surgery.

Infection is classified into three types:

1. *Early acute infection* is defined as one occurring in the first 4 weeks after surgery.

2. *Delayed with acute onset* is defined as one of acute onset of signs and symptoms of infection after several months or years of normalcy, usually as a result of hematogenous seeding from a distant process, e.g., dental manipulation.

3. *Chronic infection* is defined as one that has been present over 4 weeks characterized by insidious onset of pain; history of drainage, intermittent or present; and increased erythrocyte sedimentation rate (ESR).

DIAGNOSIS

Diagnosis of infected total hip replacement is oftentimes not difficult. Our analysis of 37

Dr. Gustilo is from the Department of Orthopaedics, Hennepin County Medical Center, Minneapolis, Minnesota. Dr. Leagogo is from the Philippine Orthopaedic Institute, Inc., Manila.

consecutive infected joint replacements revealed pain as the most common presenting problem on weight bearing and draining wound or sinus (54 percent), accompanied by fever and localized erythema. The ESR is elevated in 90 percent of cases. However, elevated white blood cell (WBC) count occurs in less than half of patients (39 percent). Carefully done, aseptic joint aspiration for culture and Gram stain study is one single reliable examination to confirm the diagnosis.[22a]

Bacteriological findings in our series (28 patients) were similar to those in other studies, with a predominance of gram-positive cocci.[23, 24] In 26 patients single bacteria grew; in seven patients, the cultures grew gram-positive and gram-negative bacteria. The common organisms were *Staphylococcus aureus* (13 cases), *Staphylococcus epidermidis* (13 cases), alpha-hemolytic *Streptococcus* (three cases), enterococcus (three cases), *Pseudomonas aeruginosa* (three cases), and *Bacillus* (two cases). Other authors have reported on the unreliability of the laboratory results for the diagnosis of infection.[20, 23] Aspiration as a diagnostic tool has produced a significant incidence of false-positive and false-negative results if not done aseptically.[22, 25] Cultures and examination performed during the surgery are more reliable, but they can also be misleading.[10, 26] Indolent infection can have a negative yield in 50 percent of cases. In our series, cultures of the fluid from preoperative aspiration of the joints in ten patients grew the involved organism and subsequently the same organism was isolated from the intraoperative specimen.

Routine and special radiography may demonstrate loosening of the prosthesis in long-standing infections in about 69 to 96 percent of cases.[4, 27] However, it is unreliable in differentiating septic from nonseptic loosening.[24]

Routine x-ray (anteroposterior and lateral) findings indicative of loosening include (1) widening of radiolucent lines, (2) endosteal scalloping and cortical thinning, (3) component sinking or migration, and (4) periosteal reaction. However, these findings are unreliable in differentiating form aseptic loosening. If the clinical symptoms, elevated ESR, and x-ray findings as described above are present, this is a strong indication of an infected total hip replacement.

In order to determine whether a painful prosthesis is loose or infected in problem cases, Fitzgerald and colleagues[28] showed that sequential technetium 99m (^{99m}Tc) and gallium 67 (^{67}Ga) bone scanning revealed 67 percent

sensitivity, 79 percent specificity, and 73 percent accuracy. The use of indium 111 (^{111}In)-labeled autologous WBCs showed 86 percent sensitivity, 100 percent specificity, and 94 percent accuracy.

The most reliable examination would be cultures and Gram stain at surgery (the patient should not be receiving preoperative antibiotics) taken from the hip joint, implants, intramedullary canal, and acetabulum after removal of components. Tissue should be sent for both culture and histologic examination. If these cultures are still negative, but the clinical picture and other laboratory findings are strongly indicative of infection, the case must be treated as an infected joint. When the prosthesis is removed and the entire cement mantle goes with it, there is strong evidence for infection.

TREATMENT (Fig. 22-1)

In early acute sepsis or delayed, acute onset, the recommended treatments are as follows:

1. Immediate arthrotomy with thorough debridement and irrigation.
2. Leave the prosthesis components unless loose.
3. Local antibiotic beads (2 to 4 weeks).
4. Systemic antibiotics (4 to 6 weeks).

After a thorough clinical and radiologic evaluation and the diagnosis of a septic hip is made, surgical debridement and irrigation must be done immediately. Usually, we follow the original surgical incision; a thorough debridement and copious irrigation are done. Cultures and Gram stain are performed immediately as soon as the joint is entered, and the patient is then given 2 grams of cephalosporin (cefamandole). The wound is thoroughly debrided of infected and necrotic tissues and copiously irrigated, varying from 5000 to 10,000 ml of normal saline solution and finished with 2000 ml of a bacitracin/polymyxin solution. The femoral head component is dislocated and examined for loosening; the acetabular component is likewise examined for loosening. The femoral head is relocated, and local tobramycin beads (60 to 90 mm) are placed in the hip joint. Two hemovac catheters are inserted without suction to allow egress of excessive hematoma and the wound is closed in layers—one in deep fascia and one for skin.

The patient is brought back to the operating room in 4 to 5 days for repeat debridement

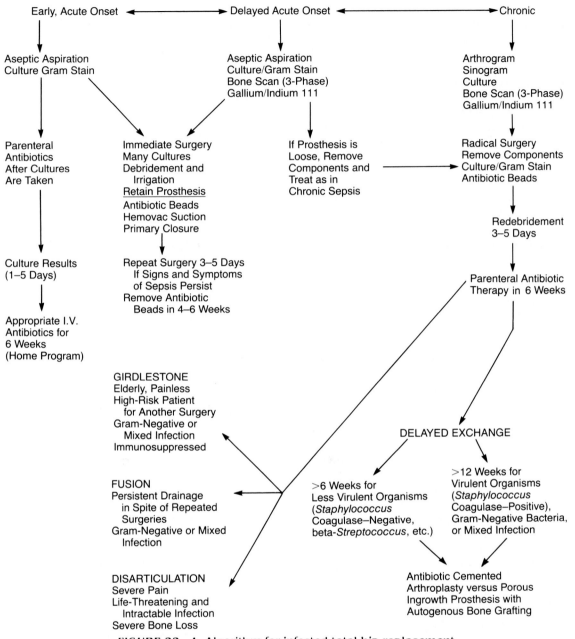

FIGURE 22–1. Algorithm for infected total hip replacement.

and irrigation if needed. The indications for repeat debridement are increasing drainage, persistent elevated temperature, and local appearance of the wound. If, at initial surgery, the hip joint is severely infected with copious purulent material, we advise leaving the wound open and coming back in 48 hours for repeat debridement, irrigation, and closure with tobramycin beads placed in the joint.

Once the bacterium is identified, in 24 to 48 hours appropriate antibiotics are selected and given in large doses for 4 to 6 weeks. No oral antibiotic afterward is recommended. The hemovac suction is usually removed in 3 to 4 days. The patient is allowed to get up with crutches after about 3 to 4 days with weight bearing as tolerated. Parenteral antibiotic therapy is continued at home through a home care program. Usually, the patient stays in the hospital for 10 to 14 days. The antibiotic beads are removed in 2 to 4 weeks.

Late Infection (Chronic) With or Without a Draining Sinus

The treatment modalities include (1) debridement and irrigation, (2) removal of all components and bone cement, (3) insertion of tobramycin beads (90 to 120 6-mm beads), (4) systemic antibiotics for 6 weeks, and (5) delayed exchange arthroplasty.

We recommend a lateral trochanteric osteotomy surgical approach in order to facilitate removal of all components and bone cement. The trochanter is retracted proximally, followed by total capsulectomy, synovectomy, and removal of dense scar and granulomatous tissue, which are commonly found around the infected hip joint. The femoral component is usually removed without much trouble, and then followed by meticulous removal of bone cement. We would recommend using a flexible light as well as C-arm x-rays to be sure all cement is removed. If all cement is not removed, Fitzgerald[28] has reported recurrent infection following delayed treatment change arthroplasty three times more if all cement has been removed. Cultures are taken from the intramedullary canal and the acetabulum after removal of the components. Then the intramedullary canal is reamed with flexible reamers until all the cement has been removed down to bleeding bone. The canal is irrigated at intervals with antibiotic solution.

The acetabular component, which is usually loose, is easily removed. All cement and granulomatous tissues are meticulously debrided. Cement protruding inside the pelvic cavity has to be removed very slowly without risking damage to blood vessels or nerves. One should consider removing it with an intrapelvic incision if it is a very large size and completely inside the pelvis. Then, acetabular reaming is performed until one sees a bleeding acetabular wall. There will still be multiple cavities where the anchoring cement plugs were before. These cavities are curetted of bone cement.

Again, the femoral canal and acetabulum are irrigated copiously with normal saline solution plus a bacitracin/polymyxin solution. Then the intramedullary canal and acetabulum are filled with 60 to 90 6-mm tobramycin beads (2.4 gm tobramycin in 40 gm of bone cement) inside the intramedullary canal; 60 to 90 6-mm beads are also inserted into the acetabulum.

Two hemovac tubes are inserted without pressure to allow egress of excess hematoma or drainage. The wound is closed in two layers at about 1 inch apart for fascia and skin. Redebridement is done in 3 to 5 days. If drainage continues to be characterized by copious, recollection of pus, if the local appearance of the wound suggests uncontrolled infection, or if the patient continues to have spiking fever and pain, the steps of surgical debridement, irrigation, and packing with tobramycin beads are repeated.

Skin traction is applied to the leg for a few days. The patient is gradually ambulated after 5 to 10 days when there is no more drainage, and hemovac suction is removed. The patient is placed on appropriate parenteral antibiotics for 4 to 6 weeks.[28-30] Routine intravenous antibiotics are continued at home through a central intravenous line by either the patient or a visiting nurse. The patient is sent home on crutches with a partial weight-bearing and an active hip exercise program.

Exchange Arthroplasty (Fig. 22-2)

Bucholz and associates[31] have had the most experience with one-stage reimplantation of the hip for infected arthroplasty, with an incidence of 77 percent good results initially, rising to 90 percent after further exchanges. Reimplantations were performed using antibiotic-impregnated cement. Carlsson and co-authors,[25] using gentamicin-impregnated cement, reported a 10 percent recurrence rate after a one-stage exchange and a 22 percent recurrence rate after a two-stage exchange. Salvati and co-workers,[32] after analyzing their experience of over 23 years, concluded that the overall results appear to be favorable with delayed exchanges in infected total hip arthroplasty.

We do not recommend immediate exchange arthroplasty. The exception is an elderly patient who cannot withstand another operation and with a less virulent single bacterial infection. Current hip revision arthroplasty reports indicate improved results with delayed exchange (Fig. 22-2).[28,32] Our surgical protocol would be to bring back the patient with gram-positive bacteria for at least 6 to 12 weeks and with gram-negative bacteria or mixed infection beyond 12 weeks. Clinically, the wound is

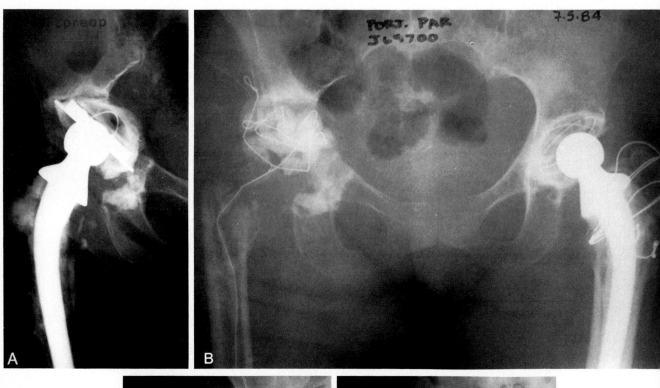

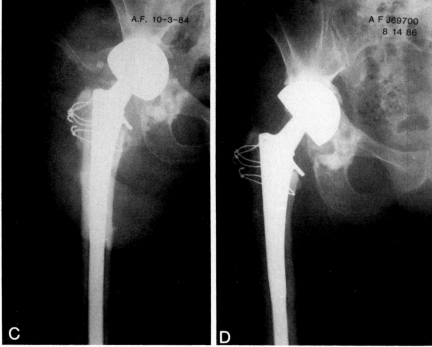

FIGURE 22–2. Delayed exchange arthroplasty.

A, A 76-year-old woman had undergone four previous operations for infected total hip replacement. She presented to the emergency room of the Hennepin County Medical Center with two draining sinuses around the hip joint of 3 years' duration. Anteroposterior (AP) x-rays of the hip showed loosening of both the acetabular and femoral components with bone loss of the acetabulum and femur.

B, Debridement and irrigation, removal of total hip component, and insertion of tobramycin beads into the acetabulum and femur were performed. The patient was placed on appropriate antibiotics for 6 weeks for *Staphylococcus* coagulase-positive, enterococcus, and *Serratia.*

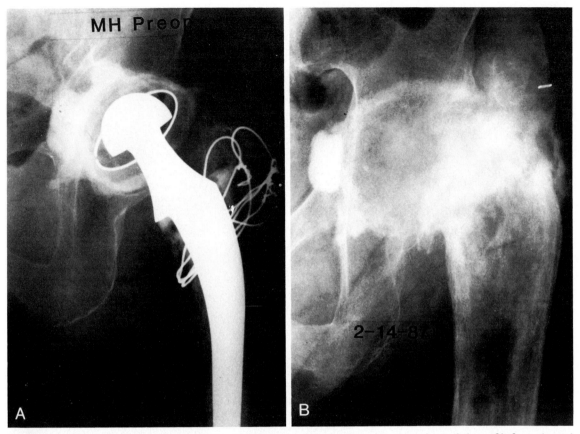

FIGURE 22–3. Resection arthroplasty. *A,* A 78-year-old woman with chronic draining of infected total hip replacement of 3 years' duration. Anteroposterior (AP) x-rays showed loosening of the femoral and acetabular component. *B,* AP x-rays showed head and neck resection after six surgical procedures to control sepsis. The patient is severely disabled and has been using a walker at all times. She primarily stays inside.

nicely healed without induration or edema and the ESR has decreased significantly and not necessarily within normal limits.

At surgery, the beads are removed, and the culture and smear are taken from the acetabulum and intramedullary canal. If Gram stain is positive, redebridement and irrigation, and probably packing the antibiotic beads again, are indicated. If the Gram stain is negative and the culture becomes positive in 24 to 48 hours, antibiotics are given for another 6 weeks. If the culture is negative at 5 days, the antibiotics are discontinued. In delayed exchange arthroplasty, aminoglycoside and cephalosporin are given for a period of 5 days until culture results are definitely known.

In the elderly patient with adequate femoral and acetabular bone stock, exchange cemented arthroplasty using antibiotic bone cement is recommended.[13, 15, 15b, 25, 33] If the prosthesis is cemented in place, the patient is allowed full weight bearing immediately. If the acetabular wall and femoral canal is deficient and thin, we recommend a cementless femoral

---

C, Delayed exchange was done 4 months later. AP x-rays showed a biologic ingrowth anatomic system (BIAS) cementless femoral component with bipolar head. Bone grafting was done for both the femur and acetabulum.

D, Two-year follow-up. AP x-rays of the hip showed reconstitution of the femur and acetabulum without recurrence of sepsis. The ESR was normal. She has no pain, but there was a loss of leg length of $\frac{3}{4}$ inch.

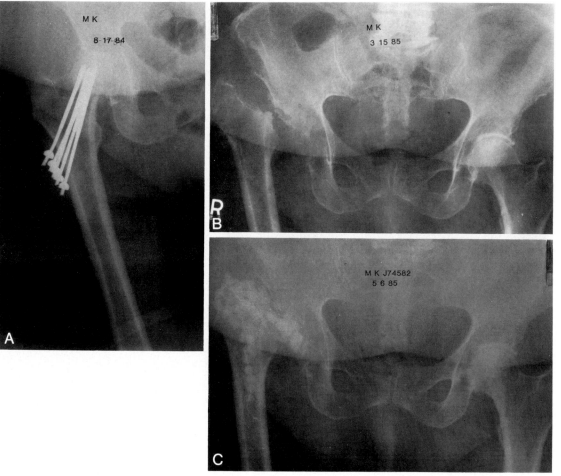

FIGURE 22–4. Girdlestone procedure.

A, A 72-year-old woman was treated with head and neck resection following infected nailing. She was placed on 6 weeks of intravenous cefazolin sodium (Ancef) for *Staphylococcus* coagulase-positive infection. Three months later, the patient was still suffering from a painful hip and drainage was still occurring.

B, Anteroposterior (AP) x-rays of the hip after second debridement and irrigation with insertion of tobramycin beads.

C, AP and lateral x-rays of the hip 18 months later with antibiotic beads still in place. The patient has been experiencing no pain, has been using a walker for long walks, and does not want any more surgery, including antibiotic bead removal.

titanium ingrowth prosthesis with bone grafting proximally, with a tight fit in the intramedullary canal. A bipolar component or acetabular ingrowth prosthesis is recommended for the acetabular wall after bone grafting with cancellous bone. The acetabular defects are grafted with cancellous bone and are impacted into the acetabular wall with reverse reaming. In very large defects, where large allograft is used, a cemented (with antibiotic) acetabular component is recommended. Screws are used to fixed the allograft to remaining acetabular wall. In some instances, two-stage arthroplasty has been done to reconstruct extensive acetab-

ular or femoral defects. If bone grafting and ingrowth prosthesis placement are done, partial weight bearing (about 30 to 40 pounds) is recommended for 6 weeks, followed by progressive weight bearing from 6 to 12 weeks.

Resection Arthroplasty (Girdlestone Procedure)

Excision arthroplasty (Figs. 22–3 and 22–4) is a reasonable joint salvage procedure for infection after total hip arthroplasty.[7, 34–36]

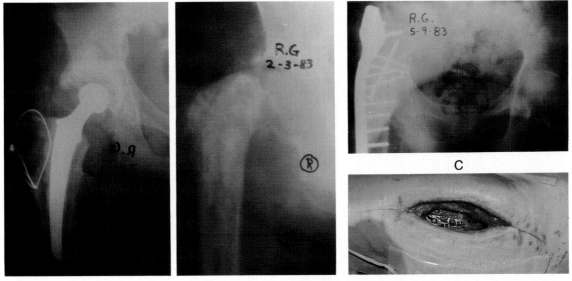

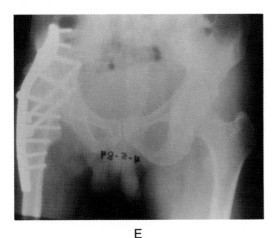
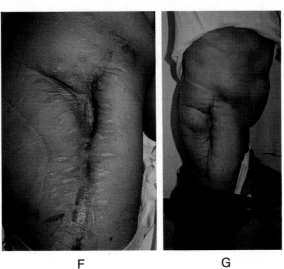

FIGURE 22–5. Arthrodesis.

A,B, A 32-year-old male kidney transplant patient with chronic draining sinus for 4 years following Girdlestone procedure for infected total hip replacement. He had undergone 15 previous operations, and the last six operations were attempts to control the infection.

C, Anteroposterior (AP) x-ray showed fusion of the hip joint with Cobra plate.

D, Wound was left open.

E, AP x-ray showed fusion of the hip joint with Cobra plate and spica cast immobilization for 3 months.

F,G, Wound has completely healed without drainage for 2 years. The patient has full ambulation with a cane for prolonged walks and has been without pain.

The indications for resection arthroplasty are virulent resistant organisms (usually gram-negative or mixed) in unhealthy, edematous, scarred soft tissue around the surgical area and severe bone loss. Excision arthroplasty is always a consideration also at the end of 6 to 12 weeks, when the patient comes back for examination. If the patient, particularly an elderly one, has no pain and does not mind using crutches or a walker for ambulation, we have left tobramycin beads indefinitely in such resection cases.

Arthrodesis (Fig. 22–5)

Arthrodesis as a salvage procedure has been performed in a limited number of cases with surprisingly high satisfactory results, as reported by Kostuik and Alexander.[37] It is indicated in recurrent failure of surgical debridement and antibiotic therapy and in the failure of one or two exchanges with persistent draining sinus. We had fused two hips with Cobra plates and accomplished a solid fusion with complete cessation of drainage and pain. However, the patient usually had $1\frac{1}{2}$ to 2 inches of leg length discrepancy.

Disarticulation

Disarticulation remains the final option for infected hip arthroplasty. This salvage procedure should be reserved for patients with life-threatening infection, severe bone loss, intractable infection, and severe pain that is unresponsive to surgical and antibiotic treatment.[38]

References

1. Hori R, Lewis J, Zimmerman J, Compere C: The number of total joint replacements in the United States. Clin Orthop 132:46, 1978.
2. James E, Hunter G, Cameron H: Total hip revision arthroplasty: does sepsis influence the results? Clin Orthop 170:88, 1982.
3. Klenerman L: The management of the infected endoprosthesis. J Bone Joint Surg 66B:645, 1984.
4. Murray WR: Use of antibiotic containing bone cement. Clin Orthop 190:89, 1984.
5. Salvati E, Chekofsky K, Brause B, Wilson P: Reimplantation in infection. Clin Orthop 170:62, 1982.
6. Andrews H, Arden G, Hart G: Deep infection after total hip replacement. J Bone Joint Surg 63B:53, 1981.
7. Connor G, Steinberg M, Heppenstal B, Balderston R: The infected hip after total hip arthroplasty. J Bone Joint Surg 66A:1391, 1984.
8. Downes E: Late infections after total hip replacement. J Bone Joint Surg 59B:42, 1977.
9. Nelson C, Green T, Porter R, Warren R: One day versus seven days of preventive antibiotic therapy in orthopedic surgery. Clin Orthop 176:258, 1983.
10. Cherney D, Amstutz H: Total hip replacement in the previously septic hip. J Bone Joint Surg 60A:1059, 1978.
11. Fitzgerald R, Jones D: Hip implant infection: treatment with resection arthroplasty and late total hip arthroplasty. Am J Med 78:225, 1985.
12. Gristina A, Kolkin J: Current concepts review: total joint replacement and sepsis. J Bone Joint Surg 65A:128, 1983.
13. Josefsson G, Lindberg L, Wiklander B: Systemic antibiotics and gentamicin-containing bone cement in the prophylaxis of postoperative infections in total hip arthroplasty. Clin Orthop 159:194, 1981.
14. Surin V, Sundholm K, Backman L: Infection after total hip replacement. J Bone Joint Surg 65B:412, 1983.
15. Torholm C, Lidgren L, Lindberg L, Kahlmeter G: Total hip joint arthroplasty with gentamicin-impregnated cement. Clin Orthop 181:99, 1983.
15a. Kavanagh B, Ilstrup D, Fitzgerald R: Revision total hip arthroplasty. J Bone Joint Surg 67A:517–526, 1985.
15b. Miley G, Schuller A, Turner R: Medical and surgical treatment of the septic hip with one stage revision arthroplasty. Clin Orthop 170:77, 1982.
16. Menon J, Thjeliesen D, Wroblewski B: Charnley low friction arthroplasty in diabetic patients. J Bone Joint Surg 65B:580, 1983.
17. Stinchfield F, Bigliani L, Neu H, Goss T, Foster C: Late hematogenous infection of total joint replacement. J Bone Joint Surg 62A:1345, 1980.
18. D'Ambrosia R, Shoji H, Heater R: Secondarily infected total joint replacements by hematogenous spread. J Bone Joint Surg 58A:450, 1976.
19. Thomas B, Moreland J, Amstutz H: Infection after total joint arthroplasty from distal extremity sepsis. Clin Orthop 181:121, 1983.
20. Callaghan J, Salvati E, Brause B, Rimnac C, Wright T: Reimplantation for salvage of the infected hip: rationale for the use of gentamicin impregnated cement and beads. The Hip: Hip Society Award Papers, St Louis, CV Mosby, 1985.
21. Artz T, Macys J, Salvati E, Jacobs B, Wilson P: Hematogenous infection of total joint replacements: a report of four cases. J Bone Joint Surg 57A:1024, 1975.
22. Donovan T, Gordon R, Nagel D: Urinary infections in total hip arthroplasty: influences of prophylactic cephalosporins and catheterization. J Bone Joint Surg 58A:1134, 1976.
22a. Patel D, Karcher A, Harris W: The role of preoperative aspiration of the hip prior to total hip replacement. The Hip: Proceedings of the Fourth Annual Open Scientific Meeting of the Hip Society. St. Louis, CV Mosby, 1976.
23. Jupiter J, Karchmer A, Lowell J, Harris W: Total hip arthroplasty in the treatment of adult hips with cement or quiescent sepsis. J Bone Joint Surg 63A:194, 1981.
24. Kamme C, Lindberg L: Aerobic and anaerobic bacteria in deep infections after total hip arthroplasty. Clin Orthop 154:201, 1981.
25. Carlsson A, Joseffson G, Lindberg L: Revision with gentamicin-impregnated cement for deep infection in total hip arthroplasties. J Bone Joint Surg 60A:1059, 1978.
26. Murray WR: Total hip replacement in non-specialized environments. The Hip: Proceedings of the Fourth Annual Open Scientific Meeting of the Hip Society. St Louis, CV Mosby, 1976.
27. Lyons C, Berquist T, Rand A, Brown M: Evaluation of radiographic hip replacement. J Bone Joint Surg 66B:168, 1984.
28. Fitzgerald R: The infected total hip arthroplasty: current concepts of treatment. The Hip: Symposium on Revision of Failed Total Hip Arthroplasty. St. Louis, CV Mosby, 1985.
29. Fremont-Smith P: Antibiotic management of septic total hip replacement: a therapeutic trial. The Hip: Proceedings of the Second Open Scientific Meeting of the Hip Society. St. Louis, CV Mosby, 1984.
30. Hughes P, Salvati E, Wilson P, Blumenfeld E: Treat-

ment of subacute sepsis of the hip by antibiotics and joint replacement criteria for diagnosis with evaluation of twenty-six cases. Clin Orthop 141:143, 1979.

31. Bucholz H, Elson R, Engelbrecht E, Lodenkamper H, Rottger J, Siegel A: Management of deep infection of total hip. J Bone Joint Surg 63B:342, 1981.

32. Salvati E, Robinson R, Zeno S, Koslin B, Brause B, Wilson P: Infection rates after 3,175 total hip and total knee replacements performed with and without a horizontal unidirectional filtered air-flow system. J Bone Joint Surg 64A:525, 1982.

33. Soto-Hall R, Saenz L, Tavernetti R, Cabaud H, Cochran T: Tobramycin in bone cement. Clin Orthop 175:60, 1983.

34. Bittar E, Petty W: Girdlestone arthroplasty for infected total hip arthroplasty. J Bone Joint Surg 65A:1087, 1983.

35. Bourne RB, Hunter GA, Rorabeck CH, Macnab JJ: A six-year follow-up of infected total hip replacement managed by Girdlestone's arthroplasty. J Bone Joint Surg 66B:340, 1984.

36. McElwaine N, Colville J: Excision arthroplasty for infected total hip replacement. J Bone Joint Surg 66B:168, 1984.

37. Kostuik J, Alexander D: Arthrodesis for failed arthroplasty. Clin Orthop 188:173, 1984.

38. Kettlekamp D: Infected total joint replacement. Arch Surg 112:552, 1977.

CHAPTER

23

Management of Infected Total Knee Replacement

INTRODUCTION

The incidence of sepsis following total knee replacement is 1 to 2 percent and is two to three times higher in patients with rheumatoid arthritis than with degenerative arthritis.[1, 2] Recent series revealed a lower infection rate (1 to 2 percent) compared to previous reports of wound sepsis in total knee replacement varying from 5 to 23 percent.[1-4] The problems inherent in infected total knee arthroplasty in contrast to total hip replacement include (1) scarcity of soft tissue around the knee joint, (2) bone loss, which makes exchange arthroplasty or fusion difficult, (3) the quadriceps and patellar tendon being vulnerable to rupture, and (4) the patella becoming vulnerable to fracture after removal of bone cement and prosthesis as it becomes very thin.

The goal in treatment of infected total knee replacement is prosthesis exchange after control or eradication of the infection, resulting in a functional knee without sepsis.

CLINICAL PICTURE, PATHOGENESIS, AND ETIOLOGY

Altered host resistance, diabetes mellitus, poor nutrition, and obesity have been mentioned as contributing factors in total joint infections.[5-7a] Patients with rheumatoid arthritis are more prone to infection because of the decreased chemotactic activity of the polymorphonuclear leukocytes.[8-11] A high percentage of patients in whom sepsis develops had previous operations on the affected joint prior to the index arthroplasty.[8, 12, 13, 13a] Concurrent sepsis from a remote site has been implicated in total hip and total knee arthroplasties.[7, 7a, 10, 14-16] Postoperatively, this can serve as a focus for hematogenous spread to the joint. Eighty percent of the etiologic organisms are *Staphylococcus* coagulase-positive and *Staphylococcus* coagulase-negative organisms.

Early Acute Infection

The cardinal signs of inflammation are usually present—pain, swelling, warmth, and redness with or without drainage. All other tests, including x-rays, are usually normal except for elevated erythrocyte sedimentation rate (ESR). Diagnosis is confirmed by aspiration, Gram stain, and culture. In the first 7 to 10 postoperative days, the differential diagnosis is *postoperative hematoma*, particularly with prophylactic anticoagulation therapy. If in doubt, aspirate the knee joint for culture and Gram stain.

Delayed with Acute Onset

Patients present with a history of getting along well for several months or years, and then suddenly acute knee pain on movement of the knee, fever, and swelling develop. The ESR may be normal, but the white blood cell (WBC) count is usually elevated. X-rays are usually normal. If there are findings of radiolucency and scalloping, probably a chronic sepsis is present that will eventually erupt. Joint aspiration for Gram stain and culture should confirm the diagnosis.

Chronic Infection

The patient usually provides a history of persistent swelling with warmth, slight redness for

From the Department of Orthopaedics, Hennepin County Medical Center, Minneapolis, Minnesota.

several weeks, nagging pain, and drainage at some time. The patient usually presents with a draining sinus. The ESR is elevated and usually there is a normal WBC count with neutrophilia. If there is a sinus tract, the diagnosis is made. If there is no drainage, joint aspiration for Gram stain and culture will confirm the diagnosis. X-rays are usually normal except for an occasional lytic change or bone loss or a periosteal elevation in cases with long duration of a draining sinus. Technetium 99m (^{99m}Tc) three-phase bone scanning, using gallium 67 (^{67}Ga) or indium 111 (^{111}In), will be positive in most cases.

TREATMENT (Fig. 23–1)

Early Infection and Delayed with Acute Onset

The knee joint is exposed through the original surgical incision for thorough debridement, synovectomy, and irrigation. Several cultures and Gram stain are taken. Intravenous antibiotics are given, after several cultures are taken at surgery, unless definite bacteriological diagnosis has been made before; appropriate antibiotic is given preoperatively. The knee joint is irrigated copiously with normal saline solution and bacitracin/polymyxin solution. The knee has to be subluxed anteriorly to have good access to the posterior joint. Both lateral and medial recesses must be debrided and irrigated. The knee joint is packed with 90 to 120 6-mm tobramycin beads. Two hemovac tubes are inserted without pressure. The wound is closed in two layers — the quadriceps tendon with interrupted suture and the skin 1 inch apart and closed loosely. Pressure dressings are applied with lateral and medial plaster splints. The hemovac is removed in 3 to 4 days when the drainage is less than 25 ml in an 8-hour period. In 10 to 14 days, the wound is inspected: if healing continues without evidence of recurrent sepsis, a knee immobilizer is applied for 5 to 6 weeks and active range of motion at intervals is started. The antibiotic

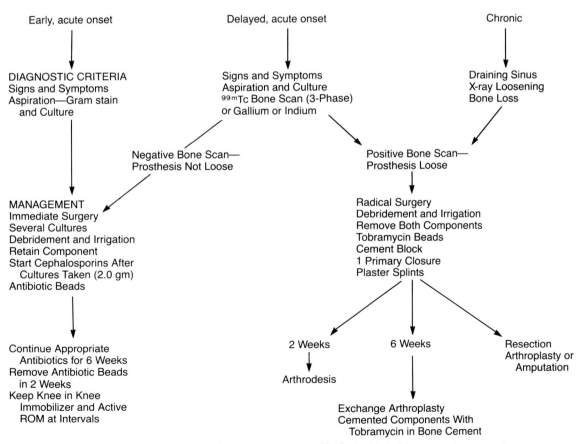

FIGURE 23–1. Algorithm for management of infected total knee replacements.

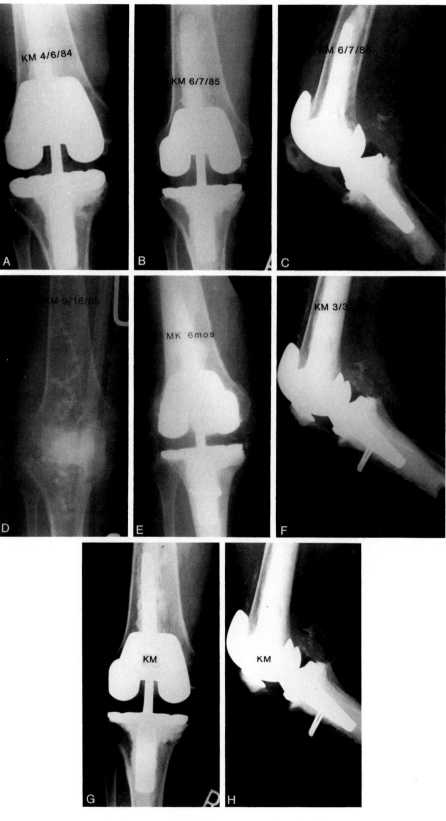

beads are removed at 2 to 4 weeks, and culture and Gram stain are again obtained. Antibiotics are given parenterally for 4 to 6 weeks.

Chronic Infection

EXCHANGE ARTHROPLASTY
(Fig. 23–2)

Immediate reimplantation of the knee prosthesis has been successful in 70 to 80 percent of cases.[17, 18]

A study by Insall and co-workers of 11 knees salvaged by a two-stage reimplantation showed no recurrence of infection in all cases after an average follow-up of 34 months.[3] Our results with this procedure have also been promising, with a success rate of 92 percent.

Radical surgery consisting of thorough debridement, total synovectomy, removal of all prosthetic components, and cement is performed. During surgery, several cultures and Gram stain should be taken from the femur and proximal tibia where the cement has been removed and also from the prosthetic component under surfaces in contact with bone and cement. Synovectomy must include the suprapatellar pouch, the lateral and medial recess, and the posterior compartment. The knee joint is copiously irrigated with normal saline solution and bacitracin/polymyxin solution. The bone cement is meticulously removed from all areas. *Tobramycin beads (90 to 120, 6 mm) are packed into the femur and proximal tibia, and the joint space maintained by a cement block with tobramycin (2.4 gm in 40 gm of bone cement).* Two hemovac tubes are inserted without pressure. Wounds are closed in two layers in an interrupted manner. Pressure dressings are applied with lateral and medial plaster splints. The hemovac suction is removed in 3 to 4 days, when drainage is less than 25 ml in an 8-hour period. At 7 to 10 days, when the wound is healing well, a cylinder cast is applied for 5 to 6 weeks. The patient is then sent home on appropriate intravenous antibiotics, depending on the culture, for a total of 6 weeks. At the end of 6 weeks, the patient is brought back to the outpatient clinic where the cast is removed and a delayed exchange knee replacement is scheduled. If there is any question at that time, the knee should be aspirated for culture. Careful planning of size and thickness of the prosthesis and solution to bone loss is undertaken to place the knee in proper ligament tension and stability.

At surgery, the tobramycin beads and cement block are removed. Culture and Gram stain specimens are taken, and the knee is redebrided and copiously irrigated using pressure lavage. Then the selected components are cemented in place with antibiotics (1.2 gm of tobramycin in 40 gm of methylmethacrylate) in the bone cement. The wound is closed in a regular manner with hemovac suction. Antibiotics are continued for 5 days until the results of the culture are definitely known. The patient is started on active range of motion immediately, usually using the continuous passive motion machine, if there is no potential problem of wound healing. If the skin is tenuous, the knee is placed in a cast for 2 weeks until the wound is completely healed. It is our experience that the range of motion is not compromised by a short period of immobilization.

How about immediate exchange at initial debridement and irrigation? Rand and co-workers[23] reported only 60 percent success with immediate exchange in contrast to zero failure of delayed exchange by Insall and associates[3] in 40 consecutive cases.

What if Gram stain is positive at surgery when you are contemplating an exchange? Our choice would be an arthrodesis; if exchange is undertaken, the patient should be placed on another 6 weeks of intravenous antibiotic therapy.

FIGURE 23–2. Delayed exchange for infected total knee replacement.

A, Infection developed in an 87-year-old rheumatoid patient after revision with custom prosthesis.

B,C, Anteroposterior (AP) and lateral x-rays 14 months later showed lucency of the tibia component. Patient had a draining sinus for 12 months.

D, Knee components were removed. Wound culture revealed *Staphylococcus* to be coagulase-positive. Antibiotic cement block and beads were inserted to maintain space. The patient was placed on appropriate intravenous antibiotic therapy for 6 weeks.

E,F, Six months after exchange replacement, the patient has been doing well without recurrence of sepsis. AP and lateral x-rays revealed components still intact without evidence of loosening.

G,H, After 18 months, she had experienced no recurrence of sepsis.

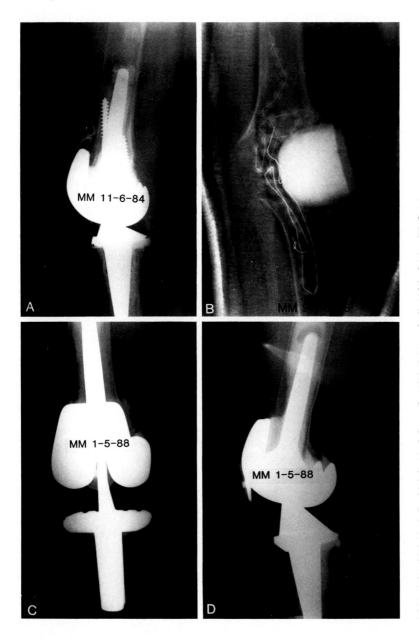

FIGURE 23-3. Delayed exchange arthroplasty and suppressive therapy.

A, Chronic infected total knee replacement for 1 year with draining sinus in a 62-year-old woman. Anteroposterior (AP) x-rays of the knee showed loosening of the tibia and femoral component.

B, Knee components were removed. Cement blocks and tobramycin beads were placed inside the joint. The leg was placed in a cylinder cast.

C,D, Delayed exchange arthroplasty was done 6 weeks later. AP and lateral x-rays of the knee at 15 months showed good position of the prosthesis. Clinically, the patient has been doing well without recurrence of sepsis. Arthrodesis would have resulted in 3 inches of shortening. Amputation was the only other alternative. If this second revision fails, the patient is willing to accept an amputation. She is receiving suppressive antibiotic therapy.

FIGURE 23-4. Arthrodesis.

A,B, Infected total knee arthroplasty of 18 months' duration and draining sinus in a 39-year-old man. Anteroposterior (AP) and lateral x-rays of the knee joint showed evidence of loosening of tibia component.

C,D, AP and lateral projections showing surgical removal of total knee components and using external fixation to maintain length with tobramycin beads to fill the space.

E,F, AP and lateral projections showed cancellous and cortical bone grafting to fill the space and maintain length.

G,H, Twelve months following fusion, including electrical stimulation, during the last 6 months there is nonunion of fusion site.

I, Closed intramedullary nailing with reaming was done.

J,K, Seven months following nailing and full weight bearing. AP and lateral x-rays showed union of the fusion site. The right leg is 1¼ inches shorter than the left leg. The patient is using a 1-inch lift in his right shoe.

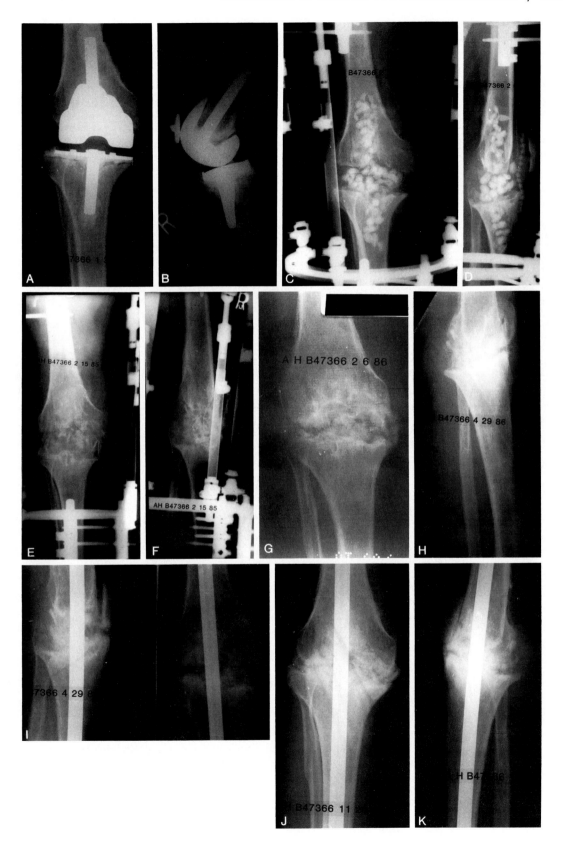

Surgical Debridement and Suppressive Antibiotic Therapy
(Fig. 23–3)

This approach is indicated in an elderly patient when revision total knee replacement has failed, or in sepsis following placement of a hinge prosthesis, when removal of the component would result in such severe bone loss that arthrodesis or resection arthroplasty or delayed exchange is not possible and the only other alternative is an above-the-knee (AK) amputation. In this particular scenario of the elderly patient or the young rheumatoid patient, surgical debridement; synovectomy without removal of components, particularly if they are not loose; insertion of tobramycin beads for 2 weeks; parenteral antibiotics for 6 weeks; and cast immobilization for 6 weeks are indicated. Following the removal of the cast and beads, a regimen of oral suppressive antibiotics is prescribed for life.

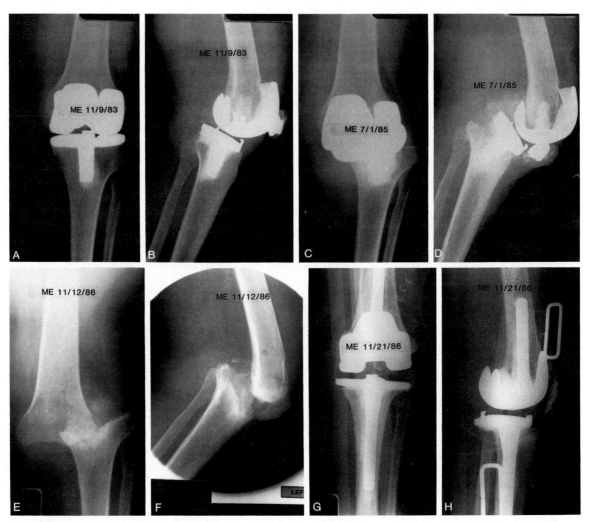

FIGURE 23–5. Resection arthroplasty.

A,B, A 68-year-old woman had a total knee replacement for degenerating arthritis. Anteroposterior (AP) and lateral x-rays showed satisfactory position of prosthesis.

C,D, Two years later, the patient presented with draining sinus and a painful knee. AP and lateral x-rays showed dislocated and loosened prosthesis.

E,F, AP and lateral x-rays of resection arthroplasty. The patient always wears a brace and is in a wheelchair primarily because of pain and instability.

G,H, AP and lateral x-rays of knee after revision with custom prosthesis. The patient has been ambulatory with a cane, and there has been no recurrence of sepsis.

Arthrodesis (Fig. 23–4)

Arthrodesis has been an accepted salvage procedure for infected arthroplasty. A variety of techniques have been reported to ensure success of the surgery.[19-24] A review of published series reveal varying success rates of fusion ranging from 17 to 88 percent.[19, 25-27] Failure was associated with lack of bone apposition, persistence of infection, and inadequate immobilization.

The indications are (1) the young patient with osteoarthritis — single joint disease, (2) a resistant organism, (3) poor skin, (4) quadriceps or patellar tendon rupture, and (5) immunosuppressed host. The surgical procedure usually consists of removal of components, and thorough total debridement and antibiotic beads. Instead of 6 weeks of waiting as in delayed exchange, we perform the arthrodesis with bone grafting in 10 to 14 days using external fixation for stabilization. The problems with arthrodesis following infected total knee replacement are a high incidence of nonunion and prolonged external immobilization (usually 10 to 12 weeks). If nonunion develops, intramedullary nailing with reaming is recommended to achieve union. Double plating may be used when nailing cannot be done because of prosthesis replacement proximally, particularly in the rheumatoid patient. The other problem in arthrodesis following septic total knee arthroplasty is marked shortening of the arthrodesed knee varying from 1 to 3 inches.

RESECTION ARTHROPLASTY
(Fig. 23–5)

According to Rand, excision arthroplasty should be reserved for the severely disabled patient with multiple joint disease and a low functional demand.[23, 28] Relief of pain and control of infection were not always afforded by this surgery. Two patients in our study had to undergo two or more debridements after removal of the prosthesis before sepsis was finally controlled.

Resection arthroplasty is indicated in a poor-risk patient, usually in the elderly patient with chronic medical problems and a low functional demand. Oftentimes, a failed arthrodesis may result in a resection arthroplasty. Overall, however, the patient has pain and cannot stand or walk for a long period of time. It is particularly disabling if the other knee is also involved.

AMPUTATION

The primary indication for amputation is uncontrollable sepsis after repeated surgical procedures. A secondary indication is an immunosuppressed host with failure to obtain wound healing and after repeated surgical failures. An AK amputation usually results with the patient confined to wheelchair. It is very seldom that a patient with an AK amputation with a good opposite leg can use an AK prosthesis.

References

1. Blin A, McBride G: Infected total knee arthroplasties. Clin Orthop 199:207, 1985.
2. Grogan T, Doney F, Rollins J, Amstutz H: Deep sepsis following total knee arthroplasty: ten year experience of the University of California at Los Angeles Medical Center. J Bone Joint Surg 68A:226, 1986.
3. Insall J, Thompson F, Brause D: Two-stage reimplantation for the salvage of infected total knee arthroplasty. J Bone Joint Surg 65A:1087, 1983.
4. Walker R, and Schurman D: Management of infected total knee arthroplasty. Clin Orthop 186:81, 1984.
5. Gristina A, Kolkin J: Current concepts review: total joint replacements in the United States. Clin Orthop 132:46, 1978.
6. Menon J, Thjelieson D, Wroblewski B: Charnley low friction arthroplasty in diabetic patients. J Bone Joint Surg 65B:580, 1983.
7. Stinchfield F, Bigliani L, Neu H, Goss T, Foster C: Late hematogenous infection of total joint replacement. J Bone Joint Surg 62A:1345, 1980.
7a. Glynn M, Sheehan J: An analysis of the causes of deep infection after hip and knee arthroplasties. Clin Orthop 101:82, 1974.
8. Andrews H, Arden G, Hart G: Deep infection after total hip replacement. J Bone Joint Surg 63B:53, 1981.
9. Cherney D, Amstutz H: Total hip replacement in the previously septic hip. J Bone Joint Surg 60A:1059, 1978.
10. D'Ambrosia R, Shoji H, Heater R: Secondarily infected total joint replacements by hematogenous spread. J Bone Joint Surg 58A:450, 1976.
11. Thomas B, Moreland J, Amstutz H: Infection after total joint arthroplasty from distal extremity sepsis. Clin Orthop 181:121, 1983.
12. Cattaghan J, Salvati E, Brause B, Rimnac C, Wright T: Reimplantation for salvage of the infected hip: rationale for the use of gentamicin impregnated cement and beads. The Hip: Hip Society Award Papers, St. Louis, CV Mosby, 1985.
13. Nelson C, Green T, Porter R, Warren R: One day versus seven days of antibiotic therapy in orthopaedic surgery. Clin Orthop 176:258, 1983.
13a. Burton D, Schurman D: Salvage of infected total joint replacements. Arch Surg 112:57, 1977.
14. Artz T, Macys J, Salvati E, Jacobs B, Wilson P: Hematogenous infection of total joint replacements: a report of four cases. J Bone Joint Surg 57A:1024, 1975.
15. Donovan T, Gordon R, Nagel D: Urinary infections

in total hip arthroplasty — influences of prophylactic cephalosporins and catheterization. J Bone Joint Surg 58A:1134, 1976.

16. Downes E: Late infections after total hip replacement. J Bone Joint Surg 59B:42, 1977.

17. Thronhill T, Dalziel R, Sledge C: Alternatives to arthrodesis for the failed total knee arthroplasty. Clin Orthop 170:131, 1982.

18. Woods G, Lionberger D, Tullos H: Failed total knee arthroplasty. Clin Orthop 173:184, 1983.

19. Broderson M, Fitzgerald R, Peterson L, Coventry M, Bryan R: Arthrodesis of the knee following failed total knee arthroplasty. J Bone Joint Surg 61A:181, 1979.

20. Frymoyer J, Hoaglund F: The role of arthrodesis in reconstruction of the knee. Clin Orthop 101:82, 1974.

21. Griend R: Arthrodesis of the knee with intramedullary fixation. Clin Orthop 181:146, 1983.

22. Johnson D, Bannister G: The outcome of infected arthroplasty of the knee. J Bone Joint Surg 68B:289, 1986.

23. Rand J, Bryan R, Morrey B, Westholm F: Management of infected total knee arthroplasty. Clin Orthop 206:75, 1986.

24. Rothacker G, Cabanela M: External fixation for arthrodesis of the knee and ankle. Clin Orthop 180:101, 1983.

25. Hagemann W, Wood G, Tullos H: Arthrodesis in failed total knee replacement. J Bone Joint Surg 60A:790, 1978.

26. Knutson K, Lindstrand A, Lidgren L: Arthrodesis for failed total knee arthroplasty. J Bone Joint Surg 67B:47, 1985.

27. Stulberg S: Arthrodesis in failed total knee replacements. Orthop Clin North Am 13:213, 1982.

28. Rand J, Bryan R: Reimplantation for the salvage of an infected total knee arthroplasty. J Bone Joint Surg 65A:1081, 1983.

John E. Lonstein, M.D.

24

Management of Postoperative Spine Infections

INTRODUCTION

An accepted complication of any spinal surgery is a postoperative infection. This can be classified as either a wound infection or disc space infection. Wound infections may follow any spinal procedure, e.g., spinal fusion, laminectomy and discectomy, or spinal decompression. A disc space infection may complicate a discogram, discectomy, or chemonucleolysis. It can also occur after an anterior spinal fusion; however, it is extremely unusual and was not found in a series of over 1000 anterior procedures.[1] This chapter discusses the occurrence, presentation, evaluation, diagnosis, and treatment of postoperative spinal wound infections and post-discectomy disc space infections.

POSTOPERATIVE WOUND INFECTIONS

Occurrence

The incidence of postoperative wound infections ranges from 3 to 10 percent.[1-4] Horwitz and Curtin reported on 531 spinal operations on 496 patients with an overall 3 percent infection rate.[2] Prophylactic antibiotics reduced the infection rate from 9.3 to 1 percent. Infections were more common if a fusion had been performed.

A large review of 7769 spinal procedures from Minneapolis and St. Paul, Minnesota, gave an overall infection rate of 2.5 percent, the majority of the procedures being spinal fusions for spinal deformity.[1] Factors related to a

From the Minnesota Spine Center, Minneapolis, Minnesota.

higher infection rate were identified. In cases performed under the age of 20, the infection rate was 1.5 percent; above the age of 20, it was 2.7 percent. The rate varied depending on the diagnosis of the spinal deformity (myelodysplasia, 7.9 percent; cerebral palsy or mental retardation, 3 percent; post polio, 2.2 percent; and idiopathic scoliosis, 1.4 percent). The use of traction was related to an increased infection rate (10.4 percent), as was the presence of previous spinal surgery (6.8 percent), especially if this had been associated with a postoperative wound infection (22 percent). The use of instrumentation was related to a higher infection rate (3.6 percent versus 1.9 percent without the use of instrumentation). On the average, the cases complicated by an infection were associated with a longer surgical procedure and greater blood loss.

The use of prophylactic antibiotics resulted in a reduction in the infection rate from 4.4 percent without antibiotic coverage to 1.2 percent with coverage. There was a reduction in all the areas noted above. This reduction is most dramatic when related to the diagnosis. In myelodysplasia the infection rate was reduced from 8.6 to 3.0 percent, and in idiopathic scoliosis it was reduced from 2.3 to 0.1 percent.

Presentation[1, 4]

As with any infectious process, the presentation of a postoperative spinal wound infection varies with the virulence of the organism, resistance of the host, and extent of the inflammatory process.

The presentation can occur early in the postoperative period or later. An early infection usually presents as a high spiking fever 2 to 5 days postoperatively. The surgical wound may be completely benign or may show swelling and erythema of the wound edges. Later presentation is with wound drainage, which may be serosanguineous to frankly purulent. This is often accompanied by localized wound separation. A rarer presentation is late after discharge from the hospital or even later with a solid arthrodesis when the first presentation of the infection is purulent drainage of a localized abscess.

Patient Evaluation

In an early infection, the patient is febrile in the immediate postoperative period. Other sources of infection (pulmonary, urinary) are investigated. The wound may appear benign, or the edges may be inflamed, edematous, and erthyematous. Gentle palpation reveals an area of tenderness. Systemic evaluation reveals a spiking fever. The erythrocyle sedimentation rate (ESR) and white blood cell (WBC) count are not in themselves diagnostic, as they are elevated in the immediate postoperative period. Baseline evaluations are obtained as rising levels indicate a continuing process; falling levels indicate that the infection is controlled.

Diagnosis

The first requirement in the diagnosis of a postoperative wound infection is a high index of suspicion. Any postoperative spiking or persistent fever must be fully investigated. The chest is examined, radiographs are made, and urine cultures are obtained. Blood cultures are ordered and taken during fever spikes.

The wound is inspected and cultures taken. After a 5-minute scrub of the wound, an aspiration is performed, localized to an area of tenderness where present. A syringe with a spinal needle is used; it is introduced a few inches lateral to the incision and directed to the area of tenderness when present. Any wound drainage is also cultured after the wound is scrubbed, thus eliminating the culture of skin bacteria. The specimen that is obtained is sent for an immediate Gram stain and also for aerobic and anaerobic cultures.

The most common organism cultured from these wound infections is *Staphylococcus aureus*. With the use of prophylactic antibiotics, two changes have occurred when an infection is present. First, the incidence of multiple organisms cultured has increased. In addition, the incidence of *Pseudomonas* cultures has increased from 17 percent prior to antibiotic coverage to 34 percent since the use of prophylactic antibiotics.[1]

Treatment

The treatment plan consists of systemic treatment and management of the wound.

Once the diagnosis has been made with a positive Gram stain or culture, treatment is instituted. When there is wound drainage or when signs are definite for the diagnosis of a wound infection, antibiotic coverage is started before a Gram stain or culture is positive. Intravenous antibiotics are given, a broad-spectrum antimicrobial of the cephalosporin group being the one initially chosen. Once the culture is obtained, the antibiotic is changed if the organism is not covered by the cephalosporins. When the antibiotic sensitivity profile is available, appropriate modification of the antibiotic coverage may be necessary. When multiple organisms are present, it is occasionally necessary to use newer antibiotics. In addition, more than one antibiotic may be necessary to give adequate antimicrobial coverage.

There are many methods available for local wound management. These include simple suture removal with wound packing, operative wound debridement with either immediate closure, delayed closure, or healing by granulation tissue.

With localized drainage or infection, it is very tempting to simply open an area of the wound on the ward, irrigate it out, and institute a program of wound irrigation and wound packing until the wound granulates in. This treatment is occasionally successful, but there are drawbacks. In most cases, the infection is not adequately treated, and persistent or recurrent drainage remains a problem. The hospitalization is prolonged, as we have found that a large proportion of these patients require subsequent surgery to treat the infection. This technique for the initial treatment of spine infections is mentioned, only to be condemned.

The best method of wound management is surgical debridement. After antibiotic therapy is instituted but before the culture results are available, the patient is taken to surgery and the wound is opened in its entirety. It is tempting, if a superficial infection is found, not to remove the fascial sutures. If only a part of the wound is infected, it is tempting not to open the whole wound. It is best to remove *all* the sutures in the muscle and fascia so that the whole surgical field is exposed to the spine, the wound being open from cranial to caudal. Any purulent material, exudate, or blood clot is sent for Gram stain and is also cultured both aerobically and anaerobically.

The wound is now debrided. All blood clots, seroma, and fluid are removed, and all necrotic tissue is debrided to normal bleeding muscle. The bone graft is carefully removed, placed in a basin, and cleaned. The wound is irrigated with copious amounts of saline or lactate solution, but the critical part of the process is the mechanical debridement of necrotic tissue. The instrumentation is not removed. Once debridement is complete, the cleaned bone graft is replaced and a decision is made regarding wound closure.

IRRIGATION AND SUCTION TUBES

If the wound is clean and healthy-appearing, primary closure is performed. Irrigation and suction tubes are inserted with two large hemovac tubes inserted deep to the fascia and two large tubes in the subcutaneous plane. One tube at each level is for ingress of the irrigating solution; the second tube is for egress and is connected to low suction. Because of the blood present in the wound after debridement, it is essential to start the irrigation and suction while the wound is being closed. This may be intermittent or a slow, continuous flow. This procedure prevents the formation of clots, which clog the system. The irrigant is saline solution without antibiotics, as adequate tissue levels are achieved with intravenous antibiotics. The irrigation-suction system is used to prevent hematoma formation—the latter being an excellent culture medium for the infecting organisms.

The wound is closed in layers by means of the same technique used in primary wound closure. Skin closure is cosmetic, with a subcuticular absorbable suture; retention sutures and mattress skin sutures are not used. Occasionally, with a low-grade localized infection with little tissue necrosis, the wound is so clean that irrigation tubes are not inserted. A hemovac drain is inserted instead. This is a very rare occurrence, and the drain should not be used if any doubt exists as to the adequacy of the debridement.

The irrigation is continued at a high level for the first 18 to 24 hours. During this period,

there is continued wound bleeding; with lower rates of irrigation, blood clots will block the system. A rate of 1000 ml/6 hours is usual, higher rates being used with marked blood tinging of the effluent. It is imperative that the irrigant and suction amounts be carefully documented. These should be equal. When discrepancies occur, they are due to obstruction of the fluid path with collection of the saline in the wound. The patency of the tubes, especially the suction tube, must be maintained. Often this problem is solved by reversing the flow; i.e., the suction tube becomes the ingress tube and vice versa. After 18 to 24 hours, the flow is reduced to 1000 ml/12 hours.

With this treatment, the patient's temperature falls and the wound is benign without tenderness or erythema. The irrigation-suction system is continued for a total of 5 to 6 days, at which time, if the infection is under control as above, all the tubes are connected to suction. The suction fluid is not cultured. With no changes in the fever or the wound after 24 hours, all the tubes are removed. The treatment of the fusion now dictates the patient's care. Ambulation and immobilization in a cast or brace now take place as in a non-infected patient. The intravenous antibiotics are continued for a total of 10 to 14 days, and oral antibiotics are then started. The WBC and ESR are checked periodically and should approach normal. Antibiotics are continued for 3 to 6 months, the exact period depending on the extent of the infection, the organism, and the wound and systemic responses.

WOUND PACKING AND DELAYED PRIMARY CLOSURE

When the wound is debrided in the operating room and is not completely healthy-looking because of significant muscle necrosis, it should not be primarily closed. This recommendation also applies to very widespread multiflora infections. In these cases, it is often difficult to differentiate healthy from necrotic tissue. The debridement is performed, and the wound is packed open. The best packing is roll-gauze (Kerlix) or vaginal packing soaked in povidone-iodine (Betadine). The wound is packed and dressed with abdominal pads and tape.

The dressing is changed in 1 to 2 days in the operating room, the timing depending on the condition of the wound. The wound is again debrided, irrigated, and repacked. This process is repeated, usually every other day for three to five changes. The appearance of granulation has not yet occurred. When the wound is clean with no evidence of infection or necrotic tissue, it is closed. Closure is performed as described above with irrigation and suction tubes. Further care is the same as above, except that antibiotic coverage is usually longer both intravenously and orally.

HEALING BY GRANULATION

With repeated dressing changes, residual infection may still be present. This rarely occurs and is found in multiflora infections or in a recurrent infection. The packing technique continues with two modifications; the dressing changes now take place on the ward, the patient being in infective isolation. The changes are performed once to twice a day. In addition, adhesive skin tapes may be needed to hold the dressings in place and to approximate the skin and subcutaneous tissue. Granulation tissue forms, and gradually the infection lessens and is controlled.

In this rare situation, the wound is allowed to granulate closed. The epithelium grows over the wound edge and must be carefully removed so that the wound can granulate from its depths, thus minimizing the area of re-epithelialized tissue. This technique is effective even in the face of exposed instrumentation. With granulation formation, the rods become covered and the wound closes.

Occasionally with smaller wounds, it is possible to perform a secondary closure. The problem with this is that tension sutures are necessary to approximate the wound, and these do not leave a cosmetic appearance. Actually, allowing healing by granulation usually gives a far superior appearance (Fig. 24–1).

After wound closure, in most cases today, recurrent infections or wound problems are unusual. These occur with a wound closed after inadequate debridement. This is usually a primary closure of a questionable wound. This also can occur after a gram-negative or multiflora infection. The systemic signs of infection persist, and the wound is edematous, erythematous, and tender. In addition, drainage may occur after removal of the tubes. Generally, the picture is one of some improvement with irrigation and suction but with a flare-up 2 to 3 days after tube removal.

In this case, the wound should be opened, as for a primary infection, and debrided. Repeat cultures are taken to exclude superinfection. The best plan now is to pack it open and allow healing by granulation. Attempts at closure in these cases is generally unsuccessful because of the recurrent and persistent infection.

The second recurrent wound problem occurs in an afebrile patient with a benign-appearing wound. There is localized wound drainage or a small area of wound separation. After a scrubbing of the area, a culture is taken. The opening is probed with a small pair of sterile forceps. In many cases, this tract goes down to the instrumentation. If the tract extends deep along the instrumentation or a pocket of purulent material drains, the whole wound needs to be reopened. Further care usually consists of packing and healing by granulation. In the rare case, the tract may pass down to the instrumentation with no extension or abscess being present. In this case, the residual wound is packed with a thin gauze strip after debridement. Continued packing occurs as the tract granulates from below. The packing should be just sufficient to keep the tract open. Overpacking makes the tract larger, and thus there is a larger area to granulate and close.

Summary

The successful treatment of a wound infection following spinal surgery depends on early diagnosis. A high index of suspicion allows the diagnosis to be made early. Wound drainage or aspirate should be cultured, and after a positive diagnosis is made, intravenous antibiotics are started. The wound is opened in its entirety and debrided and irrigated. The instrumentation is left in place, and after cleaning the bone graft is returned to the wound. Wound closure is over tubes, usually irrigation and suction, but occasionally suction only. Primary closure, delayed primary closure, or healing by granulation may be used. The exact method of closure depends on extent of the infection, the necrotic tissue in the wound, and the infecting organism. Whenever possible, a cosmetic closure is performed.

The care of the spinal fusion continues with oral antibiotics after the infection has been controlled. The fusion healing continues, but the pseudarthrosis rate after an infection is greater than in uninfected patients.

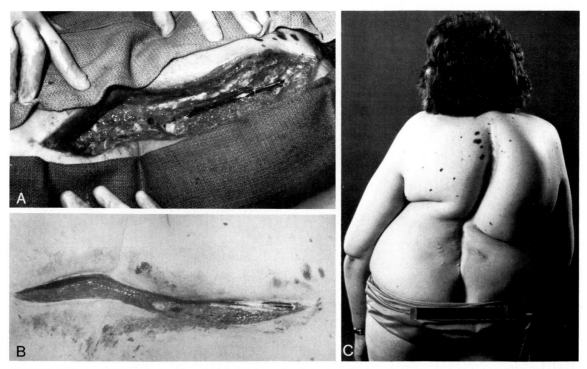

FIGURE 24–1. Wound infection following a spinal fusion for post-polio scoliosis in a 38-year-old woman.

A, Infection was diagnosed 2½ weeks after fusion. The patient was treated with debridement and closure over irrigation and suction tubes that were left in for 5 days. Four days later, there was fever with a tender wound and a positive culture of alpha *Streptococcus.* Debridement revealed necrotic fat and dead space. After debridement, the wound was packed open. The wound was redressed in the operating room. The clean wound is shown with exposed Harrington rod and granulation tissue.

B, The wound was repacked daily on the ward and gradually granulated in as shown 4 weeks later. Note the instrumentation still visible in the upper end of the wound. The patient was discharged on home care, and the wound granulated in and epithelialized.

C, A cosmetically acceptable wound is seen 10 months later.

POST-DISCECTOMY DISC SPACE INFECTION

Occurrence

Any operative approach to the disc — laminectomy, discectomy, chemonucleolysis, or discography — can be complicated by a disc space infection. Approximately 1 to 3 percent of cases of discectomy are complicated by a postoperative disc space infection.[5, 6] After chymopapain injection, the reported infection rate is lower, 0.06 to 0.08 percent.[7, 8] After discography the chance of an infection is very low.

Presentation

The presentation in these infections varies greatly. It depends on the specific infecting organism and its virulence, on the resistance of the host, and on whether the bony end plate is intact or was damaged during the surgical procedure. A mild infection presents as severe postoperative pain that gradually resolves. At the other end of the spectrum, the infection can be severe, with spread into the epidural space or into the vertebral body.

On average there is a latent period after surgery lasting days to weeks, but this is usually 7 to 12 days. After an asymptomatic period, there is the recurrence or first complaint of severe back pain. This is often accompanied by pain or cramps in the legs, abdomen, pelvic area, groin, or thighs. This often appears clinically as the same symptom complex as preoperatively. The pain is more severe and incapacitating, often resulting in voluntary bed rest. Any movement aggravates the pain.

There are no systemic signs. There is no fever or malaise. Examination shows a well-healed, non-tender, benign wound. There is marked lumbar spasm, and the pain is aggravated by slight movements. The straight leg raising is markedly restricted. Longitudinal percussion on the spine, i.e., percussion on the heel, will give severe pain. The neurological picture is unchanged.

Diagnosis

With a postoperative disc space infection, systemic signs of infection are absent. There is no fever or leukocytosis. The ESR is usually increased. At a week postoperatively, the ESR should have returned to normal; thus an increased ESR is significant, especially if it is rising.

Radiographic changes depend on the duration of symptoms.[9] Often the diagnosis is delayed, and thus radiographic changes are visible. There may be osteopenia localized to the vertebral end plate in the early stages, and later the disc space shows progressive narrowing. There is, in addition, irregularity of the subchondral end plate. These changes are better visualized using a computed tomographic (CT) scan or tomography. Magnetic resonance imaging (MRI) plays a role in the early diagnosis, as it shows the inflammation in the acute stage when radiographs are negative (Fig. 24–2). In addition, the bone scan will be positive.

A bacteriologic diagnosis is important. Blood cultures are obtained. In addition, a needle biopsy with aspiration is performed. This is best accomplished under radiographic control to ensure correct placement of the needle. This can be done under fluoroscopic or CT control. The ideal needle placement is adjacent to or into the involved subchondral bone plate. If no aspirate is obtained, it is useful to inject 1 or 2 ml of saline and then aspirate this in an effort to obtain the etiologic agent. The success of the aspiration depends on the stage of the inflammatory process that is present. In early inflammation without necrosis and purulence, the aspirate is usually negative.

Management

The management of postoperative or post-interventional disc space infections consists of antibiotics, immobilization, and drainage.

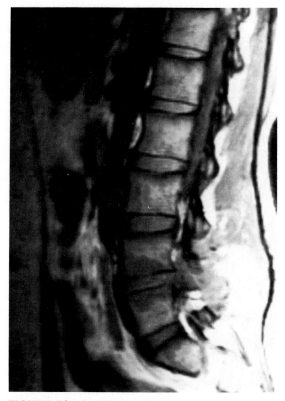

FIGURE 24–2. MRI scan taken 2 months following a laminectomy and discectomy at L4-5. Note the narrowing of the disc space and the bony changes in the end plates adjacent to the disc space.

Once the diagnosis is made (on clinical and/or bacteriologic grounds) a broad-spectrum antibiotic is started. One of the cephalosporins is usually given, initially parenterally and then orally. If a positive blood or aspirate culture has been obtained, the appropriate antibiotic is given. Because of the severe pain on movement, immobilization is necessary. Depending on the muscle spasm and pain present, this can be initial bed rest with later use of a body cast or thoracolumbosacral orthosis (TLSO) or immediate ambulation in a cast or TLSO. The ESR is followed as an indication of control of infection, antibiotics being used until this returns to normal. In 50 percent of cases, a spontaneous segmental disc space fusion occurs.[10]

In some cases, the response to treatment, i.e., antibiotics and immobilization, is poor. The infection spreads with abscess formation and osteomyelitis of the adjacent vertebra or vertebrae. This is seen clinically as a poor response to the antibiotic with persistent or increasing pain and a rising rather than falling

ESR. In addition, the radiographic changes increase with marked end plate changes showing the spread of the infection. This lack of response indicates an ongoing infection resulting from an inappropriate antibiotic and/or an already established osteomyelitis.

Surgical debridement and drainage are indicated at this stage. This has been described posteriorly or anteriorly.[11] An anterior approach allows better debridement and drainage without the danger of epidural seeding of the infection. A sympathectomy approach is used, and the appropriate disc space is entered with removal of the annulus. At the lumbosacral junction, it is usually necessary, in addition, to remove a wedge of the lower end plate of the fifth lumbar vertebra to adequately visualize the disc space. All necrotic material is debrided from the disc and end plates and are sent for Gram stain and culture. In these resistant infections, aerobic, anaerobic, and fungal cultures are performed. Once complete debridement has been carried out to bleeding bone, cancellous bone graft is inserted to ensure a fusion. Appropriate antibiotics are started parenterally, and immobilization is performed as above.

The duration of therapy—both immobilization and antibiotics—varies greatly. It depends on the infection (acute or chronic), its site (disc space above or involving the end plates), and response to therapy. The course of therapy thus can range from weeks to months. A narrow disc space is seen following the healed infection, with spontaneous fusion in 50 percent of cases.

With a high index of suspicion or pain after discectomy, discography, or chemonucleolysis injection, diagnosis can be made early, and with prompt treatment, excellent resolution of the infection will result.

References

1. Transfeldt EE, Lonstein JE, Winter RB, et al: Wound infections in elective reconstructive spinal surgery. Orthop Trans 9:128, 1985.
2. Horwitz NH, Curtin JA: Prophylactic antibiotics and wound infections following laminectomy for lumbar disc herniation. Neurosurg 43:727–731, 1978.
3. Simchen E, Stein H, Sacks TG, et al: Multivariate analysis of determinants of postoperative wound infections in orthopaedic patients. J Hosp Infect 5:137–146, 1984.
4. Taylor TKF, Dooley BJ: Antibiotics in the management of postoperative disc space infections. Aust NZ J Surg 48:74–77, 1978.
5. El-Gindi S, Aref S, Salama M, Andrew J: Infection of the intervertebral discs after operation. J Bone Joint Surg 58B:114–116, 1976.
6. LaRocca HL: Infections of the spine. Clin Neurosurg 25:296–304, 1978.
7. Agre K, Wilson RR, Brim M, McDermott MJ: Chymodiactin postmarketing surveillance. Spine 9:479–485, 1984.
8. McCulloch JA: Chemonucleolysis: experience with 2000 cases. Clin Orthop 146:128–135, 1980.
9. Allen EH, Cosgrove D, Millard FJC: The radiological changes in infections of the spine and their diagnostic value. Clin Radiol 29:31–40, 1978.
10. Thibodeau AA: Closed space infection following removal of lumbar intervertebral disc. J Bone Joint Surg 50A:400–410, 1968.
11. Garrido E: Closed irrigation suction technique in the treatment of lumbar laminectomy infection. Neurosurg 5:354–355, 1979.

Leo J. de Souza, M.B.

CHAPTER

25

Infection of the Spine

INTRODUCTION

Infection of the spine is classified as (1) *disc space infection,* classically seen in children but also encountered in adults and following disc surgery; and (2) *vertebral osteomyelitis,* most commonly seen in adults, now increasingly in the intravenous drug abuser, and occasionally in the infant.

The primary location of infection, whether in the disc space or in the vertebral body, is determined by the nature and extent of its blood supply.

The blood supply of the intervertebral disc has never been quite clear, and studies dealing with its vascular status have been relatively scanty.[1-5] However, the work of Whalen,[6] dealing with the vasculature of the developing vertebral end plate in relation to the nutrition of the disc, has thrown much light on this subject.

The annulus fibrosus and nucleus pulposus are avascular. Nutriment is brought to the disc by cartilage canals in the cartilaginous end plate, each canal consisting of an arteriole, terminal sinusoidal capillaries and venules, the vessels terminating at the hyaline cartilage – disc interface (Figs. 25 – 1 to 25 – 3). The cartilage canals originate from two sources, the arterial plexus outside the perichondrium and the nutrient artery to the vertebra. Blood-borne bacteria via the circumferentially placed cartilage canals originating in the arterial plexus could settle in the disc and give rise to primary infection. The disc could also be secondarily infected by spread along the cartilage canals from a metaphyseal locus in the vertebral body. The persistent presence of the cartilage canals in the cartilage end plates in infants and children explains the predominance of disc space infection in the young age group[7, 8]

and the much less common occurrence in the adult.[9]

The vertebral body is vascularized mainly by the nutrient artery entering the vertebral body through the nutrient foramen posteriorly. The area with maximal vascularity is the metaphysis adjacent to the anterior longitudinal ligament as a result of its being supplied both by the nutrient vessels and the peripheral arterioles.[5] If invading organisms lodge in the vertebra, it is understandably in this location. Infection spreads from here to the disc, and involvement of more than one level may occasionally be noted. Vertebral osteomyelitis is most commonly seen in adults, although it is very occasionally encountered in infants.[10]

DISC SPACE INFECTION

Children

Disc space infection is encountered classically in children, in the 11-month to 16-year age range, with a mean age of 7 years. It is not yet a very clearly understood entity and is generally presumed to be a syndrome wherein back pain is associated with disc space narrowing, fever, and an elevated erythrocyte sedimentation rate (ESR). However, it is believed to result from a hematogenous infection.[7, 8, 11-14]

There is no doubt about this pathogenesis when an organism is isolated from the affected disc space, but the mild clinical signs and symptoms, the infrequency of positive cultures (being positive only in about a third of the cases), the nonspecific changes on tissue examination, and the favorable outcome without antibiotics have led some to believe that the lesion may not be infective. In fact, Alexander[15] suggested trauma as an etiology, wherein disruption occurs at the epiphysiometaphyseal junction, resulting in disc space narrowing.

From the Department of Orthopaedic Surgery, Hennepin County Medical Center, Minneapolis, Minnesota.

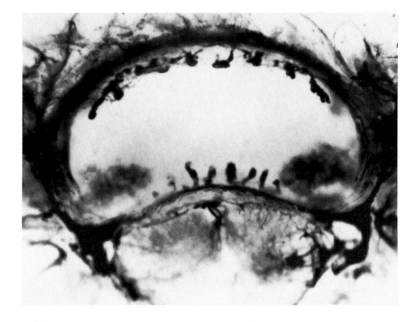

FIGURE 25–1. Transverse section of lumbar vertebrae in a newborn rabbit demonstrates the circumferential array of cartilage canals within the hyaline cartilage end plates. (Courtesy of J.L. Whalen, M.D., Ph.D.)

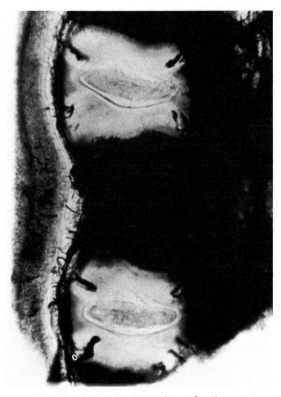

FIGURE 25–2. Sagittal section of adjacent lumbar vertebrae in a human fetus shows orientation of cartilage canals to the inner layers of the intervertebral disc. The nucleus pulposus and annulus fibrosus are clearly demarcated. The cartilage canal vessels lie completely outside the avascular intervertebral disc and have never been observed to enter disc tissue. (Courtesy of J.L. Whalen, M.D., Ph.D.)

However, the frequent presentation of malaise and fever and an elevated ESR, together with prompt response to antibiotics, seems to indicate that an infectious etiology must be operative in most, if not all, patients with the syndrome. *Staphylococcus aureus* is the organism most often isolated. The lower half of the vertebral column is most commonly involved, most particularly the lower lumbar region.

DIAGNOSIS

The outstanding symptom in the young child, 3 years of age and younger, is refusal to walk and later to stand or even sit. In the older child, about half present with low back pain, and a quarter with hip and leg pain. Abdominal pain as a presenting symptom is noted in 10 percent of the children, and meningeal irritation in another 10 percent.[16] A history of preceding illness, often upper respiratory or ear infection, or sometimes trauma, is obtained in 50 percent of the patients.

A young child prefers a recumbent position; an older child will limp. Physical findings consist of paravertebral muscle spasm and limitation of motion, with alteration of the spine configuration, usually a decrease or loss of lumbar lordosis, limitation of straight leg raising, localized tenderness at the site of the lesion, and pain on heel strike. The temperature is usually elevated, but rarely above 101° F.

Laboratory investigations should include complete blood count, ESR, and blood cul-

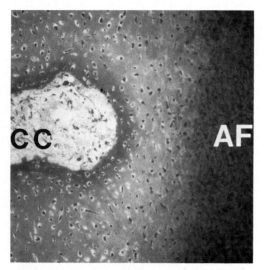

FIGURE 25-3. In a highly magnified picture (human fetus at 16 weeks), the cartilage canal (CC) can be seen to end 150 μm from the highly cellular inner layer of the annulus fibrosus (AF). (Courtesy of J.L. Whalen, M.D., Ph.D.)

ture; throat or urine cultures, and depending on epidemiological or clinical circumstances, tests for typhoid, paratyphoid and brucellosis, skin test for tuberculosis, and a chest film may be in order. The leukocyte count is usually noted to be at the upper limit of normal, but the ESR is invariably elevated to 40 to 60 mm/hr. Blood cultures are more likely to be positive in a child with acute symptoms or when the temperature is elevated to 101° F and above. The earliest roentgenographic changes take at least 3 weeks to appear from the onset of the symptoms. Narrowing of the disc space is the first radiological sign, followed by vertebral end plate haziness, irregularity, and erosion (Fig. 25-4). A bone scan helps localize the lesion much earlier and a technetium 99m (^{99m}Tc) scan is preferred at the initial screening for technical reasons, availability, and rapidity of results; should it be negative, the gallium 67 (^{67}Ga) scan should be carried out.[17, 18]

The bacteriological diagnosis is made by needle aspiration biopsy of the affected disc if it has not already been made by the blood cultures. However, it is not always necessary to resort to this diagnostic procedure, particularly since positive results are noted in only about a third, the causative organisms are usually known to be gram-positive cocci, and the response to antibiotic therapy and rest is usually satisfactory. The specific indications for needle aspiration biopsy therefore would be,

failure to respond to antibiotic therapy and rest, and in those geographic areas where unusual infections are known to be present, e.g., fungal disease, brucellosis, and tuberculosis.[8,19]

MANAGEMENT

The most important aspect of management is rest. Initially, the child is put to bed. Later, appropriate immobilization in a body cast or brace may be required if the child continues to be uncomfortable. Immobilization is then continued until back pain, muscle spasm, and local tenderness have subsided, until the ESR is down to normal limits, and until the roentgenograms indicate that no bony destruction is taking place. However, immobilization is generally not necessary for the younger child who responds to antibiotics and who walks and moves the spine comfortably, but it is often needed in the older child, who tends to have a more protracted course, lasting 2 to 3 months.[8]

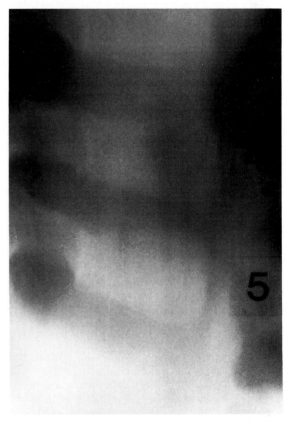

FIGURE 25-4. Radiograph of a 9-year old male child, showing narrowing of disc space at L4-L5 with irregularity and haziness of superior end plate of L5 vertebra.

Antibiotics are almost always given on the basis that the disc space lesion is the result of hematogenous infection. When the organism is cultured either from the blood or the disc space and the sensitivities are determined, the selection of the appropriate antibiotic is no problem. When no bacteriological diagnosis has been made, the selection of antibiotic is based on the fact that *S. aureus* is the most commonly isolated organism. The antibiotic most often selected, therefore, is one that is primarily anti-staphylococcal. First-generation cephalosporins or one of the penicillins effective against penicillinase-producing organisms are administered initially intravenously, later orally. Antibiotics are continued until the temperature is normal, pain has subsided, the ESR is back to normal, and radiological healing is in progress, which usually takes 4 weeks to a few months.

Antibiotics, however, are not universally used and in some centers are administered only if specific indications exist, such as a positive biopsy specimen or blood culture, clinical progression in spite of adequate immobilization, and recurrence of back pain accompanied by increased ESR or an elevated temperature.[7] Bye and Taylor[19] found no difference in the outcome of children treated by immobilization with or without antibiotics. They suggested antibiotic coverage if clinical and laboratory findings indicated a fulminating process despite enforced immobilization.

Complete clinical recovery is the usual outcome, with most patients showing residual narrowing of the disc and about 25 percent partial to complete fusion.

Adults

Although it is well known that disc space infection affects children, it is not as widely known that it can involve adults, in whom vertebral osteomyelitis is more common. Kemp and colleagues[20] outlined the differences between pyogenic infection arising primarily in the intervertebral disc and that arising primarily in the vertebral body. The two conditions shared a common etiology in that they usually occurred secondary to existing or preceding infection, but they differed in the site of involvement and in their clinical and radiological presentation. In pyogenic infections occurring primarily in the intervertebral disc in the adult, diagnosis was delayed on an average by 6 months from the onset of symptoms, which was partly due to failure to recognize the radiological signs of the lesion. The use of a bone scan is

therefore highly recommended. The disease also exhibited a marked chronicity, but the most serious feature was the high incidence of spinal cord involvement, which was probably related to the delay in diagnosis. In addition, the paraplegia complicating disc space infection was often rapid in development, more frequently irreversible, and due mainly to direct extension of the inflammatory granulations posteriorly to involve the meninges and occasionally the cord.

The radiological features were quite distinctive. The earliest change noted was decrease in the height of the disc. Progressive subchondral sclerosis associated with an increase in density of the adjacent areas of the vertebral bodies on either side of the affected disc was noted 2 to 3 months later, followed after a variable period by subchondral erosion. Approximately 50 percent of the lesions did not progress beyond this stage. Attempts at healing occurred by circumferential bone bridging. Those that did progress were characterized by "ballooning" of the disc space with erosion of the vertebral bodies (Fig. 25–5). The progressive radiologi-

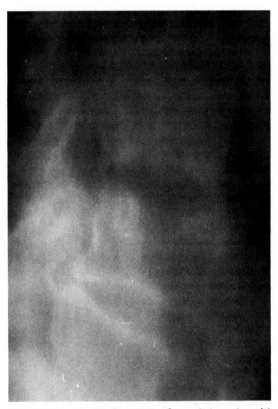

FIGURE 25–5. Radiograph of an adult male, with "ballooning" of the disc space (arrow) and erosion of the adjacent vertebrae.

cal features reflected the pathological process, wherein the infection was initially restricted to the discs with reactive changes only in the adjoining vertebrae. Only when the disease spread to involve the adjacent vertebrae as depicted in the "ballooning" were the changes consistent with osteomyelitis.

With regard to management, an aggressive approach was recommended in view of the fact that the incidence of paraplegia was very high.[20] If the condition was diagnosed early and the causative organism was identified by blood cultures or needle biopsy, conservative management with appropriate and intense antibiotic therapy was given a trial, particularly in patients in whom exploration was expected to be difficult or hazardous. If the diagnosis was overly delayed and the disease process already protracted with no bacteriological diagnosis, the lesion was explored anteriorly[9, 21, 22] for adequate debridement and decompression, and, if necessary, for fusion. In the presence of impending paraplegia, the decompressive procedure was performed as a matter of urgency.

Postoperative Infection

Infection of the intervertebral disc occasionally supervenes following the surgical procedure of discectomy. In our experience, it has been a very infrequent complication; however, the incidence is known to range from 0.75 to 2.98 percent.[23, 24]

In a typical case, the lumbar incision remains well healed and the infection is confined to the intervertebral disc. Two weeks to 2 months following the relief of the preoperative leg and back pain, a recurrence of low back pain is noted, which is severe and excruciating, aggravated by movement and out of proportion to the clinical findings. The findings are sparse excepting for marked muscle spasm. The ESR is invariably raised, and the leukocyte count invariably normal.

Staphylococcus is the most commonly encountered pathogen, although other grampositive and gram-negative organisms have been encountered. A bacteriological diagnosis can be made in more than two thirds of the patients (69.5 percent) following needle biopsy or surgery.[25]

The earliest radiographic findings noted after 4 weeks is marked narrowing of the disc space. Subsequent progression to irregularity of the adjoining end plates and reactive sclerosis is seen in about half of the cases. Spread of infection results in bone destruction, whereas healing leads to fusion or fibrous ankylosis, in approximately 6 months' time. Computed tomography (CT) would reveal changes typical of disc space infection at a much earlier date.

In magnetic resonance imaging (MRI), increased signal intensity in a postoperative disc should alert one to the presence of infection since most postoperative discs show degenerative changes and decreased signal intensity on T_2 sagittal images. The increased signal intensity should not be mistaken for a normally hydrated disc.[35]

After an attempt to obtain a bacteriological diagnosis, which includes a needle aspiration biopsy, management consists of immobilization of the lumbar spine, antibiotics, and surgery when indicated. Immobilization of the lumbar spine in a double hip spica cast results in an almost dramatic relief of pain. In the early case, 3 to 4 weeks of immobilization is adequate; in the late case, 4 to 6 weeks are required. Initially, cephalosporins are administered parenterally and, depending upon results of culture and antibiotic susceptibility tests, may be changed to more appropriate antibiotics. In the absence of a culture isolate, broad-spectrum antibiotics are given parenterally for 4 to 6 weeks (see Chapter 16 for a discussion of various alternatives). When the diagnosis is made late, antibiotics are less effective; these patients may be satisfactorily managed by immobilization alone.[26] Surgery is needed in about 25 percent of cases.[25] The indications for debridement and, if necessary, decompression and/or fusion are persistence of pain, marked systemic reaction not responding to conservative therapy, and the development of neurological complications.

Disc space infection has also been observed following the intradiscal injection of chymopapain, the infection rate ranging from 0.06 to 2.5 percent.[26a,26b,27] Bacteriological diagnosis is made by needle aspiration biopsy, and causative organisms usually are *S. aureus* and coagulase-negative staphylococci.

VERTEBRAL OSTEOMYELITIS

Adults

Once considered rare, with one or two cases being seen yearly in major medical centers, the incidence of vertebral osteomyelitis appears to be rising owing to an increase in number of elderly patients with chronic and debilitating diseases that predispose to infection.[28] Over 60 percent are aged 50 and above, and men are affected twice as often as women.[29]

The infective focus in the vertebral metaphysis adjacent to the anterior longitudinal ligament, if untreated, leads to bony destruction with collapse and kyphos, and to abscess formation, which may be paravertebral or sometimes more distant, although this occurs much less commonly than in tuberculous infection. Infection almost invariably spreads to the adjacent vertebra and the intervening disc. Contiguous posterior extension of the infection to involve the neural arch, meninges, and neural tissue may occur, with resultant complications of epidural abscess, meningitis, neurological deficits, and paraplegia. The incidence of paraplegia is estimated to be in the vicinity of 5 percent.[30]

The lumbar spine is involved most frequently and accounts for more than half the cases. The thoracic spine is involved less frequently and the cervical spine least often.

DIAGNOSIS

Preceding illness providing the primary source of infection is often located in the genitourinary tract, skin, or upper respiratory tract. In a typical presentation, the symptoms would consist of back pain, preceded by or associated with fever, chills, and general malaise. However, the onset of spinal pain could be very insidious and the systemic reaction mild or absent, making diagnosis difficult. A small number of patients may present atypically, with referred abdominal or chest pain. In addition, many of the patients will have associated chronic ailments such as urinary tract infections, diabetes, renal disease with or without dialysis, arthritis, and occult or undiagnosed malignant disease. Urinary tract pathology was found in 46.5 percent of the cumulative series of 172 patients presenting with vertebral osteomyelitis,[29] and in a study of 40 cases by Garcia and Grantham,[31] diabetes was present in 25 percent. Some of these chronic illnesses not only obscure the spinal lesion but also may predispose to it.

The classic symptoms of back pain, fever, chills, and general malaise, even when they are present, are therefore very likely to be confused with chronic illnesses commonly found in the elderly, to the extent that vertebral osteomyelitis has been termed "the great masquerader."[32] This has led, not infrequently, to error or delay in diagnosis. Common misdiagnoses have included degenerative disc disease, digestive and renal disorders with lumbar spine involvement, and cardiac or respiratory disorders with thoracic spine involvement. Occasionally, patients have undergone surgery for the correction of these presumed conditions before a correct diagnosis was made. To date, the average time from the onset of symptoms to the final accurate diagnosis has been 9 weeks.

However, in the studies that have been undertaken, most errors in diagnosis could be traced to a failure to pay proper attention to the symptom of back pain localized to the level involved.[12] Although on occasion local pain might have been overshadowed by radicular pain, it was noted in all patients.[12, 29, 31, 32a] It is therefore important to keep this presenting symptom constantly in mind as well as the entity of pyogenic infection of the spine, if it is not to be overlooked as often as it has been.

Physical examination will reveal localized tenderness at the affected spinal site, with pain on local percussion[30] or axial compression. Associated spasm and rigidity would be noted, except in lesions proximal to the tenth thoracic vertebra owing to the relative immobility of the dorsal spine.

In a protracted or untreated case, late complications of a distant abscess, kyphos deformity, neurological deficit, and paraplegia might be encountered. Paraplegia is more likely to occur in the older patient, in a patient with cervical involvement, in the presence of diabetes mellitus or rheumatoid arthritis, and when the causative organism is S. aureus.[33]

The most common pathogen in the causation of vertebral osteomyelitis is S. aureus, which is responsible for more than half of the cases. However, virtually every important clinical organism has been implicated, including a variety of bacterial species and fungi. Gram-negative organisms are encountered with increasing frequency in patients with urinary tract pathology, and Pseudomonas aeruginosa is seen in intravenous drug abusers.

As in disc space infection, the white blood cell (WBC) count is not significantly raised in any of the patients seen at the time of diagnosis. The ESR is the most helpful indicator, being raised on an average to 60 mm/hour. Blood should be obtained for culture at regular intervals over a 2-day period, as it is found to be positive either prior to the onset of the fever or when the fever is 101° F and higher. However, since patients are generally seen several weeks after the initial symptoms and the initial bacteremia, blood cultures are helpful only occasionally. Besides urine cultures, other useful tests may include serologic tests for *Salmonella* or *Brucella* infection and skin tests for tuberculosis.

The earliest radiological evidence becomes manifest 4 to 6 weeks following the onset. Edema of the paravertebral tissue is seen early, most often in the cervical spine.[12] The earliest bony changes of focal destruction occur anteriorly in the metaphysis, with mild collapse and development of kyphos, narrowing of the disc space, and involvement of the adjacent vertebra. The progressive changes will be clearly revealed by lateral tomography.[29] Paravertebral abscess will be revealed by enlargement of the retropharyngeal space in the neck, a paravertebral shadow in the thorax, and a paravertebral shadow with decrease in the definition of the psoas muscle in the lumbar spine. Healing is heralded by reactive new bone appearing at the vertebral margins with eventual bony bridging across the disc space. Fusion may eventually occur with a varying degree of angular deformity.

In the early stages, even before radiographic changes have had time to appear, the bone scan would be positive. The ^{99m}Tc scan is again preferred at the initial screening to the ^{67}Ga scan, which is resorted to in the event that the technetium scan is negative.

CT scanning also provides earlier information as well as delineates the extent and severity of the disease. In the axial views, a lytic fragmented appearance is noted in the adjacent vertebral bodies without clear differentiation of the disc. The mottled appearance is likened to that of "Swiss cheese," but the margins of the punched-out areas are irregular (Fig. 25–6). In severe cases, the defects are confluent, with destruction of large areas of the vertebral body and disc. These changes are mostly encountered in the anterior portion of the vertebral body; the posterior portion is involved when the infective lesion is progressive. Sagittal and coronal reformations confirm the destructive end plate irregularity along with the lytic changes seen in the vertebral body and the related sclerotic changes. In addition to the earlier diagnosis provided by these findings, a great advantage of the CT scan is in the demonstration of the surrounding paravertebral inflammatory soft tissue as well as epidural and neural canal changes.[34] Magnetic resonance imaging now provides depiction of even earlier manifestations of the disease, which are easier to detect and interpret, particularly in the sagittal views (Fig. 25–7).[35]

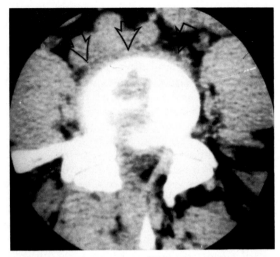

FIGURE 25–6. CT scan of lumbar vertebra showing irregular lytic areas of destruction in the end plate. The arrows point to the symmetrical almost circumferential soft tissue mass, extending from the disc margin, which is seen earlier than the end plate destruction and later regresses to normal after the discitis has cleared.

MRI T_2-weighted images show increased signal intensity in the involved disc as well as erosion and destruction of the adjacent end plates. When osteomyelitis is present, it is seen as decreased signal intensity of the marrow of the adjacent vertebral bodies on T_1-weighted images which become high signal intensity on T_2-weighted images due to the active inflammation and oedema. Sequestra present as low signal intensity lesions at the margins of the vertebra on both T_1- and T_2-weighted images. With healing, the abnormal increased signal intensity of the disc and vertebra on T_2-weighted images reverts to normal.[35]

A bacteriological diagnosis is essential for appropriate antibiotic therapy. If blood and urine cultures have been negative and antibody tests have not been helpful in identifying the pathogenic organism, a needle aspiration biopsy, and occasionally an open biopsy, are indicated. Needle biopsy is readily carried out in the lumbar spine, but there is general reluctance to using it in the thoracic spine for fear of damaging pleura and lung and in the cervical spine for fear of transgressing neurovascular structures. However, if the entry of the needle is medial to the angle of the rib[36] or if the needle is placed 4 cm from the midline, passed superior to the ribs, and kept at an angle of 35°, the pleura and lung are avoided.[37] In the cervical spine, needle biopsy of the C4 through

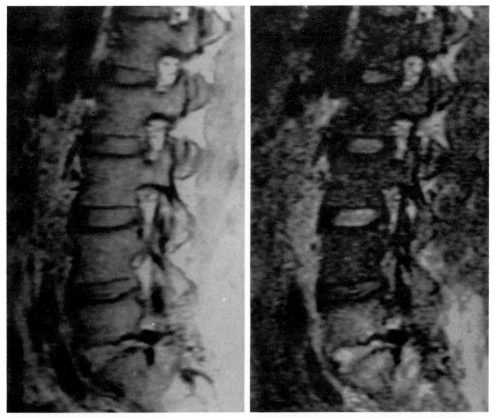

FIGURE 25–7. MRI sagittal views showing increased signal intensity on the proton density and T2-weighted images within the L5-S1 disc space were read as being due to infection, as concomitant CT scan studies showed severe destruction of the L5-S1 disc. On the T2-weighted image, the L5 and S1 vertebral bodies are of high-signal intensity in contrast to the normal low-signal intensity of the normal L3 and L4 vertebrae. This is indicative of active infection.

T1 vertebrae is carried out from a lateral approach[38] and of the first three vertebrae through an anterior or pharyngeal approach.[38] When present, a retropharyngeal or paravertebral mass in the neck is more easily accessible to aspiration.

The possible diagnostic yield for needle aspiration is approximately 68 percent.[39] If a needle biopsy is impractical or yields negative results, particularly in the presence of inconclusive clinical and radiological findings, open biopsy or surgical exploration may become essential.[30] In the lumbar and cervical spine, the anterior approach generally undertaken for the definitive treatment is employed; in the thoracic spine, a costotransversectomy is undertaken.

MANAGEMENT

With vertebral osteomyelitis being uncommon and then overlooked when encountered, it is imperative that it be constantly kept in mind when an ill patient presents with back pain (Fig. 25–8). Suspicion, an ESR determination, and a scintigram ought to help unmask "the great masquerader." Once the condition is diagnosed, management is relatively straightforward.

Patients whose condition is diagnosed in the early stages usually respond satisfactorily to rest and antibiotics. Bed rest can be supplemented by adequate orthoses: appropriate collars or braces for the cervical spine, and total contact plastic orthosis, plaster jackets, or braces for the thoracic and lumbar spine. It might occasionally be necessary to immobilize the cervical spine in skull tongs or halo to prevent collapse of the affected vertebra.[40]

Antibiotics are routinely employed once the diagnosis has been made. Ryan and Taylor[41] have suggested, however, that whereas there is a well-established case for antibiotics in acute osteomyelitis of the spine in the adult, such is

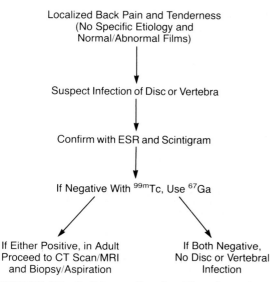

Localized Back Pain and Tenderness
(No Specific Etiology and
Normal/Abnormal Films)

↓

Suspect Infection of Disc or Vertebra

↓

Confirm with ESR and Scintigram

↓

If Negative With ^{99m}Tc, Use ^{67}Ga

If Either Positive, in Adult
Proceed to CT Scan/MRI
and Biopsy/Aspiration

If Both Negative,
No Disc or Vertebral
Infection

FIGURE 25–8. Diagnostic algorithm for spinal infection.

not the case for chronic or low-grade infective lesions, particularly of the lumbar spine.

The specific antibiotic depends on the bacteriological diagnosis. In the event of the latter not being obtained or possible, broad-spectrum antibiotics are administered promptly, with cephalosporins or penicillin with an aminoglycoside being those most commonly used (see Chapter 16 for guidelines). Antibiotics are administered intravenously for 4 to 6 weeks, depending on progress, which is monitored by the degree of pain and spasm, serial ESR determinations, and radiological changes. Patients who present in the chronic stage, whose condition is diagnosed late, or who do not respond to rest and antibiotics are more likely to need specific surgical procedures consisting of debridement, decompression, and, if necessary, stabilization of the spine. Stabilization is usually limited to one level, although on rare occasions more than one segment may need to be dealt with. Specific indications have been outlined by Leong.[42] These are (1) failure of conservative treatment to relieve symptoms and constitutional upset, (2) late presentation with significant bone erosion, (3) neurological deterioration, and (4) significant deformity. Urgent surgical intervention would be needed if paraparesis or paraplegia develops.

The approach to the spine is anterior, which is only logical as the pathology is located anteriorly. These anterior approaches have been well described.[9, 21, 22, 43, 44] Debridement consists of excision of the affected bone and disc

and the accompanying granulation tissue and abscess. In the presence of neurological complications, decompression of the dura and cord is carried out by more extensive debridement posteriorly, including excision of the posterior longitudinal ligament to fully expose and free the neurological tissue. After removal of the infected tissue, bone grafting is usually carried out to stabilize the spine, particularly if the amount of diseased tissue removed is substantial; besides, bone grafting can help improve the kyphotic deformity and expedite intervertebral fusion.[9, 45] A bone graft is best obtained from the iliac crest; the excised ribs can be used, but supplemental use of cancellous or corticocancellous bone is often required.

Results from anterior debridement and fusion have been satisfactory.[9, 32, 42, 46] In Leong's study, 25 patients treated surgically for vertebral osteomyelitis by anterior debridement and spinal fusion experienced excellent immediate relief of symptoms with no recurrences in a 3½-year follow-up. Neurological recovery was noted, with improvement of the kyphotic deformity in 16 of the 17 patients, and the fusion rate was 90 percent.[42] In patients with extensive disease and significant kyphosis deformity, a second-stage posterior instrumentation and fusion might be necessary, although this is not common.

In the past, it was customary to approach the infected area by a posterior route. The laminectomy understandably aggravated the problem, as removal of the stable uninvolved posterior elements led to subluxation of the spine and increased neural compression.[33] It was also more likely to injure the nerve tissue en route and to extend the infection to the dura. A posterior laminectomy approach, therefore, should always be avoided.

Intravenous Drug Abusers

It is practical to consider intravenous drug abusers with vertebral osteomyelitis as a separate group. The drug addict is most frequently a young male adult. The majority present with symptoms earlier than the non-addicted group and almost always with back or neck pain localized to the area of involvement. One out of ten patients with lesion in the cervical spine will present with sore throat and dysphagia. The lumbar spine is involved most often as in the general non-addicted group and accounts for more than half the cases. However, there is a much higher incidence of cervical and a much lower incidence of thoracic involvement. The cervical spine is involved in more than 25 percent, the thoracic spine in less than 5 percent.[47]

A positive bacteriological yield is obtained in more than 95 percent, gram-negative rods making up more than 80 percent of the total. The *Pseudomonas* species are predominant (66 percent) followed by *Serratia, Klebsiella,* and *Enterobacter. S. aureus,* the most common organism in the general population, is encountered much less frequently, in only 15 percent. It is not uncommon for concomitant infections, caused by the same organism, to be present at other sites.

The principles of management remain the same. Parenteral antibiotic therapy for 4 weeks or longer is successful in over 90 percent of patients; about 8 percent are known to experience relapse, and a second course of antibiotics of similar duration is regularly quite effective. Antibiotic choice is discussed in Chapter 16.

Bed rest is adequate for most patients. When the neck is involved, it is rested in a collar or brace. The lumbar spine occasionally needs to be immobilized in a brace, body cast, or total contact orthosis.

With the usually satisfactory outcome following antibiotic therapy, surgery is needed only infrequently. Open biopsy and exploration may be necessary if a bacteriological diagnosis cannot be obtained from needle aspiration biopsy, blood, or abscess cultures.

The prognosis of vertebral osteomyelitis in the intravenous drug abuser remains good. No severe permanent neurological deficits have been encountered, and no fatal outcome has been reported.[47]

Infants

Vertebral osteomyelitis has been known to occur in infants under the age of 6 months.[10] The pathology resembles adult vertebral osteomyelitis, but the infection is severe and bone destruction extensive.

The osteomyelitis is associated with septicemia usually due to *S. aureus.* Severe dissolution of the vertebral body occurs with sparing of the end plates. The ill child responds to prolonged antibiotic treatment, requiring antibiotic therapy for 3 months, with initial parenteral administration for 3 weeks. A late sequela, however, is a short segment kyphosis, which results from extensive destruction of the vertebral body.

The disease in infants is the result of severe infection of the vertebral body, as distinct from disc space infection in children, which has a generally benign course.[10]

SUMMARY

Disc space infection and vertebral osteomyelitis are distinct clinical entities and are therefore grouped accordingly. It cannot be overemphasized that localized back pain is the outstanding symptom; diagnosis will be confirmed by harboring a suspicion of the pathology and following it with ESR determinations and scintigraphic studies (Fig. 25–8).

The most common pathogen is *S. aureus,* but gram-negative organisms are frequently encountered in adult patients with urinary tract infections and *Pseudomonas* in drug abusers. A bacterial diagnosis, therefore, is essential; for the same reason, a biopsy/aspiration is very important in the adult patient.

The mainstay of treatment consists of rest and antibiotics, but surgery may be required in the adult with disc space infection, in vertebral osteomyelitis, or postoperatively.

References

1. Coventry MB, Ghormley RK, Kernohan JW: The intervertebral disc: its microscopic anatomy and pathology. Part 1. Anatomy, development and physiology. J Bone Joint Surg 27:105, 1945.
2. Mineiro JD: Coluna Vertebral Humana: alguns aspectos da sua estrulura e vascularizatoa. Lisboa, Disserrtacao de Doutoramento, 1965.
3. Smith NR: The intervertebral discs. Br J Surg 18:358, 1931.
4. Somogyi B: Blood supply of the foetal spine. Acta Morphol Sci Hung 12:261, 1964.
5. Wiley AM, Trueta J: The vascular anatomy of the spine and its relationship to pyogenic vertebral osteomyelitis. J Bone Joint Surg 41B:796, 1959.
6. Whalen JL, Parke WW, Mazur JM, Stauffer ES: The intrinsic vasculature of developing vertebral end plates and its nutritive significance to the intervertebral discs. J Pediatr Orthop 5:403, 1985.
7. Spiegel PG, Kenglo KW, Issacson AS, Wilson JC: Intervertebral disc-space inflammation in children. J Bone Joint Surg 54A:284, 1972.
8. Wenger DR, Bobechko WP, Gilday DZ: The spectrum of intervertebral disc space infection in children. J Bone Joint Surg 60A:100, 1978.
9. Kemp HBS, Jackson JW, Jeremiah JD, Cook J: Anterior fusion of the spine for infective lesions in adults. J Bone Joint Surg 55B:715, 1973.

10. Eismont FJ, Bohlman HH, Soni PL, Goldberg VM, Freehafer AA: Vertebral osteomyelitis in infants. J Bone Joint Surg 64B:32, 1982.

11. Doyle JR: Narrowing of the intervertebral disc space in children. J Bone Joint Surg 42A:1191, 1960.

12. Griffiths HED, Jones DM: Pyogenic infection of the spine. J Bone Joint Surg 53B:383, 1971.

13. Guri PG: Pyogenic osteomyelitis of the spine. J Bone Joint Surg 28:29, 1946.

14. Stone DB, Bonfiglio M: Pyogenic vertebral osteomyelitis. Arch Intern Med 112:491, 1963.

15. Alexander CJ: The aetiology of juvenile spondyloarthritis (discitis). Clin Radiol 21:178, 1970.

16. Rocco HD, Eyring EJ: Intervertebral disc infection in children. Am J Dis Child 123:448, 1972.

17. Bruschwein DA, Brown ML, McLeod RA: Gallium scintigraphy in the evaluation of disc space infection. J Nucl Med 21:925, 1980.

18. Norris S: Early diagnosis of disk space infection with 67Ga in an experimental model. Clin Orthop 144:293, 1979.

19. Bye WD, Taylor TKF: Antibiotics in the management of inflammatory lesions of the intervertebral discs in young children. Aust NZ J Surg 48:70, 1978.

20. Kemp HBS, Jackson JW, Jeremiah JD, Hall AJ: Pyogenic infections occurring primarily in intervertebral discs. J Bone Joint Surg 55B:698, 1973.

21. Hodgson AR, Stock FE: Anterior spinal fusion: a preliminary communication on the radical treatment of Pott's disease and Pott's paraplegia. Br J Surg 44:266, 1956.

22. Hodgson AR, Stock FE: Anterior spine fusion for the treatment of tuberculosis of the spine. J Bone Joint Surg 42A:295, 1960.

23. Lindholm TS, Pylkkanen P: Discitis following removal of intervertebral disc. Spine 7(6):681, 1982.

24. Pilgaard S: Discitis (closed space infection) following removal of lumbar intervertebral disc. J Bone Joint Surg 51A:713, 1969.

25. Fernand R, Lee CK: Post-laminectomy disc space infection. Clin Orthop 215, 1986.

26. Tayler TKF, Dooley BJ: Antibiotics in the management of postoperative disc space infection. Aust NZ J Surg 48:74, 1978.

26a. Agre K, Wilson RR, Brim M, McDermott MJ: Chymodiactin postmarketing surveillance. Spine 9:479, 1984.

26b. McCulloch JA: Chemonucleolysis: Experience with 2000 cases. Clin Orthop 146:128, 1980.

27. Deeb ZL, Schimel S, Daffner RH, Lupetin AR, Hryshko FG, Blakey JB: On intervertebral disk space infection after chymopapain injection. Am J Roentgenol 144:671, 1985.

28. Musher DM, Thorsteinsson SB, Minuth JN, Luchi RJ: Vertebral osteomyelitis—still a diagnostic pitfall. Arch Intern Med 136:105, 1976.

29. Kersley JB: Non-tuberculous infection of the spine. Proc R Soc Med 70:176, 1977.

30. Collert S: Osteomyelitis of the spine. Acta Orthop Scand 48:283, 1977.

31. Garcia A, Grantham SA: Hematogenous pyogenic vertebral osteomyelitis. J Bone Joint Surg 42A:429, 1960.

32. Walinski TN: Vertebral Osteomyelitis. Presented at the American Academy of Orthopaedic Surgeons, Atlanta, 1980.

32a. Digby JM, Kersley JB: Pyogenic non-tuberculous spinal infection. J Bone Joint Surg 61B:47, 1979.

33. Eismont FJ, Bohlman HH, Soni PL, Goldberg VM, Freehafer AA: Pyogenic and fungal vertebral osteomyelitis with paralysis. J Bone Joint Surg 65A:19, 1983.

34. Price AC, Allen JH, Eggers FM, Shaff MI, James Jr AE: Intervertebral disk-space infection: CT changes. Radiology 149:725, 1983.

35. Heithoff KB: Personal communication, Minneapolis, 1988.

36. Craig FS: Vertebral-body biopsy. J Bone Joint Surg 38A:93, 1956.

37. Valls J, Ottolenghi CE, Schajowicz F: Aspiration biopsy in diagnosis of lesions of vertebral bodies. JAMA 136:376, 1948.

38. Ottolenghi CE, Schajowicz F, De Schant FA: Aspiration biopsy of the cervical spine. J Bone Joint Surg 46A:715, 1964.

39. Armstrong P, Chalmers AC, Green G, Irving JD: Needle aspiration biopsy of the spine in suspected disc space infection. Br J Radiol 51:333, 1978.

40. Messer HD, Litvinoff J: Pyogenic cervical osteomyelitis. Arch Neurol 33:571, 1976.

41. Ryan MD, Taylor TKF: The bacteriological diagnosis and antibiotic treatment of haematogenous vertebral osteomyelitis in adults. Aust NZ J Surg 48:81, 1978.

42. Leong JCY: TB and adult spine infections. Spine Problems: Controversies and Update meeting, University of Minnesota, Minneapolis, July 11, 1985.

43. Kirkaldy-Willis WH, Thomas TG: The surgical approaches to the vertebral bodies. J R Coll Surg Edinb 10:109, 1965.

44. Southwick WO, Robinson RA: Surgical approaches to the vertebral bodies in the cervical and lumbar regions. J Bone Joint Surg 39A:631, 1957.

45. Shaw NE, Thomas TG: Surgical treatment of chronic infective lesions of the spine. Br Med J 1:162, 1963.

46. Emery SE, Chan DPK, Woodward HR: Pyogenic osteomyelitis—anterior debridement and fusion. First annual meeting of the Federation of Spine Associations, New Orleans, February 20, 1986.

47. Sapico FL, Montgomerie JZ: Vertebral osteomyelitis in intravenous drug abusers: report of three cases and review of the literature. Rev Infect Dis 2:196, 1980.

Raymond T. Morrissy, M.D.
Steven L. Shore, M.D.

CHAPTER

26

Septic Arthritis in Children

INTRODUCTION

Septic arthritis in childhood can result from hematogenous seeding, direct extension from bone, or direct inoculation from a puncture wound. From experimental work it is assumed that the pathology in all three is alike.[1]

In direct spread from bone or inoculation by puncture, it is obvious how the bacteria get into the joint. In the case of hematogenous spread, however, it is not as clear. Much as in the case of acute hematogenous osteomyelitis, many of the observed characteristics are not adequately explained by the assumption that hematogenous spread is all that is involved. In some situations, e.g., *Haemophilus influenzae* in the young, there is a septicemic pattern with meningeal as well as multiple joint involvement; in other children, only a single joint is involved without additional apparent illness. When a single joint is involved, it is most often the knee, followed by other joints of the lower extremity. Although trauma has been implicated as the reason,[2] there is no conclusive proof that this is a fact.

Another curious observation is that certain organisms have a predilection for the joints that varies with age. Of particular note, however, is that these are often not the organisms that affect the bone. In the case of endocarditis, it has been shown that the streptococcal cell wall has an affinity for the mucopolysaccharide in the vegetation growing on the damaged valve, thus explaining the predominance of this organism in endocarditis. Although such cell wall affinity may explain in part the prevalence of certain organisms in certain tissues, other factors, e.g., the colonization of distant tissues, must also play a large part. All of these observed facts demonstrate the complex etiology of hematogenous joint infections.

PATHOPHYSIOLOGY

Several models of septic arthritis have been described. Most rely on the direct injection of bacteria into the joint,[2-4] although septic arthritis can be produced in some animals with certain bacteria via the hematogenous route.[5, 6] Scheurmann has noted in an animal model that septic arthritis is more likely to develop in traumatized joints.[2] This is in keeping with certain risk factors that are recognized in the clinical setting: arthritis, recent trauma, or recent surgery. The synovial membrane is a unique organ in that it is very vascular, does not have a basement membrane, and produces a fluid that combines many of the components of serum with unique products of the synovium itself. The production of septic arthritis by the hematogenous route emphasizes the important role of the bacterial-host relationship, for it is apparent that most bacteremias do not result in septic arthritis.

Within a few hours of the introduction of bacteria into the joint, the bacteria will be found in the synovium. Over the next 24 to 48 hours, there will be a marked inflammatory response in the synovium, with bacteria and inflammatory cells entering the joint. If the process can be eradicated by the host or with antibiotics during this period, no changes in the cartilage appear to occur. However, as time goes on, many components of the inflammatory response begin to destroy the cartilage. This first occurs by enzymes liberated from the leukocytes. Next, the synovial cells also release destructive enzymes; eventually, the damaged cartilage itself liberates collagenase. Finally, organisms such as *Staphylococcus aureus* may

From the Scottish Rite Children's Hospital, Atlanta, Georgia.

elaborate proteolytic enzymes. In experimental models of septic arthritis, it is the ground substance that is destroyed first. This may occur as early as 5 days after the infection begins.[8] This loss is not visible to the naked eye; however, it changes the mechanical properties of the cartilage, making it more flexible.[9]

Daniel and associates[10] performed experiments in rabbit knees infected with *S. aureus* by direct inoculation. On the second day, antibiotic treatment was started. Half of the animals underwent surgical lavage of the knees at 4 and 7 days. At 4 days, thick fluid was washed from the joint; however, at 7 days, it could no longer be washed out and had to be removed manually. This material as well as synovial biopsy specimens at 7 days grew no organisms. These animals were killed at 2 and 12 weeks. At 2 weeks, matrix loss was equal in both groups; however, collagen loss was greater in the joints that were not lavaged and was termed insignificant in those that were. Of particular interest was the finding that there was still evidence of an inflammatory reaction in the animals killed at 12 weeks, 11 weeks after the joint was sterile. The exact nature and cause of this persistent inflammation are controversial and incompletely understood, probably varying with the causative organism and other host factors.

DIAGNOSIS

The symptoms and signs of joint infection vary greatly with age.

The Neonate

In the neonate, as pointed out in the discussion on osteomyelitis (see Chapter 27), the signs and symptoms may be few.[7] Affected children in this age group are often hospitalized for other reasons. Frequently, they are recognized as having sepsis but the subtle joint findings will be missed in the early stages of the infection. Because of the immature immune system in the newborn, there is a blunted inflammatory response with a consequent lack of obvious swelling or restricted motion. Diagnosis is also confounded by fat in the extremities and the mild joint contractures that are normal for this age group. As a general rule, any signs of sepsis in the neonate should also be suggestive of joint sepsis and in addition, multiple joint sepsis. Aspiration should be performed on any suspected joint. If a joint is

found to contain pus, it may be advisable to aspirate both hips because the consequences of missing a hip infection are extremely severe. In addition, an infected hip is the most likely joint to be missed on the basis of clinical examination alone.

The Infant

In infants between 2 months and walking age, the diagnosis is less difficult. The irritability caused by the pain is often noted by the parents, especially when they are changing diapers. Joint swelling and restricted joint motion are more easily noted, and discomfort is more obvious. In young infants, paralysis of a limb, usually an upper limb, may be the presenting complaint. This pseudoparalysis may be erroneously attributed to trauma.

The Child

In young children there may be a brief interlude, e.g., half a day when the child will limp, followed by refusal to walk. The more recently a child has learned to walk, the more quickly he or she may be to quit in the face of discomfort. Here, as in older children, the signs and symptoms are more easily recognized. In children who present with a gait disturbance, an infectious etiology is common. In the case of septic arthritis as well as hematogenous osteomyelitis, the initial diagnosis is often incorrect.[11]

PHYSICAL EXAMINATION

The physician must seek evidence of infection and possible predisposing causes. The orthopedic examination has two purposes: to elicit signs of infection and to determine its location. In terms of the musculoskeletal system, this means observing swelling and, less commonly, erythema; eliciting tenderness; and detecting decrease in the range of motion. The problem is that this is not always very easy, especially in younger children, particularly around the pelvis.

In young children who are irritable and crying, the examination will be impossible except for the detection of an absolute loss of motion, and even here the examiner may not be certain. In such cases, the parents can often be instructed to examine for the tenderness and restricted motion after they have quieted the child. Although this is more time-consuming, it is often rewarding.

LABORATORY STUDIES

Laboratory studies can be helpful, but may also be misleading. Although the white blood cell (WBC) count is often elevated, this is not always the case, especially in the first few days.[12] Therefore, a normal WBC count should not cause the physician to discard the diagnosis of septic arthritis. The erythrocyte sedimentation rate (ESR), on the other hand, is almost always elevated, often greatly.[13]

RADIOGRAPHS

The use of plain radiographs in suspected joint infections is both helpful and necessary. It is necessary because it can rule out a contiguous bone lesion, destruction of the joint, or a foreign body. Reports have emphasized the problems in relying on the radiograph for the diagnosis of joint sepsis. One review found that 50 percent of septic hips showed normal radiographic findings,[14] whereas another noted that older children were more likely to lack radiographic signs in septic arthritis.[13]

Despite such reports, plain radiographs can be very helpful if properly taken. Since the earliest radiographic signs are swelling in the deep soft tissue layer and obliteration of the tissue fat planes, views of the opposite extremity, positioned symmetrically to the affected extremity, will demonstrate these important findings (Fig. 26–1). The pitfalls in attempting to interpret radiographs without symmetrical positioning or comparison views have been described in the hip.[15]

BONE SCAN

Technetium bone scans do not have the same value in the evaluation of joint sepsis that they do in acute hematogenous osteomyelitis. It must be remembered that the primary value of a scan is to detect the area involved. The decreased value is not due to the fact that a good quality scan is incapable of detecting increased uptake of radioisotope in the joint; rather, the diagnosis can usually be made by a good examination of the joint motion followed by aspiration.[16] Contiguous foci of bone involvement and multiple sites of sepsis are two situations in which the scan may be useful. However, its limitations, e.g., inability to de-

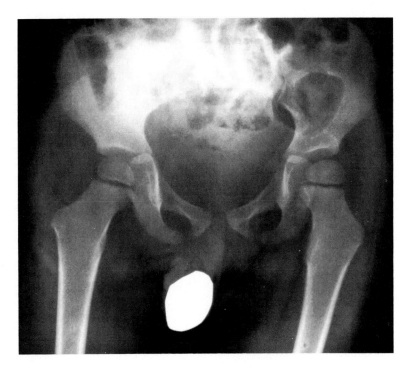

FIGURE 26–1. Anteroposterior radiograph of the pelvis of a 4-year-old child with septic arthritis of the right hip with symptoms persisting for 3 days. Although there are no changes in the bone and only questionable widening of the joint space, note the soft tissue changes that have occurred around the hip. The amount of deep soft tissue that is visible lateral to the trochanter, and the femoral neck is much greater on the patient's right side than the left, indicating deep soft tissue swelling. Also notice the swelling in the soft tissues medial to the femoral neck. The fat plains, which are easily visible around the left hip, are somewhat diminished and indistinct on the right hip. These findings are sufficient to suggest inflammation in the region of the proximal femur.

tect 50 percent of foci in the neonate, must be kept in mind.[8]

ASPIRATION

Aspiration is the diagnostic procedure of choice. It should be performed on all joints in which sepsis is a possibility. It is a test that is readily performed and one that is associated with extremely low morbidity. Aspiration can usually be done adequately with sedation and local anesthesia. However, if circumstances or physician preference warrants, the need for a general anesthesia is no excuse not to aspirate a suspected joint.

The hip is probably the most difficult joint to aspirate, especially in the young child. If pus or fluid is not obtained, the examiner cannot be certain that the needle was in the hip. To circumvent this problem, the aspiration can be done under fluoroscopy or with an image intensifier. At the time of aspiration, a small amount of dye is injected into the joint to confirm needle placement if no pus or fluid is aspirated. This can obviate an unnecessary exploration if the hip joint is not the focus of the pathology.

Proper care and testing of the aspirated material are very important. In the beginning, it may be advisable to rinse the syringe with heparin to prevent clotting of the aspirated material because clotting makes accurate analysis impossible. All material should be transported immediately to the laboratory.

CULTURES AND FLUID ANALYSIS

At a minimum, aerobic and anerobic cultures should be performed. In addition, media should be used that will support the growth of *H. influenzae* and *Neisseria gonorrhoeae*.

Next in importance is the WBC count, followed by the Gram stain. Other tests, e.g., glucose and protein, may occasionally prove valuable, but in practice seldom add to the studies already mentioned (Table 26–1). The WBC count is a generally reliable indicator of infection. However, it must be remembered that early infections may be associated with low WBC counts suggestive of a nonspecific synovitis, whereas juvenile rheumatoid arthritis fluid may reveal WBC counts above 100,000/ml.[9]

An organism causing a clinical infection will liberate antigen in the host. This may reach concentrations sufficient for detection in certain fluids. Methods to detect such antigen, e.g., counterimmunoelectrophoresis and latex agglutination, have been widely used to analyze the spinal fluid of patients with meningitis. Such methods have also been adapted to other body fluids, e.g., joint fluid, urine, and serum with variable success. When positive, they can be useful in rapid identification of the organism before cultures grow; in the event of negative cultures, they may provide the only evidence of the organism.[17, 18] Unfortunately, these methods are not useful for the detection of *S. aureus*.

DIFFERENTIAL DIAGNOSIS

The differential diagnosis of septic arthritis can be difficult, even with aspirated material to examine. Among the diagnoses that should be considered are trauma, juvenile rheumatoid arthritis, nonspecific synovitis, and rheumatic fever.

Perhaps the most common error in the diagnosis of septic arthritis is to ascribe the swelling and pain to an episode of trauma, and yet traumatic effusions are frequently seen in adolescents and occasionally in children. In most

TABLE 26–1. Synovial Fluid Analysis

Disease	White Blood Cell (WBC) Count	Percent Polymorphonuclear Leukocytes (PMNs)
Normal	<200	<25%
Traumatic	<5000 with many red blood cells	<25%
Toxic synovitis	5000–15,000	<25%
Acute rheumatic fever	10,000–15,000	50%
Juvenile rheumatoid arthritis	15,000–80,000	75%
Septic arthritis	80,000–200,000	>75%

The WBC count and percentage of PMNs present can vary in most diseases, depending on the severity and duration of the process. Overlap greater than shown in these "averages" is possible.

cases when trauma is the cause of the swelling of a joint, it takes place within 24 hours of the injury; in septic arthritis following a traumatic episode, the swelling usually begins more than 24 hours after the trauma. Depending on the nature of the injury, patients with a joint having a traumatic effusion usually experience a more comfortable range of motion than those with a septic joint.

A related and particularly vexing problem is the child who sustains a deep abrasion over the patella area and presents 2 days later with surrounding cellulitis and a joint effusion. Is the joint septic? The abrasion should be inspected closely as to depth and location to determine whether there has been entry into the joint. However, most of these are cases of cellulitis with a sympathetic effusion in the joint. These patients will be most comfortable with the knee in extension in contrast to those who have a joint infection and cannot tolerate full extension. In addition, patients with cellulitis and effusion experience a more comfortable range of motion, with the pain being localized to the area of the abrasion. If reason for doubt exists, aspiration should be performed. If aspiration is unavoidable, it may be performed through an area of cellulitis, with the recognition that antibiotics started for the cellulitis should be adequate to kill the small number of organisms that may have been introduced into the joint.

Juvenile rheumatoid arthritis (JRA) can present in much the same manner as a septic knee. Proving the adage that nothing destroys confidence like follow-up, one of the authors has operated on three "septic knees" over a 14-year period that have subsequently proved to be JRA. Although it is often felt that more than 100,000 WBCs/ml in the synovial fluid is diagnostic of JRA, this is not always so.[3] A distinguishing clinical characteristic of a patient with the knee affected by JRA is that the motion is generally more comfortable than in a patient with a septic knee. This can be even more obvious when considered in light of the large effusions characterizing joints affected with JRA. Other than this, however, the presenting picture may be indistinguishable from septic arthritis and aspiration may yield pus.

Toxic synovitis of the hip is often difficult to differentiate from *septic arthritis* of the hip. Patients may both present in the same way, with refusal to walk, and both conditions exhibit the same physical finding, indicating an inflamed hip joint. Unlike septic arthritis, however, toxic synovitis of the hip does not generally occur in children before walking age. The ESR usually is mildly elevated in toxic synovitis and greatly elevated in septic arthritis. Aspiration of the hip with synovial fluid analysis is often the only way to ensure a diagnosis of toxic synovitis. Since the consequences of delay in diagnosis and treatment of the septic hip can be very devastating, this test should not be delayed if any doubt exists.

Patients with rheumatic fever may present with a painful joint or joints, the pain usually being out of proportion to the swelling. In general, the evanescent nature of the joint symptoms and the presence of a heart murmur alert the clinician to this disorder early in its course. Detection of a heart murmur emphasizes the importance of the general physical examination.

TREATMENT

The principles of treating bone and joint infections have been discussed in the chapter on acute hematogenous osteomyelitis (AHO); see Chapter 27. This chapter discusses the application of those principles to joint infection.

As in the case of AHO, treatment goals are predicated on an understanding of the pathological process and in particular how tissue — in this case cartilage — is destroyed. As emphasized in the chapter on AHO, every effort must be made to obtain a bacteriological diagnosis before antibiotics are started. This means the gathering of all material that may yield the offending organism.

Aspiration of pus from the joint is the first step. However, in septic arthritis the cultures are positive in only 54 percent[19] to 69 percent.[13] The reasons for this are obscure. Pus is a hostile environment for the growth of organisms. In aspiration of bone in hematogenous osteomyelitis, the yield of positive cultures is about the same: 60 percent. The yield with bone biopsy is about 90 percent.[20] Although there is no evidence to indicate a higher yield with synovial biopsy, it is probably wise to send a specimen at the time of drainage. In addition, blood cultures should be obtained; these are usually positive in approximately 40 percent.[19]

In gonococcal arthritis the yield from joint cultures will be even lower than is the case with other organisms. In cases of disseminated gonococcal infection, joint cultures are positive in less than 50 percent of cases and the blood cultures are positive in less than 20 percent.[21] This means that for children with findings suggestive of gonococcal infection, whether from sexual activity or inapparent sexual molestation, cultures of suspected orifices should be performed.

Killing of the organisms that are causing the infection is one aspect of the treatment. The beginning of antibiotic therapy should not be delayed until the positive bacteriological identification of the organism. Therefore, if Gram stain does not reveal the identity of the organism, a best guess will have to be made; this is much more difficult in the case of joint sepsis due to the multiplicity of organisms that may be involved. In septic arthritis, the age of the child has the greatest bearing on the choice of initial antibiotic therapy. When age is coupled with knowledge of recent or concomitant infection, a correct guess should be possible in a high percentage of cases (Table 26–2).

The Neonate

In the neonate the organisms are the same as in AHO; as has been mentioned earlier, these two conditions frequently coexist in this age group.[7] Gram-negative enteric organism, e.g., *Escherichia coli*, group B streptococci, and *S. aureus* are all common. *Candida* is also likely, especially in neonates undergoing central venous catheterization, hyperalimentation, or prolonged antibiotic therapy.[22] A good antibiotic choice, therefore, consists of oxacillin and gentamicin unless a fungus has been identified. It bears repeating that neonates and infants

with musculoskeletal sepsis should be cared for in conjunction with an expert in infectious disease or neonatology.

The Infant

In infants younger than the age of 2 years and perhaps as old as 4 years, the two most common organisms are *H. influenzae* type B and *S. aureus*.[19, 23] Less common organisms that are found in septic arthritis in this age group are group B and group A streptococci. It is well known that most pathogenic staphylococci today are penicillin-resistant. However, it should also be realized that a significant percentage of *H. influenzae* joint sepsis seen today is caused by beta-lactamase–producing organisms. Approximately 35 percent of the clinical infections caused by *H. influenzae* in our institution are due to these organisms. Complicating this even further is the possibility of coexistent meningitis in patients with *H. influenzae* or group B streptococcal septic arthritis,[18] the symptoms of which are often minimal in this age group. With these facts known, initial therapy should be effective against resistant strains of *S. aureus* and *H. influenzae*, and the drug for *H. influenzae* should cross the blood-brain barrier. Currently, cefuroxime meets these criteria. A second alternative is a combination of chloramphenacol and a semisynthetic penicillin.

Again, it is advisable that a person knowledgeable in the treatment of infectious dis-

TABLE 26–2. Initial Antibiotic Therapy for Septic Arthritis

	Organisms	Initial Antibiotic Choices
Neonates	Group B streptococci *Staphylococcus aureus* Gram-negative coliforms	Oxacillin and gentamicin* or cefotaxime*
Infants and children 4 weeks–4 years	*S. aureus* *Haemophilus influenzae* Group B streptococci† Group A streptococci†	Cefuroxime 100–150 mg/kg/day
Children >4 years	*S. aureus* *Neisseria gonorrheae*	Oxacillin 150 mg/kg/day or cefazolin 100/mg/kg/day

* Dosages depend on age and prematurity. See discussion on acute hematogenous osteomyelitis (Chapter 27).

† Usually in a patient under 1 year of age.

eases be involved in the treatment of these young children.

The Child

In the older child, *H. influenzae* becomes less likely and *S. aureus* more likely. The advisability of using only an anti-staphylococcal drug as initial therapy depends on the treating physician's certainty that *H. influenzae* is not present.

DELIVERING THE ANTIBIOTIC: KILLING THE BACTERIA

After the antibiotic is selected, it must be delivered to the bacterial site; in septic arthritis, this means into the joint fluid or pus and the synovium. Do adequate concentrations of antibiotic enter the septic joint? Although there has been occasional opinion to the contrary, the current wisdom is that they do. In a study by Nelson, concentrations of ampicillin, methicillin, penicillin, and cephalothin were found to be in excess of the concentrations necessary to kill the usual pathogens.[24] Adequate concentrations may also be achieved by the oral route.[25] There is a second question, which has not been answered as well: Do the antibiotics work in the environment of a septic joint? The low pH and other factors in a pus-filled joint are not the optimal conditions for antibiotic action. Good experimental work in this area is lacking. However, there is evidence that it may take considerable time to sterilize a septic joint with antibiotics alone.[26]

Most investigators recommend a shorter course of antibiotic therapy for joint sepsis than for bone sepsis. This is based on empiric observation more than on well-controlled studies. Again, many factors are involved: the organism; the nature of the infection, e.g., whether there is septicemia or not; and the adequacy of the debridement, i.e., surgical drainage and lavage or repeated needle aspiration. Some organism can be treated for a lesser period. Jackson and Nelson recommend a minimum of 3 days for gonococci, 10 to 14 days for *H. influenzae,* and 21 days for *S. aureus,* coliform bacilli, and *Pseudomonas.*[27]

The caution against using intra-articular antibiotics should be emphasized. Intra-articular antibiotics are not necessary; as it has already been shown, antibiotics enter the joint in adequate concentrations. In addition, they may cause a chemical synovitis and, in the case of neomycin, may result in absorption of toxic amounts of antibiotic.

DEBRIDEMENT AND DRAINAGE

The second aspect of treatment is to remove the pus from the joint. This generally accepted principle is based on the knowledge of how cartilage is destroyed. There are three techniques for accomplishing this: arthrotomy, arthroscopy, and aspiration.

Arthrotomy

The techniques of arthrotomy may vary considerably, but their purpose is the same: to provide access to the joint adequate to allow thorough lavage. Usually, a large incision is not required; rather, a small incision that allows small retractors to be placed as an aid to the irrigation of the joint with a soft rubber catheter is sufficient (Fig. 26–2).

The question frequently arises as to the best approach to the hip joint. Tradition dictates a posterior approach. However, there are several reasons to consider an anterior approach. The major blood supply to the femoral head is in the retinaculum of the posterior part of the hip joint and may be inadvertently injured during the capsulotomy. If the hip dislocates, it will most likely do so posteriorly, and this may be made easier or irreducible by the presence of a hole in the posterior capsule. The landmarks for the surgical approach are much clearer than they are for the posterior approach, especially in a fat child with swelling. Last, dependent drainage with a drain between the skin and joint not only is unnecessary but also invites secondary infection. The anterior approach is made through a small transverse incision, separating the sartorius-tensor interval just below the anterior superior iliac spine. This leads directly onto the anterior hip capsule (Fig. 26–3).

Whether or not and how continuing drainage is achieved after the arthrotomy is often a matter of training and personal preference. A review by Patterson calls into question the need for any continuous drainage at all in the routine cases, in which surgical debridement has taken place in the first 5 days.[28] With this in mind, it probably makes little sense to leave joints open with drains in place, considering the disruption of normal joint physiology, the

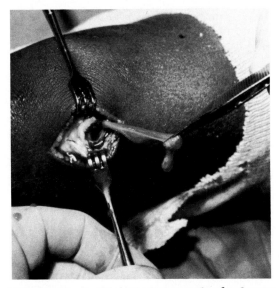

FIGURE 26–2. Clinical photograph of a 6-year-old patient with septic arthritis of the knee. The organism was *Haemophilus influenzae.* Symptoms were present for 5 days prior to drainage. Note the size of the incision. It need not be a long incision to drain the knee adequately. A small entry into the capsule, which permits irrigation and inspection with small retractors, is adequate. Note also the pus being withdrawn from the knee with the forceps. This was not removed by aspiration, could not be removed by aspiration, and is difficult to remove, even with an open drainage. This is the fibrinous exudate that accompanies the synovitis and is frequently found in septic arthritis of joints. It harbors bacteria and inflammatory products and must be removed as part of the debridement.

risk of secondary infection, and the discomfort that their manipulation causes the child. Although not proven necessary, a brief period (12 to 24 hours) of closed suction-irrigation with a physiological solution has an appeal to logic. It is a form of continuous closed debridement. This removes the fibrinous exudate, which tends to reaccumulate while the joint is inflamed. Such removal may be of value while the joint is being "sterilized" by the antibiotics, for it will prevent the loculation and sequestration of the organisms from the antibiotic in the synovial fluid.

Arthroscopy

The use of the arthroscope in draining septic joints, especially knees, has increased over the past 5 years. To date there is little published evidence on which to judge its effectiveness. In the knee it is not easy to see what advantage this technique has over a 2-cm incision when the set-up time and potential for damaging the articular cartilage in a small knee obscured with pus and hyperemic synovium are considered.

Aspiration

Repeated aspiration has had and continues to have its advocates. The exception to this is in cases of septic arthritis of the hip when surgical drainage is the universal recommendation. However, aspiration fails in one important aspect: it is an inadequate debridement (Fig. 26–2). This can be proved by first aspirating the joint and then proceeding immediately with arthrotomy. The additional pus and the fibrinous exudate that could not be removed with the needle will be apparent. This reservoir of inflammatory debris that always remains after aspiration is responsible for the continued and prolonged synovitis that is characteristic of joints treated by repeated aspiration. If these reasons should not be enough, the trauma to the patient of repeated aspiration should convince the physician that the conservative and kind course of treatment is an intelligently performed arthrotomy.

The one exception to the problems with aspiration as a treatment concerns gonococcal infections. It has been empirically observed that many joints recover very quickly after appropriate antibiotic therapy has been started and that lingering synovitis is not a problem. Many of these infections are not bacterial in origin but result from an immune reaction secondary to the disseminated gonococcal disease. Of those due to the presence of *N. gonorrhoeae* in the joint, some will resolve promptly with one aspiration and antibiotics. If fluid reaccumulates, however, arthrotomy and drainage may be necessary.

FOLLOW-UP

To date, the ideal follow-up study on septic arthritis does not exist. In view of the experimental findings of unobservable biochemical and subtle histological changes in the articular cartilage, such a study would be important. It is quite possible that the patient who does well

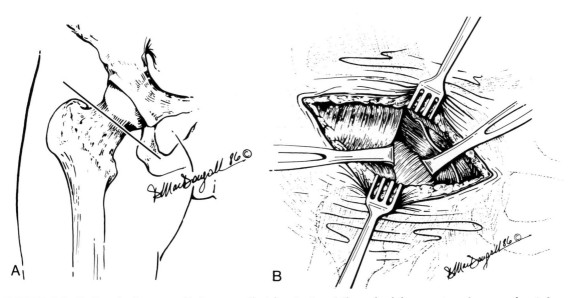

FIGURE 26–3. Surgical approach to a septic hip. *A,* An oblique incision centered approximately a thumb breadth below the anterior superior iliac spine and angles inferior and medial. This incision need not be as large as one used for open reduction of the hip. *B,* The incision is made and carried through the fat. The sartorius tensor interval is identified, and the two muscles pulled apart. The lateral border of the rectus femoris is identified and retracted medially, thus exposing the precapsular fat and the capsule of the hip joint. An incision into the capsule can then be made easily with inspection and irrigation of the hip joint.

for 20 years will not do well for 40 years. Stated another way, gross structural damage, which is rarely observed, may be only the tip of the iceberg. As noted in the discussion of pathology, the loss of matrix may occur as early as 5 days after the institution of an experimental infection. This renders the cartilage less stiff, and this in turn may result in an increased rate of wear.[29]

The importance of follow-up and the underestimation of residual damage have been emphasized in a review by Howard and coworkers.[30] They found that over half of the children thought to be normal at discharge had residual joint damage at follow-up. The hip, as has been noted in other studies, was the most frequently involved joint. *S. aureus* and *H. influenzae* were the most common associated organisms. Most follow-up studies of septic arthritis focus on the poor results seen in the hip joint and on the association with young age and delay in diagnosis and treatment.[30, 31]

References

Cited References

1. Goldenberg DL, Reed JI: Bacterial arthritis. N Engl J Med 312:764–771, 1985.

2. Schurman DJ, Mirra J, Ding A, Nagel DA: Experimental *E. coli* arthritis in the rabbit: a model of infectious and post-infectious inflammatory synovitis. J Rheumatol 4:118–128, 177.

3. Goldenberg DL, Chisholm PL, Rice PA: Experimental models of bacterial arthritis. J Rheumatol 10:5–11, 1983.

4. Johnson AH, Campbell WG, Callahan BC: Infection of rabbit knee joints after intraarticular injection of *Staphylococcus aureus.* Am J Pathol 60:165–203, 1970.

5. Lewis GW, Cluff LE: Synovitis in rabbits during bacteremia and vaccination. Bull Johns Hopkins Hosp 116:175–190, 1965.

6. Rigdon RH: Pathogenesis of arthritis following the intravenous injection of staphylococci in the adult rabbit. Am J Surg 55:553–561, 1942.

7. Fox L, Sprunt K: Neonatal osteomyelitis. Pediatrics 62:535–542, 1978.

8. Ash JM, Gilday DL: The futility of bone scanning in neonate osteomyelitis: concise communication. J Nucl Med 21:417–420, 1980.

9. Baldassare AR, Chang F, Zuckner J: Markedly raised synovial fluid leucocyte counts not associated with infectious arthritis in children. Ann Rheum Dis 37:404–409, 1978.

10. Daniel D, Akeson W, Amiel D, Ryder M, Boyer J: Lavage of septic joints in rabbits: effects of chondrolysis. J Bone Joint Surg 58A:393–395, 1976.

11. Singer JL: The causes of gait disturbance in 425 pediatric patients. Pediatr Emerg Care 1:7–10, 1985.

12. Heydemann JS, Morrissy RT: Diagnosis of bone and joint sepsis: review of 60 cases. Presented at the 53rd Annual Meeting of the American Academy of Orthopaedic Surgeons. New Orleans, February 1986.

13. Morrey BF, Bianco AJ, Rhodes KH: Septic arthritis in children. Orthop Clin North Am 6:923–934, 1975.
14. Volberg EM, Sumner TE, Abramson JS, et al: Unreliability of radiographic diagnosis of septic hip in children. Pediatrics 74:118–120, 1984.
15. Brown I: A study of the "capsular" shadow in disorders of the hip in children. J Bone Joint Surg 57B:175–179, 1975.
16. McCoy JR, Morrissy RT, Siebert J: Clinical experience with the technetium 99 scan in children. Clin Orthop 154:175–180, 1981.
17. Feigin RD, Wong M, Shackelford PG, et al: Countercurrent immunoelectrophoresis of urine as well as of CSF and blood for diagnosis of bacterial meningitis. J Pediatr 89:773–775, 1976.
18. Rotbart HA, Glode MP: *Haemophilus influenzae* type b septic arthritis in children: report of 23 cases. Pediatrics 75:254–259, 1985.
19. Nelson JD, Koontz WC: Septic arthritis in infants and children: a review of 117 cases. Pediatrics 38:966–971, 1966.
20. Waldvogel FA, Vasey H: Osteomyelitis: the past decade. N Engl J Med 303:360–370, 1980.
21. O'Brien JP, Goldenberg DL, Rice PA: Disseminated gonococcal infection: a prospective analysis of 49 patients and a review of pathophysiology and immune mechanisms. Medicine 62:395–406, 1983.
22. Svirsky-Fein S, Langer L, Milbauer B, et al: Neonatal osteomyelitis caused by *Candida tropicalis*. J Bone Joint Surg 61A:455–459, 1979.
23. Almquist EE: The changing epidemiology of septic arthritis in children. Clin Orthop 68:96–99, 1970.
24. Nelson JD: Antibiotic concentrations in septic joint effusions. N Engl J Med 284:349–353, 1971.
25. Nelson JD, Howard JB, Shelton S: Oral antibiotic therapy for skeletal infections of children. I. Antibiotic concentrations in suppurative synovial fluid. J Pediatr 92:131–134, 1978.
26. Bardenheier JA III, Morgan HC, Stamp WG: Treatment and sequelae of experimentally produced septic arthritis. Surg Gynecol Obstet 22:249–254, 1966.
27. Jackson MA, Nelson JD: Etiology and medical management of acute suppurative bone and joint infections in pediatric patients. J Pediatr Orthop 2:313–323, 1982.
28. Patterson DC: Acute suppurative arthritis in infancy and childhood. J Bone Joint Surg 52B:474–482, 1970.
29. Harris ED, Parker HG, Radin EL, Krane SM: Effects of proteolytic enzymes on structural and mechanical properties of cartilage. Arthritis Rheum 15:497–503, 1972.
30. Howard JB, Highgenboten CL, Nelson JD: Residual effects of septic arthritis in infancy and childhood. JAMA 236:932–935, 1976.
31. Fabry G, Meire E: Septic arthritis of the hip in children: poor results after late and inadequate treatment. J Pediatr Orthop 3:461–463, 1983.

Uncited References

Daniel D, Boyer J, Green S, Amiel, Akeson W: Cartilage destruction in experimentally produced *Staphylococcus aureus* joint infections: in vivo study. Surg Forum 24:479–481, 1973.
Samilson RL, Bersani FA, Watkins MB: Acute suppurative arthritis in infants and children. Pediatrics 21:798–803, 1958.

Raymond T. Morrissy, M.D.
Steven L. Shore, M.D.

CHAPTER

27

Acute Hematogenous Osteomyelitis

INTRODUCTION

Acute hematogenous osteomyelitis (AHO) is an inflammation of bone caused by bacteria that reach the bone through the hematogenous route.

Any hypothesis about the etiology of a disease should answer the known facts about that disease. There are several curious facts about AHO. It has a predilection for a certain age, usually the first decade. In adults it usually occurs in association with another disease that depresses the immune system, such as diabetes or cancer. It generally affects the most rapidly growing ends of long bones, and the lower extremity bones are the most common. The disease has a predilection for males.

ETIOLOGY

A conceptual error is to assume that bacteria are the only necessary etiologic factor in this disease. Bacteremia is an almost daily event in childhood, occurring at least 25 percent of the time after simple tooth brushing.[1] Thus, if bacteremia alone were the cause, AHO would be far more common. Some other etiologic factor must coincide with the bacteremia to cause AHO.

Further evidence for this line of reasoning is gathered from the failure of numerous investigators to produce experimental AHO in animals by the injection of organisms intravenously.[2-5] So difficult is it, in fact, that the current model for testing antibiotics is the injection of a necrosing agent, e.g., sodium

morrhuate, directly into the bone followed by the direct inoculation of bacteria.[6]

Another experimental model has been developed that utilizes trauma as an additional etiologic factor along with bacteremia. In this model, a small subclinical injury is created in the epiphyseal plate of a young rabbit's tibia. This is followed by a small dose of *Staphylococcus aureus* intravenously, which, without the injury, would not produce clinical infection. In this situation, there is an almost 100 percent incidence of AHO. In addition to providing a model that allows the study of AHO, this confirms the clinical experience that closed trauma may be the initial event in AHO in children.[7]

It should not be assumed that trauma is the only possible etiologic factor associated with bacteremia. Other factors, e.g., intercurrent illness or malnutrition, which may be associated with temporary inadequacy of immune function, are possible causes. Such alterations of immune function, as are seen in dietary deficiencies, may explain the higher frequency of AHO in the lower socioeconomic group.

All diseases are characterized by a spectrum of severity. Some diseases may be so mild as to escape detection by the methods of diagnosis used. These are said to lie below the "clinical horizon." As methods of detection improve, these are recognized and our understanding of the disease process is enlarged. This is illustrated in the experimental model of AHO, in which a bacteremia was induced that had no visible effect on the animal. Very small doses of *S. aureus* were injected and the animals observed. They showed none of the signs of systemic illness, such as weight loss, swelling, or limp, that developed in those with AHO. However, when multiple sections of the bones were

From the Scottish Rite Children's Hospital, Atlanta, Georgia.

271

done, small foci of healing osteomyelitis were occasionally seen.

Variations in this disease can also be seen in clinical examples of osteomyelitis. Several forms of hematogenous osteomyelitis are currently recognized: acute, subacute,[8] Brodie's abscess, and chronic multifocal.[9] How much these various forms are due to the changing nature of the disease, i.e., virulence of the organism and host factors, and how much is due to better diagnosis are matters for conjecture. However, the variable natural history clearly is shown in the spectrum of hematogenously caused osteomyelitis.

PATHOLOGY

A knowledge of the structural and cellular anatomy of the bone is important to an understanding of the pathophysiology because it is the one factor that makes bone infection different from soft tissue infection. The gross structure of the distal end of a bone is illustrated in Figure 27 – 1. The cortex in the metaphysis lacks the dense bone of the cortex in the diaphysis and instead is composed of a more densely organized area of trabecular bone.

The area just beneath the epiphyseal plate is composed of columns of calcified cartilage undergoing replacement by bone. Between them are the small arterioles that represent the terminal part of the interosseous circulation. Although the initial theory of Hobo[10] — which stated that bacteria lodged here because of the turbulence created in these "loops" — is frequently quoted in the literature, electron microscopy has shown these vessels to be terminal branches.[11] There are fenestrations in these small arterioles that permit the egress of cells and, presumably, bacteria. Absent from this area of the bone are any phagocytic cells. The secondary spongiosa beneath is characterized by the well-organized columns of trabecular bone, which does contain some phagocytic elements. The marrow cavity has little bone structure but is rich in phagocytic cells and other components of the reticuloendothelial system.

Hobo described the initial localization of bacteria following a bacteremia as being predominantly in the medullary cavity, with a few bacteria lodging in the sinusoids beneath the epiphyseal plate. In the first 24 hours, the bacteria were rapidly removed from the medullary cavity by the phagocytic cells. However, in

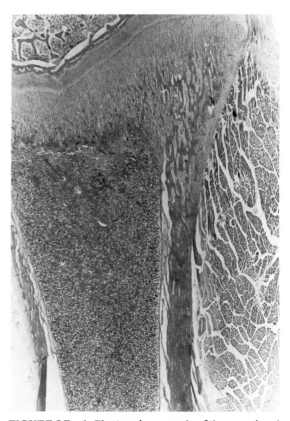

FIGURE 27 – 1. Photomicrograph of the proximal end of the immature rabbit tibia. This illustrates the transition of the thin, maze-like cortex in the metaphysis to the dense, thick cortex of the diaphysis. It can easily be seen how the periosteum is applied next to this thin metaphyseal cortex. There is no contiguous structure of bone forming the metaphyseal cortex. In addition, notice how closely the muscle is applied to and originating from the periosteum; thus, it is early involved in the edema and swelling.

the terminal sinusoids, the bacteria gradually began to multiply and to establish an infection because of the absence of phagocytic cells.

Examination of the earliest phases of developing osteomyelitis shows a picture that confirms at least part of Hobo's theory. It can be seen that at 72 hours the inflammatory process is well developed in the secondary spongiosa (Fig. 27 – 2). In some areas, it has come close to the area of the epiphyseal plate and in other areas it has not. Notice the destruction of trabecular bone behind the advancing inflammation and the preservation of bone structure between the inflammation and the epiphyseal plate beneath which the bacteria lie. A high-power view (Figs. 27 – 3 and 27 – 4) shows the

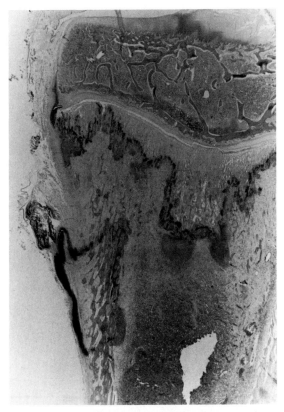

FIGURE 27 – 2. Photomicrograph of the proximal tibia of the rabbit 72 hours after the onset of acute hematogenous osteomyelitis. Notice the inflammatory response, which is moving toward the epiphysis. Note the small crack in the epiphyseal plate that is artificially produced to initiate the osteomyelitic process. Behind the inflammatory response, the bone trabeculae are destroyed. In front of the response, the bone trabeculae remain. Note also the small periosteal abscess that has developed at this early phase. (Hematoxylin and eosin, × 7.5)

location of the bacteria, the inflammatory response, and the preservation of normal architecture. Thus, it can be seen that the architectural destruction is caused by the host's own cells. The roles of the inflammatory response in both its good (destruction of bacteria) and bad (destruction of bone and cartilage) aspects are seen.

Over the next few days, the inflammatory response will move toward the area of the bacteria. The trabecular bone is resorbed during this process. If the bacteria win the race and establish a clinical infection, small abscesses develop. When the pus accumulates, it does not move down the medullary cavity, which would

appear to be the path of least resistance. This is because the inflammatory response has walled it off. The path of least resistance is through the thin metaphyseal cortex, with the result that a subperiosteal abscess will form (see Fig. 27 – 2).

On a more macroscopic level, there is an important difference between infants and children that deserves emphasis.[1] In infants, before the ossific nucleus has formed, the terminal vessels do not end at the junction of bone and cartilage but, rather, penetrate the cartilaginous epiphysis in small channels. This means that the bacteria will gain rapid access to the cartilaginous precursor of the joint. The result can be rapid destruction of the cartilaginous precursor. In addition, it explains the frequent coexistence of AHO and septic arthritis in neonates and young infants. The development of the ossific nucleus and the epiphyseal plate signals a change in the blood supply, which now enters the epiphysis through an epiphyseal artery. The epiphyseal plate will form a temporary barrier to the spread of infection from the metaphysis.

In children and adults, there are only a few areas in the skeleton where the metaphysis lies within the joint: proximal humerus, proximal femur, distal-lateral tibia, and proximal radius. This may frequently result in the coexistence of AHO and septic arthritis in older children.

DIAGNOSIS

Although the most common error in the inability to diagnose AHO is the failure to suspect it, arriving at a diagnosis can still be exceedingly difficult, even for those with considerable experience.[12] For this reason, it is important to approach every suspected case in an orderly manner. The definitive diagnosis is made when the bacteria from the bone are identified. Identification of the organism is part of the diagnosis. Because treatment cannot always be delayed in order to await positive bacteriological identification and because treatment may render a diagnosis impossible, all of the other evidence should be gathered before treatment starts.

History

Significant in the history is the duration of the musculoskeletal symptoms. This is impor-

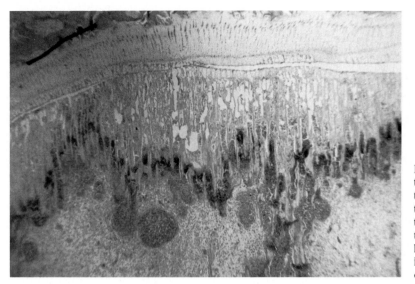

FIGURE 27 – 3. In this view of the same rabbit tibia, note the detail of the inflammatory response in respect to the bone destruction distal to it and the well-preserved bony trabeculae proximal to it. (Hematoxylin and eosin, × 40)

tant in correlation with the physical findings. An example is the differential diagnosis of AHO from cellulitis. Spreading erythema with a 24-hour history of pain is cellulitis. For osteomyelitis to cause such symptoms, the disease process would have had to be present for a much longer time, forming a subperiosteal abscess and possibly rupturing into the soft tissue.

It is, likewise, important to search for evidence of recent or concurrent infection. In a review of 60 consecutive cases of AHO and septic arthritis, it was noted that there was an associated infection in 48 percent of the patients.[12]

Physical Examination

The purpose of the orthopedic examination is to search for evidence of an infectious disease and the location of the process. The essentials are inspection for swelling and erythema, palpation for tenderness, and examination of joint motion.

Radiographs

The use of radiographs in the early diagnosis of AHO is misapplied if bone changes are

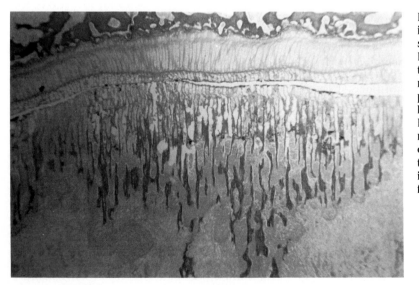

FIGURE 27 – 4. Same view as in Figure 27 – 3 using Gram's stain. Note the bacteria lodged in the proximal portion of the metaphysis beneath the crack in the epiphyseal plate. Some bacteria can also be seen lodged in the vascular channels between the calcified cartilage columns. Notice that at 72 hours they are not in close proximity to the inflammatory response.

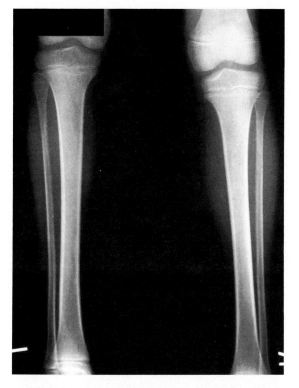

FIGURE 27 – 5. Anteroposterior views of symmetrically positioned tibias in an 8-year-old child with acute hematogenous osteomyelitis involving the right tibia. Note the deep soft tissue swelling on the right tibia in sharp contrast to that on the left. No bony involvement can be seen.

Bone Scan

The use of the bone scan in the diagnosis of AHO has been popularized to the point where it is often felt that the diagnosis cannot be made without one. The corollary of this is that a positive bone scan leads to the diagnosis of AHO. Both suppositions are incorrect. The primary value of bone scanning is to localize an area of abnormal physiology; the scan does not make a diagnosis.[14]

Whereas the plain radiograph gives an anatomic portrayal of the part by reflecting density differences or shadows, the bone scan reflects certain aspects of the physiology of the bone and soft tissues. This understanding is of fundamental importance to the correct use and interpretation of the bone scan.

The inflammation in the bone produces more changes than just the edema that is seen on the plain radiograph. Very early in the process, there is an increased blood flow to the part affected. This is reflected by an increased uptake of isotope in the early phase of the scan. Also, very early in the process, there is an increased vascularity in the area surrounding the infection, often coupled with stimulation of periosteal activity and formation of osteoid. This will be reflected in the delayed phase of the scan as a much more localized pattern of increased isotope uptake. Although the pattern of this isotope uptake is important in the interpretation of the scan, it should be viewed more as a local alteration of the physiology in the bone than as an anatomic portrayal.

In contrast to the plain radiograph, the bone scan reflects changes in bone much earlier. This is probably about the same time that swelling of the deep soft tissue layer is occurring. Therefore, if deep soft tissue swelling is identified adjacent to an area suspected of AHO by virtue of the physical examination and other laboratory data, there may be little reason for a bone scan. However, it is not always possible to identify deep soft tissue swelling, especially around the hip, pelvis, and spine. In addition, multiple foci may be suspected; however, here caution must be used. For example, in neonates, the most likely group to have multiple foci of infection, the technetium bone scan detects only about one half of the foci.[15] The bone scan is also of great value in alerting the clinician to a focus of osteomyelitis in a metaphysis adjacent to a joint swollen with either pus or fluid from a sympathetic effusion.

Interpretation of the scan is a frequent

sought. Since it usually takes at least 1 week for AHO to produce enough bone dissolution to be visible on the plain radiograph, this is not a valuable test for the prompt diagnosis of an acute condition. The real purpose of the plain radiograph is to identify soft tissue swelling.[13]

When there is inflammation in the bone, there will be edema in the adjacent deep soft tissue layer, usually the muscle. This will produce swelling, which will be noticeable in comparison to the opposite normal side (Fig. 27 – 5). As the edema spreads, the fatty layer that separates the muscle layers also becomes edematous. As the fatty layer takes on more water, its density becomes more like muscle; thus, on the plain radiograph it disappears.

Therefore, when radiographs are ordered in a case of suspected early osteomyelitis, symmetrically positioned views of the opposite extremity should also be taken and careful comparison made of the deep soft tissue layers and the fat planes.

source of error. The presence of decreased isotope uptake is just as important as increased uptake, signifying a possible area of avascularity.[16] This occurs most often in the hip, but it may also occur in other bones where the inflammatory process has disrupted the local blood supply. In typical AHO, the pattern of increased isotope uptake is an area arising from the epiphysis and extending into the metaphysis, often called "peaking" (Fig. 27–6). Diffuse patterns of uptake in an entire bone, or in a part, e.g., the foot, which is not clinically suspect, most often result from the increased vascularity in a bone that quickly follows disuse. This may occur with as little as 2 days of limping. Interpretation of the pattern of isotope uptake is important in determining its potential causes (Fig. 27–7).

Computed Tomography

Computed tomography (CT scan) is not used widely in the diagnosis of AHO. Although CT can detect changes within the bone, e.g., abscess formation, this is seldom necessary. Its primary usefulness is in the evaluation of the more subacute and chronic forms of osteomyelitis that may be confused with neoplasms and in the detection of contiguous abscesses in osteomyelitis.

Magnetic Resonance Imaging

Magnetic resonance imaging (MRI) has not been well evaluated in the diagnosis of AHO.

However, its ability to detect changes in the marrow theoretically makes it a good tool for the diagnosis of AHO. Even if it proves capable of diagnosing early AHO, its expense and availability will probably limit this technique for the foreseeable future.

Aspiration/Biopsy

All of the efforts so far have been aimed at the localization of the inflammatory process. However, the diagnosis remains unproven. When the site of the process is known, a more direct approach to the diagnosis is indicated. It should be one that will obtain material for definitive diagnosis.

This is the appropriate time for aspiration of the suspected area. Aspiration is analogous to a biopsy. It will confirm or disprove the presence of the disease process in the suspected area, it will produce material from which the diagnosis can be made, and it will help to determine the best course of treatment. In most children, and in most areas of the body, aspiration can be performed with sedation and local anesthesia. If deemed necessary, the use of a general anesthetic should not be a reason for neglecting this most important test. Likewise, aspiration will not interfere with a bone scan should it prove necessary later.[14, 17]

The most common error, next to neglecting the aspiration altogether, is to aspirate the wrong area. Frequently, in a very small child, the aspiration will be too far from the metaphysis. This may be suspected when great difficulty is found in pushing the needle

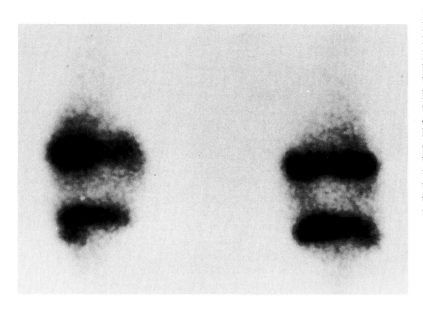

FIGURE 27–6. Technetium bone scan of a patient with a 2-day history of limping and pain in the right knee. Notice the small increase in the uptake of isotope in the lateral portion of the distal femoral epiphysis on the left. Notice also the increased uptake beginning in the metaphyseal area just proximal to this. The increased area of uptake seen in the proximal tibia on the same side is due to the overposition of the fibula.

FIGURE 27–7. Technetium polyphosphate bone scan from a 6-year-old male patient who 1 week previously had suffered a third-degree tissue loss to the posterior aspect of his heel from a bicycle spoke injury. Continuing drainage of the wound led to the suspicion of osteomyelitis, and a bone scan was obtained. Notice the atypical uptake for localized osteomyelitis of the oscalcis. The increased isotope uptake is seen in the subcortical region of the oscalcis in the same region one would expect to see early osteopenia of disuse. Note also the increased amount of uptake in the talus and the distal tibial epiphysis, also as a result of inflammation and disuse. This is not a pattern typical of osteomyelitis; this patient had cellulitis only.

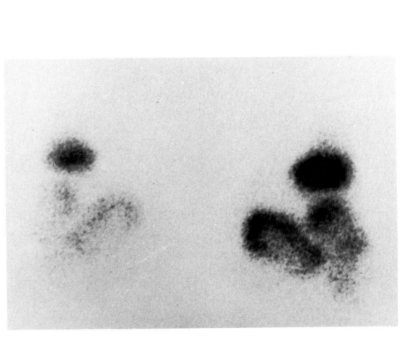

through the bone. Metaphyseal bone is soft and relatively easily penetrated by an 18-gauge or larger needle. Another error is to aspirate a swollen joint, obtain a normal or mildly inflammatory fluid, and then fail to aspirate the adjacent metaphysis, which harbors the focus of osteomyelitis that was causing the sympathetic effusion.

All material that is aspirated should be cultured. Although pus may not be found in early infections, organisms may still be present. This may also be true if the aspiration is close to, but misses, an abscess. If sufficient material is obtained, a Gram stain in addition to culture should be performed.

A perfectly executed evaluation can be ruined if the specimen is not cared for properly. Unless the specimen is to be carried directly to the bacteriologist for immediate plating, it should be placed in a suitable transport medium. Even this, however, is no excuse for delay.

TREATMENT

The historical perspective of AHO is important for two reasons. First, it demonstrates that neither surgery nor antibiotics alone constitute sufficient treatment. Second, it helps to explain why acute bone and joint sepsis receives so little attention today.

Prior to the advent and availability of antibiotics, osteomyelitis was a serious disease to be feared, as it often resulted in death, loss of limb, or severe crippling. Although it was said that surgery itself was harmful, this idea resulted more from the mortality that was higher from surgery on very ill and poorly prepared children who were given a general anesthetic than from the surgery itself. There has never been any evidence to incriminate the drainage of pus; rather, how it was drained is the question under scrutiny.

At the close of World War II, the sulfonamides and penicillin became available to the general public. This was a golden period in the treatment of many bacterial diseases that may never be seen again as pathogens continue to develop resistance to new antimicrobials. During this period, however, most bone infections were caused either by penicillin-sensitive *S. aureus* or *Streptococcus*. The juxtaposition of this "miracle" drug and sensitive organisms with the previous period explains how it could be concluded that surgery was not needed.

Throughout the 1950s and the early 1960s, as resistant organisms emerged, the picture changed. Treatment failures as well as chronic osteomyelitis increased. During the following

15 years, however, the pharmaceutical industry gained ground. Today, drugs may be seen as the winner because there is hardly any organism that cannot be killed by an antibiotic now on the market. This powerful arsenal has led to a rather cavalier approach to bone and joint sepsis. These are no longer the dreaded diseases for which there is no effective treatment, and the feeling still pervades many parts of the medical community that medical treatment alone is sufficient in all cases.

Principles

Knowing the correct treatment of a disease is not always as easy as it may seem at first. One method of determining the correct treatment is to review the literature on the subject. The difficulty here is in evaluating the accuracy of the literature, and this is especially true in clinical trials. Clinical studies on bone sepsis in the literature do not meet the rigorous standards of clinical review that would remove all doubt regarding the conclusions.[18] Therefore, although the literature provides good guidelines as to a current method, it does not prove that it is the best method for a particular case.

In a review of the literature on AHO, it is possible to find support for almost any view regarding treatment: surgery is rarely necessary,[19] surgery is usually necessary,[20] six weeks of intravenous therapy is necessary,[21] 1 week of intravenous therapy is sufficient,[22] and so on. There are so many parameters, many of them changing, in these studies that comparison of one to another is impossible.

It is, therefore, more desirable to talk in terms of the principles of treatment and to allow the clinician to apply these principles to each individual case as deemed best. There is, after all, still an art to medicine. An added bonus to this approach is that principles are one area in the treatment of infectious disease where there is a broad consensus of opinion.

The first principle is that *the organism should be identified*. Although this may not always be feasible, it is possible to make every effort to do so. This is a part of the diagnosis, and in AHO in children it should be possible in approximately 90 percent of cases.[23]

The second principle is that *the correct antibiotic should be used*, i.e., one that will kill the causative organism. The application of this principle is marred by a serious problem; it is often not possible to identify the organism for 24 hours and to know its sensitivity for an additional 24 hours. Treatment cannot be delayed until all questions are answered with certainty. Calculated guesses — the art — will have to be made before the organism is positively known — the science.

The art in applying this second principle is to gather the facts in a particular case that will narrow the possibilities and lead to the correct conclusion. A history of a recent or concurrent infection is often helpful, especially when coupled with knowledge of the organisms commonly associated with that particular infection. Current knowledge of the epidemiology of the infection is also helpful, e.g., neonatal infections occurring in a nursery population. Material obtained from aspiration is particularly helpful if organisms can be identified on a Gram stain.

Once the possible organisms are identified, it is necessary to know their sensitivities. In this situation, guessing should always be supplemented by a current knowledge of various sensitivity patterns in a particular area, whether it be a nursery or hospital.

In AHO, approximately 75 percent of the cases will be due to *S. aureus*. This general prevalence of *S. aureus* lessens in neonates and to some extent in children younger than 5 years of age.[24-26] Among the newborn and younger infants, until 2 to 3 months the streptococci and the gram-negative enteric rods are more likely to be present. In previously normal children over 4 years of age, *S. aureus* is probably the causative organism in greater than 90 percent of cases. In such circumstances, a semisynthetic penicillin or first-generation cephalosporin is the drug of choice.

Based on these considerations, infants (other than neonates) and children should be treated initially for osteomyelitis with oxacillin (150 mg/kg/day) intravenously. For the penicillin-allergic patient, cefazolin (100 mg/kg/day) should be used. For the rare patient allergic to both penicillins and cephalosporins, clindamycin (25 to 40 mg/kg/day) or vancomycin (40 mg/kg/day) can be used effectively.

For the full-term neonate with osteomyelitis, initial therapy should cover *S. aureus*, group B streptococci, and gram-negative enteric rods. Therefore, a good choice for initial antibiotics would be oxacillin (100 mg/kg/day every 8 hours from birth to 7 days of age, and 150 mg/kg/day divided every 6 hours for older neonates) and gentamicin (5 mg/kg/day divided every 12 hours from birth to 7 days of age, and 7.5 mg/kg/day divided every 8 hours for older neonates). An alternative would be cefotaxime alone (100 mg/kg/day divided every 12 hours from birth to 7 days and 150 mg/kg/day divided every 8 hours for older neonates).

The third principle is that *the antibiotic must be delivered to the organism in sufficient concentration to kill the organism.* It is this principle that is the most difficult to apply and where the most controversy arises. There are several questions that are usually asked in regard to getting the antibiotics to the organisms:

1. Do they penetrate into the area of the infection, including pus?

2. How long is it necessary to administer the antibiotics?

3. By which route should they be given?

There are also a couple of questions that are rarely asked that are equally important:

1. Do the antibiotics work in the area of the infection?

2. Is killing the organisms the only goal in the treatment of bacterial infections?

3. Are live organisms necessary for tissue destruction?

ANTIBIOTIC PENETRATION

A subject long debated was whether or not antibiotics penetrated bone as well as soft tissue. The accumulated evidence to date indicates that in the case of cancellous bone, antibiotics in current use penetrate very well, achieving levels close to serum levels.[27-29] Unlike the blood-brain barrier, the blood-bone barrier is not a serious obstacle to antibiotic penetration. In all of these studies, methodological problems involved in extracting and measuring the antibiotic from the bone must be considered. In addition to the ability to penetrate bone, it also appears that antibiotics have the ability to penetrate pus.[30]

Penetration into cortical bone may be more difficult and less certain in clinical situations. Cortical bone derives the outer one third of its blood supply from the periosteal vessels and the inner two thirds from the medullary blood supply. Unlike soft tissue, cortical bone is not characterized by a capillary connection between its afferent and efferent systems. Much of the nutrient supply and, presumably, the antibiotics reaches the osteocytes and other areas of bone through the fluid in the canalicular system.[9] This tenuous route of nutrition in cortical bone is easily disrupted by infection. Along with the slower turnover of cortical bone, this helps to explain the chronic nature of cortical bone infections.

The question that has not been adequately answered, however, is: Do antibiotics work in the region of an infection, especially in pus? The low pH and other factors present in an abscess do not appear to be the ideal medium for antibiotic effectiveness. It is known that the aminoglycosides do not work in such an environment, but little study has been done with other antibiotics.[31, 32]

ROUTE OF ADMINISTRATION

The route by which the antibiotic is administered is not the important issue; what is critical is that *adequate serum levels be achieved.* This is the essential consideration in using oral antibiotics for skeletal infections. It is unlikely that the dying organisms will know or care how the antibiotic got to them.

In the majority of cases, it is possible to achieve adequate serum concentrations of the commonly used antibiotics through the oral route. This has been demonstrated experimentally.[27, 33] Numerous clinical trials have been conducted over the past decade demonstrating that oral therapy can be successful[34-37] and demonstrating the causes of failure, e.g., lack of compliance[34] and inadequate dosage.[33]

Because the vagaries of intestinal absorption are such that adequate serum levels cannot be guaranteed in every case by doubling or even tripling the "normal" oral dose, it is essential to document that adequate serum levels are being achieved. Since levels of antibiotic in vascularized bone are similar to the levels in the serum for most commonly used antibiotics, it is sufficient to demonstrate that adequate serum levels are achieved. This can be done by testing for the minimal inhibitory concentration (MIC) or the minimal bactericidal concentration (MBC). If a pathogen is not identified from the patient, a standard laboratory strain of the suspected organism can be used. Generally, a peak MBC level of 1 : 8 or greater is aimed for, although this is based on information from the treatment of subacute bacterial endocarditis. Such a high ratio may not be necessary in bone sepsis.

The second potential problem with oral administration is compliance. Most doctors are personally aware of the difficulty in taking medications several times per day without error. This problem is compounded when giving terrible-tasting liquids to small children.

This has been identified as one of the main problems with compliance in oral antibiotic therapy. Taste is one reason why some may prefer to use cephalosporins instead of semisynthetic penicillins when treating a staphylococcal infection because the former are usually more palatable than the latter.

From this discussion, guidelines for the use of oral antibiotics in the treatment of bone sepsis can be derived: (1) the organism should be known and its sensitivities identified, (2) the patient's condition should be improving, (3) the parents should be judged to be reliable, (4) the patient should be able to tolerate the drug without vomiting or diarrhea, and (5) adequate serum levels of the drug must be documented.

DURATION

The duration of antibiotic therapy is another controversy that the literature has done little to resolve. Many of the large series come from medical centers and have an atypical patient mix. A good example of this is the often quoted series of Waldvogle and colleagues.[38] The patients in this study were different from the average patient with AHO; they were a difficult and complicated group transferred to a large teaching medical center. The recommendation that 6 weeks of intravenous antibiotic is necessary may not be valid in the light of current knowledge about oral administration, and any conclusion reached in this group of patients should be transferred only with extreme caution to an entirely different group of patients, e.g., those who are seen in a typical orthopedic practice and whose disease may have a very different history.

This question as to the duration of therapy has no proven correct answer. It seems likely, from a knowledge of the pathophysiology of the disease process, that there are probably a great many variables in each case. One obvious example would be whether or not surgical debridement is performed to reduce the size of the inoculum and to remove necrotic tissue. What is needed are guidelines to help individualize therapy, rather than rigid rules that may result in overtreatment or undertreatment.

With these considerations in mind, it is recommended that an appropriate antibiotic be given intravenously for 5 to 7 days. If patients respond clinically in a prompt fashion to this, with or without the aid of drainage, they can then be given an oral antibiotic regimen for an additional 3 weeks. The peak serum bactericidal levels should be at least 1 : 8. For infants and younger children, when an antibiotic suspension is required for *S. aureus* infection, cephalexin (100 mg/kg/day) is used because of its better taste. For older patients who can swallow capsules, dicloxacillin (100 mg/kg/day) is generally used. For penicillin-allergic individuals (not anaphylaxis), cephalexin can be used, with the maximum dose being 3 gm/day. For the unusual patient who is allergic to both penicillins and cephalosporins, clindamycin (25 to 40 mg/kg/day) is an excellent therapeutic choice and is well tolerated orally. Adequate serum levels must be ensured and the dose adjusted if necessary.

For the difficult patient with extensive bone involvement, slow clinical progress, or need for extensive surgery, longer-term intravenous antibiotic therapy should be used, 3 to 6 weeks commonly being necessary. If normal venous access is impossible, a central venous catheter will be necessary. Home intravenous therapy in the older child and the adolescent is practical and can considerably reduce the hospital stay and cost. Antibiotic therapy should be continued until all clinical signs of infection have disappeared and the erythrocyte sedimentation rate (ESR) has returned to near normal.

In the authors' experience and that of others,[39] the ESR is not a good indicator of disease activity during the first week of therapy. The ESR lags behind the clinical response by about 1 week. However, failure of the ESR to fall after the first 7 to 10 days should make one suspicious of a continuation of the disease process. In our experience, this problem has been most common in children in whom surgical debridement of an abscess has not been performed or in whom the initial extent of the osteomyelitis was not fully appreciated and the debridement was inadequate.

SURGERY

One of the most difficult questions to resolve is: When is surgery necessary? Again, it is relatively easy to find support in the literature for any option, since there are so many variables. A better starting point is to consider the pathology and the goals of treatment and then to decide if surgery is helpful.

In the treatment of infectious disease, it is often assumed that killing the organisms is not only the paramount goal but also the only goal. However, the physician has another concern that is not completely linked to the killing of the organisms—and that is to stop tissue destruction.

It has been pointed out that the physical destruction of the tissue is done largely by the host itself, no doubt under the influence of the bacteria. This destruction is mediated through the complex phenomenon called the *inflammatory response*. The exact mechanisms for this response in bone have not been well studied. They are much better understood in cartilage and are explained in the discussion on septic arthritis (see Chapter 26). It is sufficient to say at this point that live bacteria are not necessary for all of the destructive aspects of the inflammatory response; dead bacteria and other bacterial products that remain after they are killed are sufficient in themselves.

The amount of necrotic material and bacterial debris remaining at the time of bacterial killing differs with each case—one of many variables that illustrates the difficulty of deriving scientific data from patient studies. Clearing this debris is the job of the host inflammatory response. It is a complex and incompletely understood response that may take days or weeks to remove foreign and necrotic material. Although the role of the inflammatory response has been understood only in modern times, physicians for centuries have understood the desirability of draining an abscess based on clinical experience.

Understanding the harmful effect of the inflammatory response makes it easier to understand the main role of surgery in AHO. Surgery is for debridement. It is an augmentation of the host response. It reduces the inoculum and removes necrotic and avascular bone, dead bacteria, and other harmful bacterial products. Surgery has the potential to do in 1 hour what it may take the host days or weeks to do. In such cases, it speeds resolution of the disease process, allowing an earlier and safer switch to oral antibiotics and decreasing hospital time.

Is surgery always indicated? Not in all cases. It is certainly essential when pus is found on aspiration, which would signify an abscess. It is indicated when radiographic changes of osteomyelitis are seen, because pus, necrotic material and chronic inflammation are present at this stage of the disease. If none of the aforementioned circumstances is present, a trial of intravenous antibiotic therapy is appropriate after all material has been collected in an effort to obtain a culture of the organism.

A more difficult situation is encountered when none of these conditions pertains yet the patient fails to respond to antibiotic therapy.

Two possibilities exist: the wrong antibiotic may have been selected, a problem that can be ruled out if the organism and its sensitivity has been identified; or, more likely, an unrecognized abscess is present. In the patient who fails to show a significant response, i.e., decreased fever, swelling, or tenderness within 36 to 48 hours, a renewed search for an occult abscess should be started. If an abscess has been positively identified, surgical drainage of this area is the conservative (although surgical) course of treatment.

In most cases, this is not an extensive operation. A small, well-placed incision should suffice. The periosteum is incised, with a narrow width of periosteum elevated around the metaphysis, to be sure that any subperiosteal pus is identified. A drill hole of appropriate size ($\frac{1}{4}$ to $\frac{1}{2}$ inch) is made in the cortex. A curette is used to remove the necrotic, pus-filled cancellous bone. The hole may be enlarged with a rongeur if the osteomyelitis is more extensive. In some patients in whom the condition has been neglected, or in children who have an immune deficiency, the pus may fill the medullary canal. In such cases, a strip of cortex may be removed from one epiphyseal plate to the other and the medullary canal curetted. Although this may seem radical, the bone will heal rapidly in a child, provided that the infection is controlled.

It is the authors' preference in most routine cases to close the wound over irrigation suction tubes. If this irrigation system is to work, the outflow tube must be placed in a cavity that has been well debrided, and the tube must be large; all of this is necessary so that the tube does not become blocked with debris. This system is best thought of as a closed and continuous debridement. Only physiological solutions should be used. Antibiotics should not be added: they are not necessary, they can be very irritating, and some (e.g., neomycin) can be absorbed in toxic amounts. Last, this irrigation system should not remain in place for longer than 48 hours because superinfection may result. In many cases, closed suction may be sufficient. The decision of whether or not to leave the wound open is made by the surgeon, but with the correct antibiotic and adequate debridement it does not seem necessary in the usual case.

COMPLICATIONS

Complications from AHO in childhood are, fortunately, not common. Chronic osteomyelitis is distinctly rare in childhood; when present, it can usually be eradicated. This is in part due to the rapid turnover of bone in childhood. When this is combined with modern techniques of bone resection and grafting, cure is usually possible.

Pathological fracture can occur. It can be minimized by taking measures that will enforce the proper protection of the bone during healing. Children cannot be assumed to be reliable in complying with non–weight bearing when this is considered necessary. Fear of pathological fracture should not limit debridement when it is necessary. In children, a bone with a large defect but free of infection will heal more rapidly than an infected bone with continued infection.

Most complications associated with osteomyelitis occur in the neonate and result from associated joint infection.[40]

References

1. Everett ED, Hirschman JV: Transient bacteria and endocarditis prophylaxis: a review. Medicine 56:61–77, 1977.
2. Hamblen DL: Hyperbaric oxygenation: its effects on experimental staphylococcal osteomyelitis in rats. J Bone Joint Surg 50A:1129–1141, 1968.
3. Robertson DE: Acute hematogenous osteomyelitis. J Bone Joint Surg 20:34–47, 1938.
4. Scheman L, Janota M, Lewin P: The production of experimental osteomyelitis. JAMA 117:1525–1529, 1941.
5. Starr CL: Acute hematogenous osteomyelitis. Arch Surg 4:567–587, 1922.
6. Norden CW: Experimental osteomyelitis. I. A description of the model. J Infect Dis 122:410–418, 1970.
7. Morrissy RT, Haynes DW: Acute hematogenous osteomyelitis: a model with trauma as an etiologic agent. Presented at the 51st Annual Meeting of the American Academy of Orthopaedic Surgeons, Atlanta, February 1983.
8. Green NE, Beauchamp RD, Griffin PP: Primary subacute epiphyseal osteomyelitis. J Bone Joint Surg 63A:107–114, 1981.
9. Rhinelander FW: Effects of medullary nailing on the normal blood supply of diaphyseal cortex. In American Academy of Orthopaedic Surgeons: Instructional Course Lectures, Vol. 22. St. Louis, CV Mosby Co, 1973.
10. Hobo T: Zur pathogenese de akuten haematogenen osteomyelitis, mit berucksichtigung der vitalfarbungs lehre. Translated by Astride Seifen, M.D. Acta Scholar Medicinalis Kioto 4:1–29, 1921.
11. Schenk RK, Wiener J, Spiro D: Fine structural aspects of vascular invasion of the tibial epiphyseal plate of growing rats. Acta Anat 69:1–17, 1968.
12. Heydemann JS, Morrissy RT: Diagnosis of bone and joint sepsis: review of 60 cases. Presented at the 53rd annual meeting of the American Academy of Orthopaedic Surgeons, New Orleans, February 1986.
13. Capitanio MA, Kirkpatrick JA: Early roentgen observations in acute osteomyelitis. Am J Roentgenol Radium Ther Nucl Med 108:488–496, 1970.
14. McCoy JR, Morrissy RT, Seibert J: Clinical experi-
ence with the technetium 99 scan in children. Clin Orthop 154:175–180, 1981.
15. Ash JM, Gilday DL: The futility of bone scanning in neonatal osteomyelitis: concise communication. J Nucl Med 21:417–420, 1980.
16. Berkowitz ID, Wenzel W: Normal technetium bone scans in patients with acute osteomyelitis. Am J Dis Child 134:828–830, 1980.
17. Canale ST, Harkness RM, Thomas PA, Massie JD: Does aspiration of bones and joints affect results of later bone scanning? J Pediatr Orthop 5:23–26, 1985.
18. Rudicel S, Esdaile J: The randomized clinical trial in orthopaedics: obligation or option? J Bone Joint Surg 67A(8):1284–1293, 1985.
19. Blockey NJ, Watson JT: Acute osteomyelitis in children. J Bone Joint Surg 52B(1):77–87, 1970.
20. Mollan RAB, Piggot J: Acute osteomyelitis in children. J Bone Joint Surg 59B(1):2–7, 1977.
21. Waldvogle FA, Vasey H: Osteomyelitis: the past decade. N Engl J Med 303:360–370, 1980.
22. Kolyvas E, Ahronheim G, Marks MI, Glenhill R, Owen H, Rosenthall L: Oral antibiotic therapy of skeletal infections in children. Pediatrics 65(5):867–871, 1980.
23. Waldvogle FA, Medoff G, Swartz MN: Osteomyelitis: clinical features, therapeutic considerations and unusual aspects. Springfield, Ill, Charles C Thomas, 1971.
24. Dich VO, Nelson JD, Haltalin C: Osteomyelitis in infants and children. Am J Dis Child 129:1273–1278, 1975.
25. Jackson MA, Nelson JD: Etiology and medical management of acute suppurative bone and joint infection in pediatric patients. J Pediatr Orthop 2:313–323, 1983.
26. Winters JL, Cahen I: Acute hematogenous osteomyelitis. J Bone Joint Surg 42A:691–704, 1960.
27. Bloom JD, Fitzgerald RH Jr, Washington JA, Kelly PJ: The transcapillary passage and interstitial fluid concentration of penicillin in canine bone. J Bone Joint Surg 62A(7):1168–1175, 1980.
28. Lunke RJ, Fitzgerald H Jr, Washington JA: Pharmacokinetics of cefamandole in osseous tissue. Antimicrobial agents and chemotherapy 19(5):851–858, 1981.
29. Wiggins DE, Nelson CL, Clark R, Thompson CH: Concentration of antibiotic in normal bone after intravenous injection. J Bone Joint Surg 60A(1):93–96, 1978.
30. Tetzlaff TR, Howard JB, McCracken GH, Calderon E, Larrondo J: Antibiotic concentrations in pus and bone of children with osteomyelitis. J Pediatr 92(1):135–140, 1978.
31. Bryan LE, Van den Elzen HM: Streptomycin accumulation in susceptible and resistant strains of Escherichia coli and Pseudomonas aeruginosa. Antimicrob Agents Chemother 9:928–938, 1976.
32. Bryant RE, Hammond D: Interaction of purulent material with antibiotics used to treat Pseudomonas infections. Antimicrob Agents Chemother 6:702–707, 1974.
33. Nelson JD, Howard JB, Shelton S: Oral antibiotic therapy for skeletal infections of children. I. Antibiotic concentrations in suppurative synovial fluid. J Pediatr 92:131–134, 1978.
34. Bryson YJ, Connor JD, Leuers M, Giammona ST: High dose dicloxacillin treatment of acute staphylococcal osteomyelitis in children. J Pediatr 94:673–675, 1979.
35. Feigin RD, Pickering LK, Anderson D, Keeney RD,

Shackelford PG: Clindamycin treatment of osteomyelitis and septic arthritis in children. Pediatrics 55:213–223, 1975.

36. Green JF: Cloxacillin in treatment of acute osteomyelitis. Br Med J 2:414–416, 1967.

37. Tetzlaff TR, McCracken GH Jr, Nelson JD: Oral antibiotic therapy for skeletal infections of children. II. Therapy of osteomyelitis and suppurative arthritis. J Pediatr 92:485–490, 1978.

38. Waldvogle FA, Medhoff G, Swartz MN: Osteomyelitis: a review of clinical features, therapeutic considerations and unusual aspects. N Engl J Med 282:198–207, 260–266, 316–323, 1970.

39. Nelson JD, Bucholz RW, Kusmiesz H, Shelton S: Benefits and risks of sequential parenteral-oral cephalosporin therapy for suppurative bone and joint infections. J Pediatr Orthop 2:255–262, 1982.

40. Bergdahl S, Ekengren K, Eriksson M: Neonatal hematogenous osteomyelitis: risk factors for long-term sequelae. J Pediatr Orthop 5:564–568, 1985.

Margaret L. Simpson, M.D.

28

Septic Arthritis in Adults

PATHOPHYSIOLOGY

Suppurative arthritis results from bacterial invasion of the joint space. Hematogenous bacterial inoculation of the synovium is the most common event resulting in suppurative arthritis. Because the synovium is extremely vascular and lacks a basement membrane, easy access of blood-borne bacteria to the synovial space is achieved. Suppurative arthritis may also occur because of direct extension from a contiguous site (osteomyelitis) or from direct inoculation (intra-articular injection, surgical procedure).[1] A previous joint problem predisposes that particular joint to a suppurative arthritis.[2]

In experimental bacterial arthritis, the initial synovial response occurs within 24 to 48 hours of bacterial inoculation.[3] First, a polymorphonuclear leukocyte infiltration occurs with vascular congestion and lining cell proliferation. As the bacteria multiply, a purulent joint effusion develops. Within 7 days, chronic and sometimes irreversible synovial changes may begin to occur. Further destruction of the joint and bone may develop because of the release of proteolytic enzymes from the polymorphonuclear leukocytes. In addition, necrosis caused by direct pressure of the arthritis process also increases the local damage. Later, proliferating synovial cells enhance enzymatic digestion and invade the cartilage-bone matrix.

Local as well as systemic host factors may determine those individuals in whom septic arthritis develops during a bacteremic or local infectious process. The administration of oral or intra-articular corticosteroids is a significant predisposing factor for the development of septic arthritis. A history of pre-existing arthritis (rheumatoid arthritis or osteoarthritis) or trauma to a joint may be obtained in 30 percent of the cases. Extra-articular sites of infection are found in up to 50 percent of adults with septic arthritis.[2, 4] Other systemic predisposing factors include diabetes mellitus, the presence of a malignancy, and complement deficiencies or immunologic abnormalities.[1]

Septic arthritis is monoarticular in almost 90 percent of cases.[2] Persons with polyarticular suppurative arthritis are more likely to be elderly, to have received systemic corticosteroids, or to have a history of rheumatoid arthritis.[4]

The joint most frequently involved by a bacterial process in adults is the knee (40 to 50 percent), followed by the hip (20 to 25 percent), ankle (10 to 15 percent), and elbow (10 to 15 percent),[5, 6] with other diarthrodial joints less frequently involved. The synarthrodial sacroiliac and sternoclavicular joints are unusual sites of infection, seen more in the intravenous drug user.[7, 8]

CLINICAL PRESENTATION AND LABORATORY EVALUATION

Almost all patients present with a painful joint, and the majority also have swelling, heat, and erythema of the joint. Range of motion of the involved joint is markedly decreased. Fever is present in 80 percent of patients but is usually of low grade and commonly is not accompanied by shaking chills or other signs of sepsis.[4] Peripheral leukocytosis occurs in only half of the patients.[4] An elevated erthrocyte sedimentation rate (ESR) is frequently found.[1] The average duration of symptoms before diagnosis is 14 days.

Evaluation of the synovial fluid is necessary when septic arthritis is in the differential diag-

From the Hennepin County Medical Center, University of Minnesota, Minneapolis, Minnesota.

nosis. Synovial fluid analysis reveals a substantial inflammatory response in the vast majority of cases. The mean synovial fluid leukocyte count usually approaches 100,000 cells/mm³ with over 85 percent of the cells being polymorphonuclear leukocytes.[1, 4] In the small number of patients with a low initial synovial fluid white blood cell (WBC) count, a repeat examination within 24 hours almost always demonstrates a more impressive leukocytosis. Crystalline arthritis may also cause a moderate synovial fluid leukocytosis, and a search for crystals should be performed on the joint fluid.

A Gram stain smear of synovial fluid is positive in 65 percent of cases.[4] The rate of positive stain varies with the microbial agent causing the septic arthritis. With staphylococcal infections, the organism will be demonstrated on a Gram stain in 75 percent of cases. However, only 50 percent of those infected with gram-negative bacilli and fewer than 25 percent of patients with gonococcal arthritis will reveal the organisms on a Gram stain.[1]

Aerobic and anaerobic cultures should be performed on synovial fluid from patients with suspected septic arthritis. Synovial fluid cultures are positive in almost all cases of septic arthritis, if *Neisseria gonorrhoeae* is excluded. Previous antibiotic therapy before the synovial fluid is obtained may cause the culture to be negative. Blood cultures are positive in 50 percent of nongonococcal septic arthritis.[4] Blood cultures should be obtained in all persons thought to have a suppurative arthritis.

In studies including infectious arthritis caused by *N. gonorrhoeae*, over 50 percent of the cases will be caused by this organism.[1, 9] Persons presenting with gonococcal arthritis are usually young, healthy adults with no other predisposing factors for an infectious arthritis. Initial migratory polyarthralgias is a common previous complaint. Approximately 60 percent of the patients with disseminated gonococcal infection will have fever, dermatitis, and tenosynovitis. The remaining 30 to 40 percent will present with a classic monoarticular arthritis. Meningococcal arthritis, although seen less frequently, may present with the same clinical picture as disseminated gonococcal infection.[1] With *N. gonorrhoeae* infections, blood and joint fluid cultures may be negative. The possible primary sites of infection (cervix, urethra, rectum, pharynx) should be cultured.

Staphylococcus aureus is the predominant organism isolated in nongonococcal arthritis, causing 40 to 70 percent of suppurative arthritis.[4, 6] In septic arthritis occurring in rheuma-

toid arthritis, 80 percent of the cases are caused by *S. aureus*.[10] *Streptococcus* species are also a significant source of problems for persons with septic arthritis. All the *Streptococcus* species (*S. pneumoniae*, *S. viridans*, groupable *Streptococcus* strains and enterococcus) account for approximately 25 percent of cases of septic arthritis. Gram-negative bacilli have become an increasingly important etiology of septic arthritis during the last 20 years.[10] Predisposing factors for gram-negative bacilli septic arthritis are similar to gram-negative bacilli bacteremia. The most common gram-negative bacillus isolated in a septic joint is *Escherichia coli*. In septic arthritis occurring in intravenous drug users, *Pseudomonas aeruginosa* is a common isolate.[7] In the hospitalized patient who develops nosocomial septic arthritis, *S. aureus* and a wide range of gram-negative bacilli may be the causative microbial etiologic factors. In adults *Hemophilus influenzae* has been increasingly recognized as an etiologic factor in septic arthritis.[11] Anaerobic bacteria are less common microbial isolates in septic arthritis. Polymicrobial bacterial cultures of synovial fluid occur in fewer than 10 percent of those with septic arthritis.[9]

THERAPY

Parenterally administered antibiotics have been found to achieve adequate bactericidal levels in infected joint fluid.[12] Intra-articular antibiotics do not need to be administered and actually may induce a chemical synovitis.[13]

The Gram stain will frequently assist in directing the presumptive antimicrobial regimen. Gram-positive cocci in clusters are indicative of *S. aureus*, necessitating the use of penicillinase-resistant penicillin (12 gm/day of nafcillin or oxacillin). A first-generation cephalosporin (cefazolin, 6 gm/day) may also be used for *S. aureus*. Whenever gram-positive cocci are found on the Gram stain, initial antibiotic coverage needs to include *S. aureus*. If streptococci are cultured from the joint fluid, penicillin (12 to 24 million units/day) is the antibiotic utilized. If gram-negative bacilli are initially seen in a nonhospitalized patient, a third-generation cephalosporin (cefotaxime, 6 to 12 gm/day, or ceftriaxone 2 gm/day) is appropriate for initial therapy. This regimen will also provide coverage for *Haemophilus influenzae*. For many gram-negative bacilli, a third-generation cephalosporin will provide adequate coverage if the organism is sensitive in vitro to the agent. For persons receiving immunosuppressive agents or in whom the septic arthritis develops during hospitalization, coverage for *P. aeruginosa* needs to be included with an aminoglycoside pending identification of the organism. This group of patients also needs antimicrobial coverage of *S. aureus* if Gram stain has not revealed an organism. Initial antimicrobial coverage aimed at *S. aureus* and *P. aeruginosa* needs to be utilized in intravenous drug users pending identification of the microbial etiology. In a young, sexually active adult with no organisms found on the Gram stain, antimicrobial coverage should be primarily for gonococcal arthritis with penicillin (12 million units/day).

Duration of therapy varies depending on the organism isolated. For *N. gonorrhoeae*, 10 to 14 days of therapy is adequate. After parenteral antibiotics are begun for gonococcal arthritis, oral antibiotics (ampicillin, tetracycline) may be given when a good clinical result has been achieved to complete the course of treatment. For *S. aureus* and gram-negative bacilli, 4 to 6 weeks of the appropriate parenteral antimicrobial regimen needs to be administered. Patients with a slow clinical response or who are immunosuppressed in any manner will require a 6-week course of therapy for *S. aureus* or gram-negative bacilli.[14] If streptococci or *Haemophilus* species are isolated, a 2- to 3-week course of parenteral antibiotics is usually adequate.[6] The use of oral antibiotics in septic arthritis necessitates monitoring of serum levels to ascertain efficacious levels. Oral antimicrobial therapy for septic arthritis has not been well studied.

As part of the therapeutic regimen, adequate joint drainage of the purulent effusion needs to be performed. In most joints, repeated needle aspiration may be performed as the effusion accumulates.[1] If the joint fluid is not demonstrating a decline in polymorphonuclear leukocytes or repeated bacterial cultures show growth, open surgical drainage is needed. If loculated fluid is present or joint aspirations cannot adequately drain the joint, surgery needs to be performed. Because of the difficulty of performing adequate aspiration of joint fluid with infections of the hip or shoulder, early surgical drainage is recommended if either of these joints is infected.[1] If a coexistent osteomyelitis is present, open surgical drainage is necessary. During the acute phase of the septic arthritis process, the joint should be immobilized.

The response to treatment of septic arthritis depends on several variables. Results are not as good in patients who have had symptoms for more than 1 week before the initiation of therapy compared with those who have had symptoms for a shorter period before treatment.[4] The microbial etiology is also a determining factor in the final result. Complete joint recovery is very high in joints with streptococcal and gonococcal arthritis. Fifty percent of infected joints will be affected by persistent problems when *S. aureus* is the cause, and 67 percent of joints infected with gram-negative bacilli will show residual damage.[4] The rapidity with which synovial fluid sterility is achieved also affects the outcome of joint function.[15] In patients with good joint outcome, the synovial fluid culture remained positive, with a mean of 2.4 days; in patients with poor results, the mean was 8.2 days.

Septic arthritis needs to be in the differential when a patient presents with a painful joint. Because of altered host response in many patients, an infected joint may not always be swollen and erythematous. An arthrocentesis needs to be performed on any joint in which an infection may be occurring to provide a diagnosis as well as to delineate the necessary therapeutic regimen.

References

1. Goldenberg DL, Reed JI: Bacterial arthritis. N Engl J Med 312:764, 1985.
2. Kelly PJ, Martin WJ, Coventry MB: Bacterial (suppurative) arthritis in the adult. J Bone Joint Surg 52A:1595, 1970.
3. Johnson AH, Campbell WG Jr, Callahan BC: Infection of rabbit knee joints after an intra-articular injection of *Staphylococcus aureus*. Am J Pathol 60:165, 1970.
4. Goldenberg DL, Cohen AS: Acute infectious arthritis: a review of patients with nongonococcal joint infections (with emphasis on therapy and prognosis). Am J Med 60:369, 1976.
5. Rosenthal J, Bole GG, Robinson WD: Acute nongonococcal infectious arthritis: evaluation of risk factors, therapy and outcome. Arthritis Rheum 22:889, 1980.
6. Smith JW: Infectious arthritis. In Mandell GL, Douglas RG, Bennett JE, eds: Principles and Practice of Infectious Diseases. John Wiley & Sons, Inc. New York, 1985, p 697.
7. Gifford DB, Patzakis M, Ivler D, et al: Septic arthritis due to *Pseudomonas* in heroin addicts. J Bone Joint Surg 57A:631, 1975.

8. Bayer AS, Chow AW, Louie JS, Nies KM, Guze LB: Gram-negative bacillary septic arthritis: clinical, radiographic, therapeutic and prognostic features. Semin Arthritis Rheum 7:123, 1977.

9. Sharp JT, Lidsky MD, Duffy J, Duncan MW: Infectious arthritis. Arch Intern Med 139:1125, 1979.

10. Mitchell WS, Brooks PM, Stevenson RD, Buchanan WW: Septic arthritis in patients with rheumatoid disease: a still underdiagnosed complication. J Rheumatol 3:124, 1976.

11. Borenstein DG, Simon GL: *Hemophilus influenzae* septic arthritis in adults: a report of four cases and a review of the literature. Medicine 65:191, 1986.

12. Nelson JD: Antibiotic concentrations in septic joint effusions. N Engl J Med 284:349, 1971.

13. Argen J, Wilson CH Jr, Wood P: Suppurative arteritis. Arch Intern Med 117:661, 1966.

14. Bacterial arthritis. Lancet 2:721, 1986.

15. Ho G Jr, Su EY: Therapy for septic arthritis. JAMA 247:797, 1982.

Peter A. Schlesinger, M.D.

CHAPTER

29

Nonsuppurative Infectious Arthritis

INTRODUCTION

Infectious agents are an important cause of nonsuppurative arthritic syndromes in adults and children. Unlike the case of pyogenic septic arthritis, however, direct invasion of the joint by these agents is not uniformly seen. The classes of organisms involved, the pathogenetic mechanisms, and the clinical manifestations show considerable diversity. In addition to those diseases in which a specific infection is known to be prerequisite, such as rheumatic fever, viral etiologies are being actively sought in such chronic inflammatory arthritides as rheumatoid arthritis and systemic lupus erythematosus. In rheumatoid arthritis, for example, there is evidence that antecedent Epstein-Barr viral infection exerts a permissive, if not causative, role.[1] However, the remainder of this chapter focuses on syndromes of established or strongly suspected infectious etiology.

PATHOPHYSIOLOGY

Regarding the pathophysiology of the nonsuppurative arthritides, two principal mechanisms are operative. The first is direct invasion of the joint by a nonpyogenic organism. Among the viral infections, only rubella has been isolated from the synovial fluid of multiple patients; herpes and enteroviruses have been occasionally recovered.[2, 3] Chronic Lyme arthritis is most likely due to the persistence of small numbers of the causative spirochete, *Borrelia burgdorferi,* in the synovium, where they can be visualized in perivascular sites.[4]

From the Hennepin County Medical Center, Minneapolis, Minnesota.

The second, and more common, mechanism is that of a "reactive arthritis." Defined broadly, it represents a *sterile* synovitis occurring in association with an infection elsewhere in the body, usually at mucosal surfaces.[5, 6] Examples are rheumatic fever and sexually acquired reactive arthritis. A latent period between acquisition of the triggering infection and the subsequent arthritis is compatible with the notion that the host's immune response to that infection is responsible for the arthritis. Furthermore, certain host cell surface antigens, coded for within the major histocompatibility complex (MHC), are associated with some reactive arthritides, suggesting that the host immune response is genetically conditioned. The immune response may be either *cell-mediated,* as measured by T-lymphocyte transformation, or *humoral,* through the production of antibodies. The debated concept of "molecular mimicry" holds that a cellular or humoral immune response against microbial structures or products cross-reacts with certain host tissues. Evidence for such a mechanism has been adduced for both rheumatic fever[7] (e.g., shared cross-reacting antigens between streptococcal M protein and human heart sarcolemmal membrane protein) and for arthritis following certain enteric bacterial infections.[8]

Finally, certain syndromes do not follow either of the above models. The arthritis associated with the prodromal phase of hepatitis B infection[9] or with bacterial endocarditis[10] is likely due to circulating immune complexes, without evidence of an exaggerated or otherwise abnormal host immune response. Hepatitis B closely resembles the experimental model of "one-shot serum sickness."[11] Several weeks after hepatitis B viral acquisition, a certain ratio of hepatitis B surface antigen (HBsAg) to antibody (anti-HBs) occurs, in "antigen excess," leading to the development of circulating immune complexes. These immune complexes bind complement and are presumably responsible for the clinical manifestations of arthritis and urticaria. Later, as HBsAg levels fall, the arthritis resolves. Arthritis in the setting of disseminated gonococcal infection (see Chapter 28) may involve both bacterial replication within the joint and immune complex mechanisms.[12]

Hepatitis B

Hepatitis B viral infection remains a frequent cause of acute arthritis in adults. Despite the advent of a highly effective vaccine, hepatitis B is still seen in intravenous drug users, sexual contacts of hepatitis B carriers, and certain high-risk medical personnel, among others. The frequency of arthritis in patients with hepatitis B is approximately 20 percent.[2, 3, 13] There are several possible clinical outcomes after acquisition of the hepatitis B virus (Table 29–1).

The pattern of the arthritis is usually symmetrical and polyarticular, with a predilection for the fingers.[2, 3, 13] The onset is typically abrupt, with an additive or migratory course. The degree of objective inflammation is variable, and periarticular involvement may occur. A rash commonly accompanies the arthritis; it can be urticarial, maculopapular, or petechial. Although constitutional symptoms, such as malaise and anorexia, are frequent, the arthritis-dermatitis phase usually precedes overt hepatic involvement. The onset of jaundice often coincides with resolution of the arthritis. Anicteric cases also occur. The duration of the arthritis is usually brief (days to weeks); it can be treated symptomatically with salicylates or other nonsteroidal anti-inflammatory drugs (NSAIDs). Diagnosis is based on an appropriate clinical syndrome accompanied by a positive blood test for HBsAg. The peripheral leukocyte count and erythrocyte sedimentation rate (ESR) are frequently normal.

Infection with hepatitis B virus is also associated with a number of other syndromes, including nephropathy, "essential" mixed cryoglobulinemia, and systemic necrotizing vasculitis; these have been reviewed elsewhere.[13]

Rubella and Other Viruses

Arthritis occurs in both naturally acquired rubella or following immunization with a live attenuated rubella vaccine.[2, 3] In each case, arthritis is more likely to develop in postpubescent patients, especially females; over one third of adult women receiving the vaccine are affected. The synovitis is symmetrical and usually affects the hands, wrists, and knees. Carpal tunnel syndrome and tenosynovitis are common. Other features of rubella, including the typical rash, low-grade fever, malaise, and posterior cervical lymphadenopathy, are usually present. Cases of radiculoneuropathy affecting the arms or legs have been described following rubella vaccination.[14]

The duration of rubella-associated or rubella vaccine-associated arthritis is usually brief, and the treatment is symptomatic. Rubella virus does appear to have tropism for joints, and there are reports of its isolation from the synovial fluid of patients with chronic arthritis.[15, 16] The significance of this observation is unclear.

A number of common viral infections, such as mumps and others caused by the herpesvirus family, are occasionally associated with arthritis.[2, 3] Infections with certain arboviruses, seen outside the United States, commonly cause arthritis.[2, 3]

Lyme Disease

Lyme disease is a newly recognized tick-borne spirochetal infection. Untreated, it can

---

TABLE 29–1. Sequelae to Hepatitis B Virus Infection*

Hepatic
Acute
  1. Asymptomatic infection, with development of anti-HBs
  2. Asymptomatic infection with carrier state developing
  3. Acute hepatitis, with resolution or hepatic failure
Chronic
  1. Chronic active hepatitis
  2. Chronic persistent hepatitis
  3. Postnecrotic cirrhosis
  4. Hepatocellular carcinoma

Extrahepatic
  1. Arthritis/dermatitis
  2. Nephropathy
  3. Essential mixed cryoglobulinemia
  4. Systemic vasculitis

* From Inman RD: Rheumatic manifestations of hepatitis B virus infection. Semin Arthritis Rheum 11:407, 1982.

cause acute attacks of arthritis, or more rarely, chronic destructive arthritis. The incidence of Lyme disease appears to be increasing, especially in endemic areas of the northeastern and north central United States, where it is transmitted by *Ixodes dammini* or related ixodid ticks.[17]

CLINICAL FEATURES

The clinical manifestations of Lyme disease can be divided into three stages.[18, 19]

Cutaneous (Stage 1). Stage 1 disease occurs during periods of tick activity (usually April to November), when the causative spirochete, *Borrelia burgdorferi,* is injected into the skin by an infected tick. From several days to a month later, a characteristic skin lesion, erythema migrans (formerly, erythema chronicum migrans), develops at the site of the tick bite.[18-20] Erythema migrans begins as a small red macule or papule that expands to become annular. The edge of a lesion usually remains bright red; the center often shows clearing but may become indurated, vesicular, or necrotic. Secondary skin lesions may develop at distant sites. Stage 1 disease is often accompanied by systemic signs and symptoms suggesting a flulike or meningitis-like illness. Untreated, erythema migrans usually resolves over days to weeks.

Cardiac or Neurologic (Stage 2). A minority of patients go on to experience cardiac or neurological sequelae (stage 2), including atrioventricular heart block, meningoencephalitis, and Bell's palsy. These manifestations are usually self-limited.

Arthritic (Stage 3). Stage 3 disease develops in about 60 percent of initially untreated patients, weeks to months later, consisting of discrete attacks of oligoarticular inflammatory arthritis, each attack usually lasting a few weeks.[19] The knee is the most frequently affected joint. In some of these patients, a chronic erosive synovitis with pannus formation develops.

DIAGNOSIS

The diagnosis of Lyme disease is predominantly clinical. The presence of erythema migrans is virtually pathognomonic. Serologic studies for antibodies to *B. burgdorferi* are adjunctive; results are frequently normal during the first several weeks of illness.[19]

TREATMENT

Antibiotic therapy is indicated in order to shorten the course of stage 1 disease and to prevent major late disease manifestations. Tetracycline, 250 mg, or phenoxymethyl penicillin, 500 mg, four times a day for 10 to 20 days, is the drug of choice; erythromycin is a slightly less effective alternative in penicillin-allergic children or pregnant women.[19] For neurological involvement or stage 3 arthritis, a longer course of antibiotics is needed, with either parenteral penicillin or oral tetracycline; the optimal regimen remains undefined.[21] Parenteral ceftriaxone has shown promise in refractory disease.[21a] NSAIDs provide symptomatic relief for arthritic attacks. Patients with chronic synovitis occasionally require synovectomy.

Bacterial Endocarditis

Musculoskeletal involvement in patients with bacterial endocarditis is common. Manifestations include arthralgias, arthritis, myalgias, diffuse low back pain, and vertebral osteomyelitis.[22, 23] In one series of 26 patients with arthritis, 22 (85 percent) had arthritis prior to the diagnosis of endocarditis.[22] One to three joints are most often affected. Monoarticular arthritis of a joint rarely affected in primary septic arthritis, such as the sternoclavicular or acromioclavicular, should increase the clinical suspicion of bacterial endocarditis. The synovial fluid is inflammatory but is almost always culture-negative. The arthritis is likely immune complex–mediated, secondary to antibodies combining with bacterial antigens, although septic emboli from the heart may occur as well. Parenteral antibiotic therapy for the endocarditis leads to resolution of the arthritis. Repeated arthrocentesis or arthrotomy, once a frankly septic joint is excluded, is rarely required.

Rheumatic Fever

The incidence of acute rheumatic fever declined dramatically in developed countries over the past century. Yet rheumatic fever and chronic rheumatic heart disease remain a serious public health issue in developing tropical and subtropical countries. Because of the large numbers of recent immigrants to the United States from Asia and Latin America, and because of the milder or non-existent extra-articular disease features in the adult, alertness to the possibility of rheumatic fever remains important.

The diagnosis of acute rheumatic fever in the adult will usually depend on the findings of inflammatory polyarthritis, fever, and elevated ESR in the setting of a recent group A beta-hemolytic streptococcal pharyngitis as documented by throat culture and/or an elevated titer of antistreptolysin O (ASO) or other streptococcal antibody.[24, 25] The arthritis is variably described as migratory or additive, but in almost all cases the onset is abrupt, severe, and large-joint, lower extremity predominant. Overlying erythema and periarticular involvement are common.[25] Synovial fluid aspirates are mildly to moderately inflammatory with a wide range of leukocyte counts. The arthritis and fever usually remit dramatically in response to salicylates or other NSAIDs.

Other manifestations of acute rheumatic fever in the adult are less common. Active carditis occurs in 15 to 35 percent of patients, usually in the setting of pre-existent rheumatic heart disease.[24, 26] New murmurs are not always present, and isolated pericarditis or congestive heart failure may occur.[26] Erythema marginatum is uncommon in the adult; subcutaneous nodules and chorea are virtually never seen.

Treatment of acute rheumatic fever involves anti-rheumatic therapy with salicylates or NSAIDs and eradication of pharyngeal group A streptococci with antibiotics. Prophylaxis against reinfection is determined by an individual's risk of carditis.

Reiter's Syndrome and Reactive Arthritis

Historically, a relationship between arthritis and antecedent venereal or enteric infection was noted as early as the eighteenth century. However, until recently, the absence of effective antimicrobial therapy and the inability to distinguish gout from those conditions led to diagnostic confusion. In patients with gonorrhea and arthritis, eradication of the gonococci did not necessarily terminate or attenuate the arthritis, suggesting an additional triggering mechanism for the latter. We now recognize the categories of "sexually acquired reactive arthritis" and "enterocolitic reactive arthritis," for which a number of triggering microbial agents have been implicated (see Pathophysiology earlier in this chapter).[5, 6] The term

"Reiter's syndrome" is a subset of these reactive arthritides, displaying a triad of arthritis, urethritis, and conjunctivitis. Sometimes the expression "incomplete Reiter's" is applied to patients with characteristic arthritic manifestations who do not exhibit the complete triad. Patients with these reactive arthritides have an increased likelihood of carrying the tissue antigen HLA-B27.[27] Historically thought to be a disease of men, sexually acquired reactive arthritis also affects women, although the diagnosis is more easily missed.

In terms of specific initiating infection, *Chlamydia trachomatis* has been strongly implicated for sexually acquired reactive arthritis.[5, 6, 28] In such patients, the history of a new sexual partner and/or the presence of *C. trachomatis* in the genital tract is frequently linked with disease onset. Furthermore, there was an overall stronger host immune response to *C. trachomatis* in men with nondiarrheal Reiter's syndrome in contrast to men with uncomplicated nongonococcal urethritis.[28] For enteric reactive arthritis, implicated organisms include certain *Salmonella* and *Shigella* strains, *Yersinia enterocolitica, Campylobacter jejuni,* and possibly *Clostridium difficile.*[5, 6, 29]

The joint manifestations of these reactive arthritides are remarkably consistent from patient to patient (Table 29–2). They are typically nonmigratory, oligoarticular, asymmetrical, and lower extremity predominant.[5, 6] There is a strong predilection for inflammation at tendinous insertions (entheses), particularly the Achilles tendon. Also characteristic is dactylitis or periostitis along the shafts of the phalanges, giving rise to a "sausage" finger or toe. Sacroiliitis and spondylitis may occur as well.

Extra-articular involvement is common.[5, 6] Urethritis, from clinically severe to asymptomatic, is frequent. It is seen in enteric reactive arthritis as well and can occur in the absence of a definable urethral infection. Patients with conjunctivitis and oral ulcers are usually asymptomatic. The skin lesions of keratodermia blennorrhagica begin as vesicles and then develop hyperkeratotic crusts; they most frequently involve the palms, soles, and glans penis (balanitis).

The cornerstone of medical therapy in these patients is NSAIDs, such as indomethacin, sulindac, or naproxen. Relatively high doses, such as indomethacin, 150 to 200 mg/day, are often required for relief. Salicylates, unlike their action in viral arthritis or rheumatic fever, are often ineffective. Intra-articular in-

TABLE 29–2. Clinical Features of Joint Involvement in Reactive B27-Associated Arthritis*

1. Asymmetric distribution
2. Predilection for large joints
3. Joints involved in rapid succession
4. Lower extremities affected in 80 to 90 percent
5. Upper extremities affected in about 50 percent
6. Typically an oligoarthritis
7. Enthesopathy (insertional tendinitis) in 30 to 50 percent
8. Low back pain in 20 to 30 percent

* From Aho K, Leirisalo-Repo M, Repo H: Reactive arthritis. Clin Rheum Dis 11:33, 1985.

jections of a corticosteroid preparation may be necessary if a particular joint is refractory to NSAID therapy. The arthritis usually remits after several weeks to months, but may become chronic. Antibiotic therapy for chlamydial urethritis, usually with a tetracycline, is given to the patient and sexual partner, not to shorten the course of the arthritis, but to eradicate the carrier state and to prevent genital tract sequelae, especially in females.[30] Generally, antibiotic therapy is not required in enteric reactive arthritis (other than *C. difficile*), since the infection is usually self-limiting.

Reactive arthritis bearing similarities to the aforementioned syndromes is sometimes seen in association with hidradenitis suppurativa or acne conglobata,[31] following jejunal-ileal bypass,[32] and in inflammatory bowel or Whipple's disease.[32]

DIAGNOSTIC CONSIDERATIONS

When should one suspect a nonsuppurative arthritis related to an infectious agent? Generally, involvement of more than one joint by an inflammatory process makes a septic process less likely. Examination of synovial fluid for cell counts and crystals and synovial fluid culture are nonetheless indicated for both monoarthritis and polyarthritis in a previously unaffected patient. If inflammatory synovial fluid is present and if a septic or crystal-induced arthritis has been reasonably excluded, arthritis related to a nonsuppurative infection is a consideration. In some cases, the associated infection is readily apparent, as in Reiter's syndrome following a *Salmonella*-induced diarrheal illness. However, the infection may be subtle, such as with preicteric hepatitis B or an asymptomatic chlamydial urethritis.

Two guidelines are helpful. First, the arthri-

TABLE 29–3. Differential Diagnosis of Nonsuppurative Infectious Arthritis

Disease	Historical Clues and Symptoms	Signs	Laboratory Tests
Hepatitis B	History of exposure	Urticaria	Hepatitis B surface antigen (HBsAg)
Rubella or rubella vaccine	History of exposure Recent vaccination	Morbilliform rash Lymphadenopathy	—
Lyme disease	History of tick bite Residence in endemic area History of erythema migrans	Erythema migrans Meningoencephalitis Cranial neuritis Radiculoneuritis	Lyme disease serology (antibodies to *Borrelia burgdorferi*)
Bacterial endocarditis	Intravenous drug abuse Diseased/prosthetic heart valve	New murmur Embolic phenomena Splenomegaly	Blood culture
Acute rheumatic fever	History of streptococcal pharyngitis History of prior rheumatic fever or rheumatic heart disease	Carditis (uncommon) Erythema marginatum (rare)	Antistreptolysin O or other streptococcal antibody Throat culture for beta-hemolytic group A streptococcus
Sexually acquired reactive arthritis (Reiter's syndrome)	History of new sexual partner Urethral discharge Dysuria	Dactylitis Tendinitis Conjunctivitis Oral ulcers Urethritis Keratodermia blennorrhagica	Urethral or cervical smear for *Chlamydia trachomatis* (direct fluorescent antibody)
Enteric reactive arthritis (Reiter's syndrome)	History of diarrheal illness and/or travel	Same as for sexually acquired reactive arthritis	Stool culture

tis associated with infections is usually of *acute* onset. Synovitis in the setting of rheumatoid arthritis or systemic lupus erythematosus commonly develops more insidiously. Second, extra-articular manifestations, especially cutaneous, are frequently present. Table 29–3 lists distinguishing historical features, symptoms, signs, and laboratory tests for the entities discussed. It should be noted that the "standard" rheumatological tests such as those for rheumatoid factor (RF) and antinuclear antibodies (FANA) are frequently not helpful in evaluating an acute arthritic illness of short duration. If no precise rheumatological diagnosis can be made at the initial visit, the patient can often be treated symptomatically, provided that care has been taken to exclude entities requiring immediate specific treatment, such as bacterial endocarditis. Often the arthritis resolves, and medications can be successfully discontinued. In the case of persistent synovitis, other symptoms, signs, or laboratory abnormalities may later emerge that allow one to arrive at a specific diagnosis.

References

1. Fox RI, Lotz M, Rhodes G: Epstein-Barr virus in rheumatoid arthritis. Clin Rheum Dis 11:665, 1985.
2. Steere AC, Malawista SE: Viral arthritis. In McCarty DJ, ed: Arthritis and Allied Conditions, 10th ed. Philadelphia, Lea & Febiger, 1985.
3. Schnitzer TJ: Viral arthritis. In Kelley WN, Harris ED Jr, Ruddy S, Sledge CB, eds: Textbook of Rheumatology, 2nd ed. Philadelphia, WB Saunders Co, 1985.
4. Johnston YE, Duray PH, Steere AC, et al: Lyme arthritis: spirochetes found in synovial microangiopathic lesions. Am J Pathol 118:26, 1985.
5. Aho K, Leirisalo-Repo M, Repo H: Reactive arthritis. Clin Rheum Dis 11:25, 1985.
6. Keat A: Reiter's syndrome and reactive arthritis in perspective. N Engl J Med 309:1606, 1983.
7. Williams RC Jr: Molecular mimicry and rheumatic fever. Clin Rheum Dis 11:573, 1985.
8. Kono DH, Ogasawara M, Effros RB, Park MS, Waldord RL, Yu DTY: Ye-1, a monoclonal antibody that cross-reacts with HLA-B27 lymphoblastoid cell lines and an arthritis causing bacteria. Clin Exp Immunol 61:503, 1985.
9. Alpert E, Schur PH, Isselbacher KJ: Sequential changes of serum complement in HAA related arthritis. N Engl J Med 287:103, 1972.
10. Bayer AS, Theofilopoulos AN, Eisenberg R, Dixon FJ, Guze LB: Circulating immune complexes in infective endocarditis. N Engl J Med 295:1500, 1976.
11. Dixon FJ, Vazquez JJ, Weigle WO, Cochrane C: Pathogenesis of serum sickness. Arch Pathol 65:18, 1958.
12. Masi AT, Eisenstein BI: Disseminated gonococcal infection (DGI) and gonococcal arthritis (GCA): II. Clinical manifestations, diagnosis, complications, treatment, and prevention. Semin Arthritis Rheum 10:173, 1981.
13. Inman RD: Rheumatic manifestations of hepatitis B virus infection. Semin Arthritis Rheum 11:406, 1982.
14. Schaffner W, Fleet WF, Kilroy AW, et al: Polyneuropathy following rubella immunization. Am J Dis Child 127:684, 1974.
15. Grahame R, Armstrong R, Simmons NA, Mims CA, Wilton JMA, Laurent R: Isolation of rubella virus from synovial fluid in five cases of seronegative arthritis. Lancet 2:649, 1981.
16. Chantler JK, Ford DK, Tingle AJ: Persistent rubella infection and rubella-associated arthritis. Lancet 1:1323, 1982.
17. Steere AC, Malawista SE: Cases of Lyme disease in the United States: locations correlated with distribution of *Ixodes dammini.* Ann Intern Med 91:730, 1979.
18. Steere AC, Malawista SE, Hardin JA, Ruddy S, Askenase PW, Andiman WA: Erythema chronicum migrans and Lyme arthritis: the enlarging clinical spectrum. Ann Intern Med 86:685, 1977.
19. Steere AC, Malawista SE: Lyme disease. In McCarty DJ, ed: Arthritis and Allied Conditions, 10th ed. Philadelphia, Lea & Febiger, 1985.
20. Steere AC, Bartenhagen NH, Craft JE, et al: The early clinical manifestations of Lyme disease. Ann Intern Med 99:76, 1983.
21. Steere AC, Green J, Schoen RT, et al: Successful parenteral penicillin therapy of established Lyme arthritis. N Engl J Med 312:869, 1985.
21a. Dattwyler RJ, Halperin JJ, Pass H, Luft BJ: Ceftriaxone as effective therapy in refractory Lyme disease. J Infect Dis 155:1322, 1987.
22. Churchill MA Jr, Geraci JE, Hunder GG: Musculoskeletal manifestations of bacterial endocarditis. Ann Intern Med 87:754, 1977.
23. Thomas PH, Allal J, Bontoux D, et al: Rheumatological manifestations of infective endocarditis. Ann Rheum Dis 43:716, 1984.
24. Barnert AL, Terry EE, Persellin RH: Acute rheumatic fever in adults. JAMA 232:925, 1975.
25. McDanald EC, Weisman MH: Articular manifestations of rheumatic fever in adults. Ann Intern Med 89:917, 1978.
26. Ben-Dov I, Berry E: Acute rheumatic fever in adults over the age of 45 years: an analysis of 23 patients together with a review of the literature. Semin Arthritis Rheum 10:100, 1980.
27. Brewerton DA, Caffrey M, Nicholls A, Walters D, Oates JK, James DCO: Reiter's disease and HL-A27. Lancet 2:996, 1973.
28. Martin DH, Pollock S, Kuo CC, Wang SP, Brunham RC, Holmes KK: *Chlamydia trachomatis* infections in men with Reiter's syndrome. Ann Intern Med 100:207, 1984.
29. Lofgren RP, Tadlock LM, Soltis RD: Acute oligoarthritis associated with *Clostridium difficile* pseudomembranous colitis. Arch Intern Med 144:617, 1984.
30. Stamm WE, Holmes KK: *Chlamydia trachomatis* infections of the adult. In Holmes KK, Mardh P, Sparling PF, Wiesner PJ, eds: Sexually Transmitted Diseases. New York, McGraw-Hill, Inc, 1984.
31. Rosner IA, Richter DE, Huettner TL, Kuffner GH, Wisnieski JJ, Burg CG: Spondyloarthropathy associated with hidradenitis suppurativa and acne conglobata. Ann Intern Med 97:520, 1982.
32. Good AE, Utsinger PD: Enteropathic arthritis. In Kelley WN, Harris ED Jr, Ruddy S, Sledge CB, eds: Textbook of Rheumatology, 2nd ed. Philadelphia, WB Saunders Co, 1985.

George Peltier, M.D.

30

Sacral Pressure Sores

INTRODUCTION

By any surgeon's definition, the pressure sore is one of the greatest nuisances of modern medical care. The pressure sore complicates surgery, delays discharge, is untreatable in many cases, and even confuses the nomenclature for diagnosis. The frequently used descriptive word "decubitus," which is often misused, is reserved only for the sore that develops with the patient in a recumbent position. A pressure sore is therefore defined as the necrosis of soft tissue and bone over a protuberance of the skeletal system where prolonged pressure has been exerted from any cause.

The epidemiology of pressure sores has been studied extensively by Petersen and Bittmann.[1] These investigators found an incidence of 43.1 patients with sores per 100,000 in Danish hospitals and nursing homes. Sixty percent of the patients had a sacral ulcer, the most frequently encountered sore. Thirty-six percent of those with sacral sores were wheelchair patients in whom the ulcer undoubtedly developed in bed.

The classic sacral decubitus ulcer arises from pressure placed on the sacrum from being supine on a hard surface for an excessive period of time. In head injury patients and those who have taken a drug overdose, acute pressure sores frequently develop prior to arrival at the hospital. We have seen this in patients who have suffered a hip fracture and have been trapped by their injury on the floor of their home. This type of pressure ulcer has developed in patients undergoing surgery while lying on the firm operating table surface in association with the low tissue perfusion.

CLASSIFICATION

We have adopted the classification system proposed by Daniels and co-workers for the severity of the sacral ulcer[2]:

Grade I. A skin area of erythema or induration overlying a bony prominence, i.e., an incipient pressure sore.

Grade II. A skin area of superficial ulceration extending into the dermis.

Grade III. An ulcer extending into the subcutaneous tissue, but not into muscle.

Grade IV. A deep ulcer extending through muscle down to the bony prominence.

Grade V. An extensive ulcer with widespread extension along bursae or into joints or body cavities.

Radiation is another cause of sacral pressure sores. The pelvis is a frequent site for applying therapeutic external radiation, and frequently the posterior port rests directly on the sacral bone. Minimal pressure then causes necrosis of the overlying skin and infection develops.

Thermal injury is a frequent cause of sacral ulceration, and the exact mechanisms are varied. The electric light is a popular method of treating chronically irritated perineal skin. The light helps dry the surface of the skin and warms the skin, thus increasing local blood flow. However, the heat of the bulb can cause severe injury if it comes in contact with the skin of the patient. Malfunctioning heating pads are a source for sacral injury because a low heat over an extended period of time may cause a deep burn. These burns are exacerbated by the pressure induced by a hard surface or the stiff wiring of the heating pad. The cautery ground plate can malfunction and cause severe burns. A cautery ground pad should never be placed over the bony sacrum of any patient. Pooling of blood around the cautery pad can also cause a severe burn.

From the Hennepin County Medical Center, Minneapolis, Minnesota.

TREATMENT

Treatment of the sacral pressure sore is one of the most complex medical problems that we face (Table 30–1). Our principal concern is the prevention of the initial occurrence of any changes at all in the sacral skin, and therefore high-risk patients must be identified. Any unconscious patient is a likely candidate for a sacral pressure sore. These patients cannot perform any spontaneous movements or change their body positions. An example is the anesthetized patient undergoing a lengthy operation. Foam pads or water-filled gloves should be used to protect bony prominences. Friction in moving the patient from bed to cart should be avoided because this can cause a blister or Grade II injury. Anemia has been shown to be a predisposing factor in the formation of pressure sores. Pressure changes in the skin are very likely to develop in any debilitated patient, even though these individuals are able to move their extremities and are able to sense that pressure is occurring. Chronic urine and fecal soilage irritates the skin and makes the skin more sensitive to the insults of pressure. Once rupture of the skin occurs, the opportunistic fecal flora are at hand to invade tissue.

The relief of pressure is very important in prevention of the pressure sore, and a variety of therapeutic beds are used for this purpose. High-risk patients should be placed on these beds prior to the development of a pressure sore and not just after the nurse has noted changes over the sacrum. Once changes have occurred, pressure sores are very likely to develop in other locations and application of the therapeutic beds is mandatory. High-risk patients must still be rotated on an every-2-hour schedule, or patients must be awakened and must change their own position at regular in-

tervals. Total dependence on the therapeutic beds is not at all advisable.

In spite of the best possible preventive medical care, the sacral pressure sore can appear and direct treatment may be undertaken. The Daniels Grade I or incipient pressure sore of the sacrum appears as an area of erythema, and the patient may complain of soreness. Immediate steps should be taken to prevent any pressure from being applied to the sacral area until the erythema clears.

Daniels Grade II pressure sores necessitate local treatment in addition to relieving all pressure. We have used semipermeable transparent adhesive dressings very successfully for the lightly secreting wound. For heavy drainage, an absorbent dressing containing gauze or a similar material is required. The new collagen topical dressings and their close relatives also are very useful. Treatment is much like that for burns because the patient must be pushed into positive nitrogen balance and be given vitamin and mineral supplementation. In these cases, wound cultures are only valuable if the wound becomes secondarily infected.

Infection severely complicates the clinical course because the Grade I and II pressure sores frequently convert quickly to deeper wounds. Grade III sores require debridement to control infection, and this may be accomplished using three general methods. Necrotic tissue may be surgically removed until living tissue is approached. Wet to dry saline packs have been a classic method of passive debridement, and these remain a useful, gentle method for cleaning a wound. Last, there are several chemical and enzymatic methods of wound debridement that may be selected.

Sacral pressure sores may lead to systemic infection and sepsis, causing death; this arises in the Grade III, IV, and V ulcers (Fig. 30–1). Certainly, intravenous antibiotic therapy cannot cure a sacral pressure sore, but carefully selected antibiotics are helpful in controlling systemic infection, curing concurrent infection and preventing septicemia.[3] Galpin and colleagues[4] reviewed 21 patients in whom sepsis developed solely as a result of decubitus ulcers and found that 13, or 62 percent, of the infections arose from sacral ulcers. The mortality rate of sepsis from a sacral ulcer was 47 percent and was largely due to *Bacteroides fragilis.* Among the patients who underwent surgical debridement, the mortality rate was only 26 percent. Contamination of the sacral ulcer with fecal flora is universal so that antibiotic

TABLE 30–1. Treatment of Sacral Pressure Sores

Class	Treatment
I Skin erythema	Local care and relief of pressure
II Skin necrosis	Local care and relief of pressure
III Subcutaneous tissue loss	Debridement and surgical closure
IV Exposed bone	Debridement and surgical closure
V Bone necrosis	Debridement, bone resection, flap closure

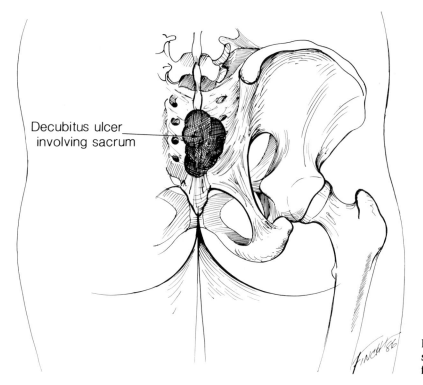

Decubitus ulcer involving sacrum

FIGURE 30-1. Sacral pressure sore in an irradiated field.

treatment should cover the anaerobic spectrum and enteric gram-negative organisms.

SURGERY

The surgical closure of the sacral pressure sore can be accomplished by the careful selection of the patient and a judicious selection of an operative procedure in the Grade III, IV, and V ulcers. The acute nature of the sacral ulcer must be controlled, and the ulcer must be converted to a chronic wound. All debridement must be completed, and the ulcer must be starting to heal spontaneously. The situation that caused the ulcer must be corrected. This usually means altering the social situation for a patient, but in many cases this is an insurmountable problem. Certainly, for a patient who has a rapidly terminal illness, a large flap closure should not be chosen. Patients who neglect their self-care should neither undergo surgery nor have extensive rehabilitation prior to or with surgery. Candidates for surgery should be in positive nitrogen balance, and any metabolic deficiencies should be corrected. Patients must be able to commit several weeks to the task of very careful positioning themselves following surgery.

Multiple operations are now available for surgical closure of the sacral pressure sore once a patient has been properly prepared.[5, 6] Primary closure of the ulcers of the sacrum is usually impossible because of the lack of distensibility of the tissue. Skin grafts can successfully close the wound but are not resilient enough in the long run to stand up to pressure. Therefore, most of the sacral ulcers in the Daniels Grades III, IV, and V are closed with a random or a musculocutaneous flap brought in from the buttock area. All of the bursa and all of the necrotic bone must be completely excised. Random rotational flaps have been used routinely for the small sacral ulcer, but the large or massive ulcer has been approachable using only the gluteus maximus musculocutaneous flap. Rotating skin with sensibility into an area of anesthetic skin occasionally is a very useful procedure.

The gluteus maximus muscle provides the basis for all of the musculocutaneous flaps for closing the sacral ulcer.[5, 7, 8] The muscle flap has been employed for closing pressure sores for three reasons. The muscle is used as a carrier for a segment of skin providing a resurfacing flap that resists necrosis. Second, the muscle provides new blood supply to nourish the bone and lymphatics to control infection. Last,

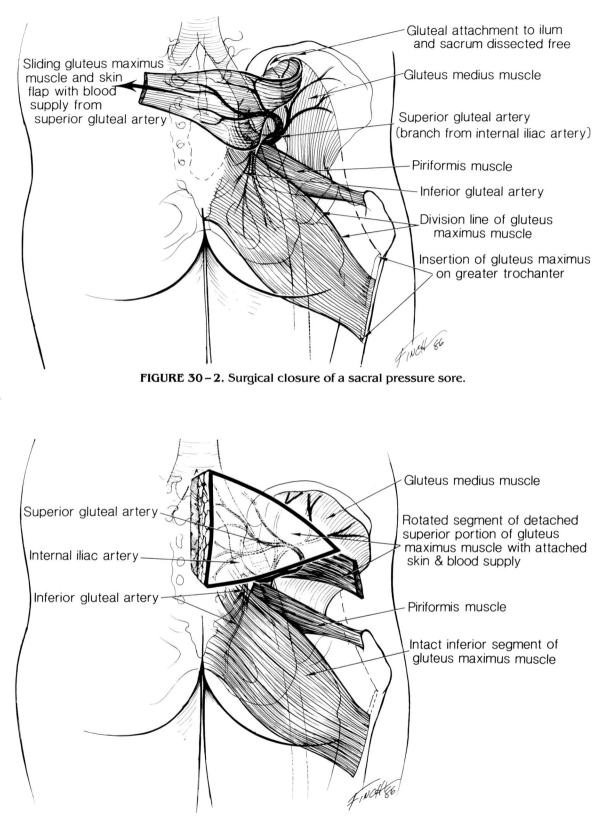

Sliding gluteus maximus muscle and skin flap with blood supply from superior gluteal artery

Gluteal attachment to ilum and sacrum dissected free

Gluteus medius muscle

Superior gluteal artery (branch from internal iliac artery)

Piriformis muscle

Inferior gluteal artery

Division line of gluteus maximus muscle

Insertion of gluteus maximus on greater trochanter

FIGURE 30–2. Surgical closure of a sacral pressure sore.

Gluteus medius muscle

Superior gluteal artery

Internal iliac artery

Inferior gluteal artery

Rotated segment of detached superior portion of gluteus maximus muscle with attached skin & blood supply

Piriformis muscle

Intact inferior segment of gluteus maximus muscle

FIGURE 30–3. Sacral ulcer pictured in Figure 30–1 now closed with bilateral gluteus maximus musculocutaneous flaps.

the muscle provides padding to protect the bony prominences for a few months after surgery. Nola and Vistnes[9] have demonstrated that there is a significant reduction of bulk when a muscle is released from its insertion and transposed. Also, the transposed muscle is more sensitive to pressure than the skin muscle flap; thus, the patient must be very careful not to re-ulcerate these flaps. The gluteus maximus is a thick, flat muscle that obtains its blood supply from the superior and inferior gluteal arteries (Fig. 30–2). This muscle therefore can be split into a superior and inferior portion. The entire muscle cannot be sacrificed in an ambulatory patient, but the superior portion of the muscle carries a large enough flap to close a defect (Fig. 30–3). In a paraplegic patient, the entirety of both muscles may be used to pad and resurface the sacrum.[10]

When the gluteus flap has been raised, it must be brought into the defect without any tension on the closure (Fig. 30–3). Almost always, both gluteus flaps are required for a tension-free closure in the midline over the sacrum. The entire bursa should be excised so that fresh tissue will heal against fresh tissue. The bony prominences and any soft bone must be removed. If osteomyelitis has been demonstrated, the wound should be irrigated with appropriate antibiotic fluids and methylmethacrylate antibiotic beads should be left in the wounds in a manner similar to that for operating on any other form of osteomyelitis. On occasion, in Daniels Grade V patients, we have used homograft to hold the beads in place on a flat surface of bone and have delayed the actual flap rotation for a week. The wound should be liberally drained to prevent accumulations of fluid or blood from developing. The drains are left in until drainage is totally absent. Ambulation should be started at 2 weeks, and during that period the patient should be maintained on a pressure-relieving bed. Only minimal pressure should be applied to the sacrum during the 2-week period. A rehabilitation program is very useful at this time to aid in the future prevention of pressure sore recurrence.

SUMMARY

The cost of the sacral pressure sore is extremely high both in dollars and in lives. The best treatment for this disease is prevention, and every effort must be made to prevent the occurrence of pressure sores and to treat them at a very early stage. The patient likely to be at risk must be identified, and the appropriate preventive measures must be instituted.

References

1. Petersen NC, Bittmann S: The epidemiology of pressure sores. Scand J Plast Reconstr Surg 5:62–66, 1971.
2. Daniels RK, Hall EJ, MacLeod MK: Pressure sores: a reappraisal. Ann Plast Surg 3:55–63, 1979.
3. Lamon JD, Alexander E: Secondary closure of decubitus ulcers with the aid of penicillin. JAMA 127:396, 1945.
4. Galpin JE, Chow AW, Bayer AS, et al: Sepsis associated with decubitus ulcers. Am J Med 61:346–350, 1976.
5. Minami RT, Mills R, Pardoe R: Gluteus maximus myocutaneous flaps for repair of pressure sores. Plast Reconstr Surg 60:242–249, 1977.
6. Shively RE, Schafer ME, Kernahan DA: The spread of sensibility into previously anesthetic skin following intercostal flap transfer in a paraplegic. Ann Plast Surg 5:396–400, 1980.
7. Maruyama Y, Nakajima H, Wada M, et al: A gluteus maximus myocutaneous island flap for the repair of a sacral decubitus ulcer. Br J Plast Surg 33:150–155, 1980.
8. Scheflan M, Nahai F, Bostwick J: Gluteus maximus island musculocutaneous flap for closure of sacral and ischial ulcers. Plast Reconstr Surg 68:533–538, 1981.
9. Nola GT, Vistnes LM: Differential response of skin and muscle in the experimental production of pressure sores. Plast Reconstr Surg 66:728–733, 1980.
10. Ramirez OM, Orlando JC, Hurwitz DJ: The sliding gluteus maximus myocutaneous flap: its relevance in ambulatory patients. Plast Reconstr Surg 74:68–75, 1984.

Joseph E. Clinton, M.D.

CHAPTER

31

Puncture Wounds by Inanimate Objects and Mammalian Bite

INTRODUCTION

A puncture wound to the extremity is an innocuous-appearing injury that may result in protracted disability, multiple surgical procedures, and life-threatening infection. The initial appearance of the wound belies its potential for complication. Proper initial management of the injury must occur with consideration of factors predisposing to complications. Wounding mechanism, degree of bacterial contamination, inoculation of deep structures with debris and organisms, time since injury, and host factors all play a role in determining the management strategy.

This chapter focuses on puncture wounds to the extremities caused by inanimate objects and mammalian bites. The wounding mechanism is of prime importance. Types of super-infection and long term-complication vary according to the mechanism. General management principles for each type of wound are discussed. Tetanus and rabies prophylaxis, as well as antibiotic therapy for the wound that is already infected, are addressed.

SCOPE OF THE PROBLEM

Significance of Mechanism

The term "puncture" implies a hole or depression produced by a perforating object. The wounding object may be any pointed object capable of piercing the skin. Whether that object is a nail from a construction site; a nail in a barnyard; or a tooth of a dog, cat, rat, bat, or human is an important consideration. The mi-

From the Hennepin County Medical Center, Minneapolis, Minnesota.

croorganisms and debris inoculated into the victim's tissue greatly impact the potential for complication.

Clinical Features

The actual appearance of the wound gives little information of the wounding mechanism. Puncture wound depth is difficult to assess on physical examination. Wounds of similar appearance function differently, depending on the degree of contamination by bacteria and foreign material, injury to deep structures, and ability of the wound to drain externally. A common feature of puncture wounds of various mechanisms is poor wound drainage. Contamination at the time of injury is often inaccessible to surface cleansing maneuvers. Failure to irrigate and debride the wound properly often allows bacteria to proliferate in deep structures.

WOUNDS CAUSED BY INANIMATE OBJECTS

Puncture Wound of the Foot

The classic example of innocence in wound appearance is an injury caused by puncture of the sole of the foot produced by stepping on an unseen nail. Acute, superficial examination of the wound reveals little information. Local tenderness is present surrounding a puncture wound. Dirt may be present on skin edges but often is not. The intuitive management strategy is to clean the skin, reassure patients, instruct them in signs of infection, and send them home to await further developments.

Unfortunately, further developments may come in the form of serious complications. An infection rate of 10 percent has been reported in a series of more than 2500 patients with puncture wounds of the foot,[1] where the deep structures are of major concern (Fig. 31–1). Entry of the nail into any of the joint spaces may result in septic arthritis.[2] Cartilaginous or bony injury can easily lead to osteochondritis or osteomyelitis, often as a result of *Pseudomonas aeruginosa*[3-6] or other ubiquitous soil and water inhabitants. Debris carried deep into the wound may result in a foreign body inflammatory response as the body tries to rid itself of the offending agent. The clinician should understand and anticipate the complications mentioned. Anticipation of complications often allows it to be avoided or, when it occurs, contributes to an awareness that will ensure rapid and effective management.

Complications of Foot Puncture

Historical information is important to risk assessment in the foot puncture wound. Wounding agent, location of the wounding incident, depth of the wound, and general health status of the host are questions of concern. Shoes worn at the time of injury may be important. Comparison of the nail to the depth of the shoe worn may provide an idea of the depth of the wound.

Pseudomonas osteomyelitis is a well-recognized complication of this injury.[4-5] The athletic shoe often becomes colonized by *P. aeru-*

ginosa, presumably as a result of moisture produced by perspiration.[6] Cultures of layers of athletic shoes have shown the foam layer of the sole to be the most likely source of the infection.[6] The association of athletic shoes with this infection has prompted the descriptive term "sneaker osteo" for the condition.

Retained foreign body must always be considered. Soft-tissue radiography can aid in localization of radiodense items such as metal and glass. A retained wooden or other radiolucent foreign body cannot be apparent on the radiograph, and exploration may be demanded when the possibility exists.[7]

The wounding environment is an important historical consideration. A barnyard injury must be handled more aggressively than a construction site injury. The potential contamination with gas-forming organisms or tetanus, particularly from manure, must prompt thorough debridement and establishment of drainage in affected wounds.

Host factors increase risk of complication. The diabetic patient and the patient with peripheral vascular insufficiency of other etiology face greater risks from puncture wounds than do healthy people. Clinical decisions in regard to these patients should err on the side of aggressive management with the expectation of development of infection.

MAMMALIAN BITE INJURY

A common cause of puncture wound is the bite injury. Once again, complications are related to the wounding agent and the mechanism of injury, its location, and host factors. Mammalian bite injuries are categorized into those produced by (1) domestic pets (dogs, cats), (2) humans, and (3) wild animals.

Domestic Animal Bites

It is estimated that 500 to 700 bites per 100,000 population occur per year in the United States.[8] The majority of the victims are children, with infants younger than 1 year of age being at greatest risk of fatal injury. Eighty to 90 percent of bites are inflicted by the domestic dog. Cats produce 5 to 10 percent of the injuries and rodents, 2 to 3 percent.[9]

The risk of infection seems to be greater in the cat bite wound than the dog bite. Dog bites have been reported to be complicated by infection in 5 to 30 percent of cases, whereas

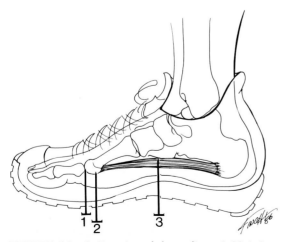

FIGURE 31–1. Puncture injury sites. *1,* Metatarsal-phalangeal joint. *2,* Cartilage of metatarsal head. *C,* Plantar fascia.

TABLE 31–1. Factors Increasing Infection Risk in Mammalian Bites

1. Wounds of the extremities
2. Wounds unable to be irrigated or debrided
3. Cat and primate bites
4. Age older than 50 years
5. Asplenism, alcoholism, diabetes
6. Immunosuppression, steroid therapy
7. Peripheral vascular insufficiency

complication by infection in cat bites may be as high as 30 to 50 percent.[10] Several factors that increase the risk of infection of the bite wound have been identified (Table 31–1).[10, 11]

Human Bites

It is the bite of our own species that carries the greatest risk of infection. The mechanism of injury and the bacterial flora involved may be responsible to the degree of disability associated with the human bite injury.

Seventy-three percent of human bite wounds are inflicted during aggressive behavior. The upper extremity predominates as the site of the injury, with 61 percent of human bites occurring there, according to one study.[12] Other common sites include the head and neck (15 percent), thorax and abdomen (11 percent), and lower extremities (9 percent).[12]

Forty-one percent of human bites are of the "fight-bite" variety sustained when a fist strikes the mouth of an opponent during a fight.[13] It is important to understand the danger associated with the wounding mechanism. Puncture of the extensor tendon over the metacarpal phalangeal joint is frequently associated with this injury (Fig. 31–2A,B). Risk of penetration of the joint itself is significant. When the hand is in the resting position, the inoculated portion of the tendon retracts proximal to the skin wound, thereby effectively sealing the bacteria in the soft tissue of the hand (Fig. 31–2C).

Human saliva may contain 10^8 bacteria/ml with up to 42 pathogens.[14] Bacteria identified in wounds include *Streptococcus viridans* group in 85 percent, group A beta-hemolytic streptococci in 35 percent, *Staphylococcus aureus* and *Staphylococcus epidermidis* in 40 percent and *Eikenella corrodens* in 30 percent.[15] Infection with any of these organisms is possible. Transmission of viral hepatitis from human bite has

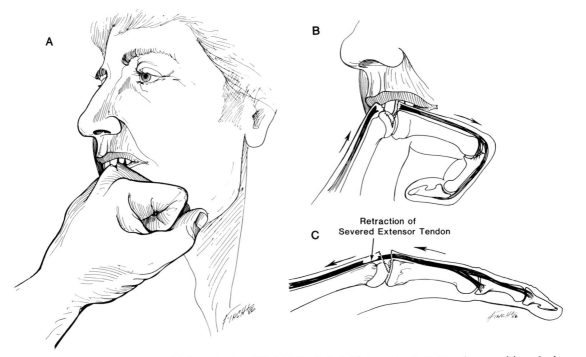

Retraction of Severed Extensor Tendon

FIGURE 31–2. Mechanism of injury during "fight-bite." *A,* Initial contact. *B,* Tendon position during injury. *C,* Tendon injury site with hand at rest.

been documented.[16] The risk must be considered and precautions taken when significant risk is found for hepatitis exposure in this fashion. No other viral disease transmission has been clearly identified as a common risk in human bite wounds.

Wild Animal Bites

The foremost concern in wild animal bite injury is that the biting animal may have been rabid. Fear of transmission of the deadly virus to the human host is often the overriding consideration. The risk of bacterial infection from wild animal bites is no greater and is probably less than it is from domestic animal bites.[17]

Knowledge of the circumstances of the bite, the animal species, and the geographic location will often simplify the rabies analysis. An unprovoked attack by a wild carnivore (e.g., skunk, bat, raccoon, bobcat, coyote, fox) creates a set of circumstances with the highest likelihood for rabies transmission. Rodents and lagomorphs rarely carry rabies and have not been documented as having transmitted human rabies.[17, 18]

WOUND MANAGEMENT

The course of the wound to healing or infection and complication is usually determined by its initial management. Irrigation method, adequacy of debridement, closure decisions, infection in the high-risk wound. Wound management considerations outweigh prophylactic antibiotics as determinants of future well-being of the wound.

Copious irrigation of wounds with saline is the standard approach to initial wound management. Infection rates in bite wounds are doubled in those that cannot be irrigated.[11] Bacteria clearance is improved over that achieved with low-pressure irrigation by using pulsatile irrigation such as that produced with a Water-Pik device.[19] It is clear that high-pressure irrigation is superior to low pressure in its ability to cleanse and disinfect wounds.[20] A reasonable approach recommended for bite wounds is to irrigate with at least 150 cc normal saline using a syringe with a 19-gauge catheter to provide pressure irrigation.[11]

Irrigation with solutions other than saline has been recommended by various authors. Hexachlorophene detergent has been recommended to fight infection.[21] However, the tissue toxicity of detergents has been demonstrated to be detrimental to wound healing. One percent povidone-iodine solution has decreased the incidence of wound infection when placed into surgical wounds without harming tissues.[22] In contrast, the 10 percent solution or the scrub solution of povidone-iodine is tissue toxic and should not be used as a soak or wound cleanser.[23, 24] Pluonic F-68, a detergent without antibacterial activity, has been demonstrated to be a nontoxic detergent used in the past.[25, 26] Benzalkonium chloride has been recommended for use in wounds considered at risk for rabies contamination. A safe course seems to be to clean contaminated skin with a detergent solution, if necessary, and to irrigate the wound with saline and/or 1 percent povidone-iodine with a syringe and 19-gauge needle.

Debridement of all bite and puncture wounds is an important and often poorly performed procedure. The most prudent recommendation is to excise the wound margins in all cases. Important objectives are accomplished by doing so; exploration of the wound, removal of deep debris and foreign bodies, and drainage are facilitated and contused wound edges are removed as a breeding ground for bacteria. The wound can be left open to heal safely by secondary intention in most cases. Faust and associates described a method for opening a puncture wound by trimming skin edges where the wound was cleansed of debris and left open after wound margins were excised.[21] The approach is a reasonable routine management protocol for puncture wounds to the foot.

Careful exploration of the wound is mandatory to find occult foreign bodies and injuries to important deep structures such as tendons and joint capsules. Soft tissue radiography should be considered part of routine exploration when a foreign body of an extremity is suspected. The radiograph will uncover surprisingly small foreign bodies in some instances. It is also an aid for removal of the offending agent by allowing localization through the use of crossed needles and hemostats.[27, 28]

A high index of suspicion is necessary to diagnose tendon injuries early when wounds overlie them. Involvement of the extensor tendons of the hand in fight-bite injuries to the metacarpal-phalangeal joint area are the most common example of this type of injury. (Fig. 31–2). The victim's tooth is seen to violate the skin over a joint (Fig. 31–2A), then the tendon

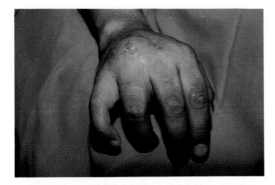

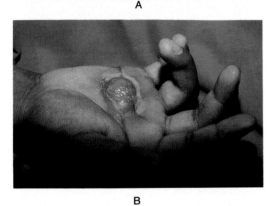

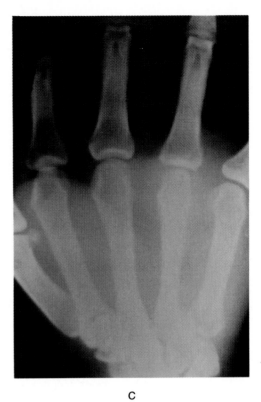

FIGURE 31–3. Osteomyelitis and soft tissue infection 2 months after "fight-bite" injury. *A,* Dorsum of hand. *B,* Volar aspect of hand. *C,* Sclerosis of fourth metacarpal.

and possibly the joint itself. (see Fig. 31–2*B,C*) Examination of the wound in the resting position will reveal an apparently intact tendon (see Fig. 31–2*C*). However, examination of the wound in the fisted position reveals the rent in the tendon and the possibility of joint involvement. Tendons must be examined throughout the entire range of motion before their integrity is declared. The failure to do this may lead to fight-bite injury and infectious complication (Fig. 31–3). This patient is suffering from complication of a fight-bite injury sustained 2 months prior to this photograph. In addition to the obvious soft tissue infection, there is osteomyelitis of the fourth metacarpal bone.

Whenever possible, bite wounds should be left open to heal by secondary intention. This is particularly true in bite wounds to the extremities. An open wound allows drainage and minimizes risk of secondary infection.

Occasionally, wounds must be closed for cosmetic reasons. Cosmetic concerns usually arise in reference to facial wounds. Fortunately, the risk of infection is lower in facial wounds than it is for the extremity wound, and closure can be safely carried out after thorough irrigation and debridement.[29, 30]

The objectives of dressing any wound are to protect it from further contamination from the environment, provide an environment conducive to rapid healing, and to assist in wound cleansing by the debriding action of dressing changes. Hand dressings usually have the additional objective of immobilization of the affected hand.

A simply applied dressing that is changed daily is sufficient for puncture wounds of the foot and for bites that do not overlie tendons. Hand injuries should be immobilized with a bulky dressing in the position of function. Frequency of changes should be at least daily. If the wound is infected and draining, dressing change should occur two to four times per day.

Antibiotic Management

One of the most common mistakes in puncture and bite wound management is to use prophylactic antibiotics as a substitute for good wound management. Antibiotics have a place in some of these injuries, but they will not pardon a poorly cleansed wound.

The key to success in inanimate puncture wound management is debridement with removal of foreign material. Prophylactic antibiotics should be withheld unless the wound is grossly contaminated. When gross contamination does exist, a broad-spectrum antibiotic should be used, pending results of wound culture.[31]

Puncture wound of the foot may be complicated by infection in 10 percent of cases.[21] *P. aeruginosa* has been identified as a common infecting agent in foot puncture injuries. Typically, infection with this agent presents at a mean 6 days (range 2 to 21 days) following injury.[3] Osteomyelitis infection may present months after the initial puncture injury.[32, 33] Once present, these infections must be managed by aggressive combined surgical and antibiotic therapy. There is no evidence that prophylaxis lessens the incidence of this complication.

The incidence of infection following mammalian bite injury varies according to the species involved. There is some evidence that prophylactic antibiotics are of benefit in cat bite wounds and in high-risk dog bites.[11, 34-36] Patients with human bite injuries are commonly considered candidates for prophylactic antibi-

TABLE 31–3. Initial Antibiotic Therapy for Puncture and Bite Wounds

Recommended Antibiotic Prophylaxis/Treatment*

1. Treat all cat bites and human bites.
2. Treat dog bites older than 8 hours.
3. Treat hand bites.
4. Treat deep punctures.
5. Treat immunosuppressed host.

Recommended Antibiotics for Human Bites†

1. Amoxicillin plus clavulanic acid (Augmentin)
2. Penicillinase-resistant penicillin plus penicillin V (for *Pasteurella multocida* and anaerobes.)
3. Erythromycin or tetracycline.

* Data from Trott A: Care of mammalian bites. Pediatr Infect Dis J 6:8–10, 1987.

† Data from Feder HM, et al: Review of 59 patients hospitalized with animal bites. Pediatr Infect Dis J 6:24–28, 1987; Trott, 1987; and Guba et al: The selection of antibiotics for human bites of the hand. Plast Reconstr Surg 56:538–541, 1976.

otics because of the high degree of bacterial contamination and severity of associated complications.[37-40]

Common offending organisms in mammalian bites include the aerobic and anaerobic organisms of the skin of the victim and the mouth of the biting animal (Table 31–2).[41, 42] Although *viridans* group streptococci and *S. aureus* are the most common organisms found in infected wounds, it is clear that many other organisms must be considered during therapy. Organisms specific to the animal bite are *Pasteurella multocida*, *P. fluorescens* group, and M-5. *Bacteroides* sp. seems to be more commonly seen in human bites.[39-41]

Specific antibiotic recommendations vary, depending upon the type of wound (Table 31–3).[39, 40, 43] The frequency of *S. aureus* in infected wounds would seem to favor the use of a penicillinase-resistant penicillin, such as oxacillin or a cephalosporin, for therapy of these injuries. However, the significantly decreased activity of these penicillins against many of the other organisms, such as *P. multocida* and *Bacteroides* sp., requires that penicillin V be added to the oxacillin. Penicillin V should also be added when a cephalosporin (usually first-generation) is used. A more favorable regimen may be to simply use amoxicillin plus clavulanic acid (Augmentin). Clavulanic acid is a beta-lactamase inhibitor that increases the spectrum of amoxicillin. Alternative therapy in penicillin-allergic patients is to use tetracycline (adults only) or erythromycin.[39]

TABLE 31–2. Common Organisms Isolated from Bite Wounds*

Aerobic	Dog, Cat	Human
Streptococci	x	x
Staphylococcus aureus	x	x
Staphylococcus epidermidis	x	x
Neisseria sp.	x	x
Corynebacterium	x	x
Pasteurella multocida	x	
Eikenella corrodens		x
Klebsiella pneumoniae		x
Pseudomonas fluorescens	x	
M-5	x	
Haemophilus parainfluenzae		x
Haemophilus aphrophilus	x	
Anaerobic		
Peptococcus sp.	x	x
Veillonella sp.	x	x
Bifidobacterium sp.		x
Bacteroides sp.	x	x

* From Feder HM, et al: Review of 59 patients hospitalized with animal bites. Pediatr Infect Dis J 6:24–28, 1987.

TABLE 31–4. Criteria for Hospitalization of Bite-Injured Patients*

1. Signs of systemic toxicity or underlying medical problems
2. Cellulitis and lymphangitis
3. Abscess
4. Osteomyelitis
5. Moderate to marked edema
6. Penetration of joint capsule
7. Inability of patient to provide adequate wound and follow-up care.

* From Chainard RN, D'Ambrosia RD: Human bite infections of the hand. J Bone Joint Surg 59:416–418, 1977.

Mammalian bites, once clinically infected, also necessitate aggressive management. Hospitalization should be considered when cellulitis is present following a bite wound. Surgical debridement and drainage are often necessary. Criteria for hospitalization of human bite injuries were identified by Chuinard and D'Ambrosia in 1977 and are listed in Table 31–4.[44] Management of the infected patient

TABLE 31–5. Tetanus Prophylaxis: Summary Guide in Routine Wound Management, United States, 1985*

History of Adsorbed Tetanus	Clean, Minor Wounds		All Other Wounds†	
	Td‡	TIG	Td‡	TIG
Unknown or < three	Yes	No	Yes	Yes
> or = three§	No‖	No	No¶	No

* Based on Recommendation of the Immunization Practices Advisory Committee (ACIP): Diphtheria, tetanus, and pertussis: guidelines for vaccine prophylaxis and other preventive measures. MMWR 34:422, 1985.

† Such as, but not limited to, wounds contaminated with dirt, feces, soil, saliva, etc.: puncture wounds; avulsions; and wounds resulting from missiles, crushing, burns, and frostbite.

‡ For children younger than 7 years old; diphtheria-tetanus-pertussis (DTP) (DT, if pertussis vaccine is contraindicated) is preferred to tetanus toxoid alone. For persons 7 years old and older, Td is preferred to tetanus toxoid alone.

§ If only three doses of *fluid* toxoid have been received, a fourth dose of toxoid, preferably an adsorbed toxoid, should be given.

‖ Yes, if more than 10 years since last dose.

¶ Yes, if more than 5 years since last dose. (More frequent boosters are not needed and can accentuate side effects.)

Abbreviations: Td = Tetanus-diphtheria; TIG = tetanus immune globulin.

as an outpatient is valid with a reliable patient if no tendon or neurovascular involvement or cellulitis is present. Follow-up to ensure reinspection and redressing within first 48 hours is necessary.[44] Peeples and co-authors found that 67 percent of these patients could be successfully managed on an ambulatory basis.[45]

Tetanus Prophylaxis

Tetanus prophylaxis is an important consideration in the treatment of all puncture wounds, whatever the cause. An annual average of 90 cases of tetanus per year has occurred over the past decade. Forty percent of persons over 60 of age or older lack protective antitoxins.[46]

Recommendations for the dosage and type of toxoid and antitoxin to be used vary with the type of wound and prior immunization (Table 31–5). It is recommended that adults routinely receive booster tetanus-diphtheria (Td) immunizations at mid-decade ages (15, 25, 35, 45 years and so on) to prevent development of an inadequately immunized state. If boosters are given as part of wound management before 10 years have elapsed, the next booster is recommended 10 years later.

Rabies Prophylaxis

In the United States, rabies in humans has decreased from an average of 22 cases per year in 1946 to 1950 to zero to five cases per year since 1960. Each year 25,000 people receive prophylaxis in the United States.[18] Recommendations for prophylaxis vary according to animal species and condition at the time of attack (Table 31–6).[18]

Hepatitis Prophylaxis

Transmission of hepatitis B (HBV) from a "bite wound" has been documented.[16] Prophylaxis using hepatitis B immune globulin (HBIG) should be considered in patients receiving a "bite wound" from a person with a high risk of hepatitis B. Populations considered at high risk as a source for hepatitis B infection include (1) immigrants from areas of high hepatitis virus endemicity (especially Southeast Asia), (2) clients in institutions for the mentally retarded, (3) intravenous drug abusers, (4) homosexual/bisexual men, (5)

TABLE 31–6. Rabies Post-exposure Prophylaxis, July 1984*

The following recommendations are only a guide. In applying them, take into account the animal species involved, the circumstances of the bite or other exposure, the vaccination status of the animal, and presence of rabies in the region. Local or state public health officials should be consulted if questions arise about the need for rabies prophylaxis.

Animal Species	Condition of Animal at Time of Attack	Treatment of Exposed Person†
Domestic Dog and cat	Healthy and available for 10 days of observation	None, unless animal develops rabies‡
	Rabid or suspected	RIG§ and HDCV
	Unknown (escaped)	Consult public health officials. If treatment is indicated, give RIG§ and HDCV
Wild Skunk, bat, fox, coyote, raccoon, bobcat and other carnivores	Regard as rabid unless proven negative by laboratory tests‖	RIG§ and HDCV
Other Livestock, rodents, and lago-morphs (rabbits and hares)	Consider individually. Local and state public health officials should be consulted on questions about the need for rabies prophylaxis. Bites of squirrels, hamsters, guinea pigs, gerbils, chipmunks, rats, mice, other rodents, rabbits, and hares almost never call for antirabies prophylaxis.	

* Based on Recommendation of the Immunization Practices Advisory Committee (ACIP): Rabies prevention — United States, 1984. MMWR 33:397, 1984.

† *All bites and wounds should immediately be thoroughly cleansed with soap and water.* If antirabies treatment is indicated, both RIG and HDCV should be given as soon as possible, *regardless* of the interval from exposure. Local reactions to vaccines are common and do not contraindicate continuing treatment. Discontinue vaccine if fluorescent-antibody tests of the animal are negative.

‡ During the usual holding period of 10 days, begin treatment with RIG and HDCV at the first sign of rabies in a dog or cat that has bitten someone. The symptomatic animal should be killed immediately and tested.

§ If RIG is not available, use antirabies serum, equine (ARS). Do not use more than the recommended dosage.

‖ The animal should be killed and tested as soon as possible. Holding for observation is not recommended.

Abbreviations: RIG = Rabies immune globulin; HDCV = human diploid cell rabies vaccine.

TABLE 31–7. Hepatitis B Prophylaxis: Recommendations for Hepatitis B Prophylaxis Following Percutaneous Exposure*

Source	Exposed Person	
	Unvaccinated	Vaccinated
HBsAg-positive	1. HBIG × 1 immediately† 2. Initiate HB vaccine series‡	1. Test exposed person for anti-HBs 2. If inadequate antibody,§ HBIG (×1) immediately plus HB vaccine booster dose
Known source High-risk HBsAg-positive	1. Initiate HB vaccine 2. Test source for HBsAG; if source positive, HBIG × 1	1. Test source for HBsAg only if exposed is vaccine nonresponder; if source HBsAg-positive, give HBIG × 1 immediately plus HB vaccine booster dose
Low-risk HBsAg-positive	Initiate HB vaccine series	Nothing required
Unknown source	Initiate HB vaccine series	Nothing required

* Based on Recommendations for preventing transmission of infection with human T-lymphotropic virus type III lymphadenopathy–associated virus in the workplace. MMWR 34:331, 1985.)

† HBIG dose — 0.06 ml/kg IM.

‡ HB vaccine dose — 20 μ-g IM for adults; 10 μ-g IM for infants or children under 10 years of age. First dose within 1 week; second and third doses, 1 and 6 months later.

§ Less than 10 SRU by radioimmunoassay negative by enzyme immunoassay.

Abbreviations: HB = Hepatitis B; HBIG = hepatitis B immune globulin; IM = intramuscularly.

household contacts of HBV carriers, and (6) patients of hemodialysis units.[47]

Recommendations for hepatitis B prophylaxis include vaccine and/or HBIG, depending upon exposure factors (Table 31–7).[47] These guidelines should also be applied to human bite wounds or needle sticks involving high risk population groups.

Acquired Immunodeficiency Syndrome (AIDS) Prophylaxis

The risk of transmission of human immunodeficiency virus (HIV) through a bite wound is unknown. The inoculum of the HIV necessary to produce HIV infection appears to be much greater than that required of HBV to produce hepatitis.[48] When a bite wound inflicted by a person with HIV infection is brought to attention, the best course is to cleanse and debride the wound promptly. As of this writing, there has been one case report of presumed HIV transmission attributed to bite injury.[49] Evidence indicates that the virus is unlikely to be transmitted by saliva, but presence of bleeding gingiva may allow serum transfer from an infected patient.

SUMMARY

The innocuous puncture wound may produce severe consequences when improperly managed. Thorough history of mechanism is mandatory. Consideration of potential involvement of deep structures is mandatory before a treatment regimen is prescribed. Thorough cleansing and debridement are required for all wounds. Prophylactic antibiotics, antitoxin, and antiviral treatment should be administered as determined by the mechanism and extent of injury.

References

1. Houston AN, Roy WA, Faust RA: Tetanus prophylaxis in the treatment of puncture wounds of patients in the deep South. J Trauma 2:439, 1962.
2. Chusid MJ, Jacobs WM, Sty JR: *Pseudomonas* arthritis following puncture wounds of the foot. J Pediatr 94(3):429–431, 1979.
3. Jacobs RF, Adelman L, Sack CM, et al: Management of *Pseudomonas* osteochondritis complicating puncture wounds of the foot. Pediatrics 69:432–435, 1982.
4. Siebert WI, Dewan S, Williams TW Jr: *Pseudomonas* puncture wound osteomyelitis in adults. Am J Med Sci 283:83–88, 1982.
5. Graham GS, Gregory DW: *Pseudomonas aeruginosa* causing osteomyelitis after puncture wounds of the foot. South Med J 77(10):1228–1230, 1984.
6. Fisher MC, Goldsmith JF, Gilligan PH: Sneakers as a source of *Pseudomonas aeruginosa* in children with osteomyelitis following puncture wounds. J Pediatr 106:608–609, 1985.
7. Cracchiolo A: Wooden foreign bodies in the foot. Am J Surg 140:585–587, 1980.
8. Berzon D, DeHoff J: Medical costs and other aspects of dog bites in Baltimore. Public Health Rep 39:377–381, 1974.
9. Scarcella JV: Management of bites. Ohio State Med J 65:25–31, 1969.
10. Callaham M: Human and animal bites. Topics Emerg Med 4(1):1–15, 1982.
11. Callaham M: Prophylactic antibiotics in common dog bite wounds: a controlled study. Ann Emerg Med 9(8):410–414, 1980.
12. Marr JS, Beck AM, Lugo JA Jr: An epidemiologic study of the human bite. Public Health Rep 94:514–521, 1979.
13. Malinowski RW, Strate RG, Perry JF Jr, et al: The management of human bite injuries of the hand. J Trauma 19:655–659, 1979.
14. Heinrich JJ, Fichandler BC, Krizek RJ, et al: Emergency treatment of bites and stings. 2. Human bites. J Emerg Nurs 2:21–24, 1976.
15. Goldstein EJ, Citron DM, Wield B, et al: Bacteriology of human and animal bite wounds. J Clin Microbiol 8:667–672, 1978.
16. MacQuarrie MB, Forghani B, Wolochow DA: Hepatitis B transmitted by a human bite. JAMA 230(5):723–724, 1974.
17. Ordog GJ: Rat bites: fifty cases. Ann Emerg Med 14(2):126–130, 1985.
18. Recommendation of the Immunization Practices Advisory Committee (ACIP): Rabies prevention—United States, 1984. MMWR 33:393–402, 407–408, 1984.
19. Brown LL, Shelton HT, Bornside GH, Cohn I Jr et al: Evaluation of wound irrigation by pulsatile jet and conventional methods. Ann Surg 187(2):170–173, 1978.
20. Stevenson T, Thacker JG, Rodeheaver GT, et al: Cleansing the traumatic wound by high pressure irrigation. JACEP 5:17–21, 1976.
21. Faust RA, Roy WA, Ewin DM, Espenan PA, Brown JE: Management and tetanus prophylaxis in the treatment of puncture wounds. Am Surg 38(4):198–204, 1972.
22. Vijanto J: Disinfection of surgical wounds without inhibition of normal wound healing. Arch Surg 115:253, 1980.
23. Rodeheaver G, Bellamy W, Kody M, et al: Bactericidal activity and toxicity of iodine-containing solutions in wounds. Arch Surg 117(2):181, 1982.
24. Sindelar WF, Mason GR: Irrigation of subcutaneous tissue with povidone-iodine solution for prevention of surgical wound infections. Surg Gynecol Obstet 148(2):227, 1979.
25. Rodeheaver GT, Kurtz L, Kircher BJ, Edlich RF: Pluronic F-68: a promising new skin wound cleanser. Ann Emerg Med 9(11):572–579, 1980.
26. Bryant CA, Rodenheaver GT, Reem EM, et al: Search

for a nontoxic surgical scrub solution for periorbital lacerations. Ann Emerg Med 13(5):317–321, 1984.

27. Tandberg D: Glass in the hand and foot: will an x-ray film show it? JAMA 248(15):1872, 1982.

28. Pond GD, Lindsey D: Localization of cactus, glass and other foreign bodies in soft tissues. Ariz Med 34(10):700, 1977.

29. Callaham ML: Treatment of common dog bites: infection risk factors. JACEP 7(3):83–87, 1978.

30. Torphy DE, Ray CG: *Pasturella multocida* in dog and cat infections. Pediatrics 43:295–297, 1969.

31. Riegler JF, Routson GW: Complications of deep puncture wounds of the foot. J Trauma 19(1):18–22, 1979.

32. Fitzgerald RH, Cowan JDE: Puncture wounds of the foot. Orthop Clin North Am 6(4):965–971, 1975.

33. Peterson HA, Tressler HA, Lang AG, Johnson EW: Fracture conference: puncture wounds of the foot. Minn Med 56:787–794, 1973.

34. Elenbaas RM, McNabney WK, Robinson WA: Evaluation of prophylactic oxacillin in cat bite wounds. Ann Emerg Med 13:155–157, 1984.

35. Rosen RA: The use of antibiotics in the initial management of recent dog-bite wounds. Am J Emerg Med 3(1):19–23, 1985.

36. Elenbaas RM, McNabney WK, Robinson WA: Prophylactic oxacillin in dog bite wounds. Ann Emerg Med 11:248–251, 1982.

37. House HC, Morris D: Bites of the hand. Md State Med J 26:88–94, 1977.

38. Mann RJ, Hoffeld TA, Farmer CB: Human bites of the hand: twenty years of experience. J Hand Surg 2:97–104, 1977.

39. Feder HM, Shanley JD, Barbera JA: Review of 59 patients hospitalized with animal bites. Pediatr Infect Dis J 6:24–28, 1987.

40. Trott A: Care of mammalian bites. Pediatr Infect Dis J 6:8–10, 1987.

41. Brook I: Microbiology of human and animal bite wounds in children. Pediatr Infect Dis J 6:29–32, 1987.

42. Bilos ZJ, Kucharchuk A, Metzger W: *Eikenella corrodens* in human bites. Clin Orthop 134:320–324, 1978.

43. Guba AM Jr, Mulliken JB, Hoopes JE: The selection of antibiotics for human bites of the hand. Plast Reconstr Surg 56:538–541, 1976.

44. Chuinard RN, D'Ambrosia RD: Human bite infections of the hand. J Bone Joint Surg 59:416–418, 1977.

45. Peeples E, Boswick JA Jr, Scott FA: Wounds of the hand contaminated by human or animal saliva. J Trauma 20:383–389, 1980.

46. Recommendation of the Immunization Practices Advisory Committee (ACIP): Diphtheria, tetanus, and pertussis: guidelines for vaccine prophylaxis and other preventive measures. MMWR 34:405–414, 419–426, 1985.

47. Recommendation of the Immunization Practices Advisory Committee (ACIP): Recommendations for protection against viral hepatitis. MMWR 34:681–686, 691–695, 1985.

48. Recommendations for preventing transmission of infection with human T-lymphotropic virus type III/lymphadenopathy–associated virus in the workplace MMWR 34:681–686, 691–695, 1985.

49. Transmission of HIV by human bite [news]. Lancet 2(8557):522, 1987.

Index

Note: Page numbers in *italics* refer to illustrations; page numbers followed by *t* refer to tables.